Governing HIV in China

HIV and AIDS have long been problematized in the People's Republic of China as objects of governance in political frameworks and institutions. The state's attitudes towards health programs have, nevertheless, changed significantly during the 21st century. Pilot programs at the beginning of the century, which focused on underground sex workers, have now developed into the roll-out of a nationwide program, with supportive legislation and broadcast media publicity.

This book therefore examines China's evolving AIDS response, providing an up-to-date investigation into the positions and practices of the state. It explains the origins, rationales and implementation of initiatives focused on female sex workers and explores the extension of such initiatives to include other populations identified as key to ending the AIDS epidemic, especially homosexual men and rural-to-urban migrant labourers. Ultimately, through an analysis of the different approaches to the governance of commercial sex and sexual health, *Governing HIV in China* concludes by considering the challenges raised by China's commitment to the United Nations' vision of ending AIDS as a global health threat by 2030.

This book will be useful for students and scholars of Social Policy, Public Health Policy and Chinese Studies.

Elaine Jeffreys is Professor in the School of International Studies at the University of Technology Sydney, Australia.

SU Gang is Research Associate in the School of International Studies at the University of Technology Sydney, Australia.

Routledge Studies on China in Transition
Series Editor: David S. G. Goodman

For a full list of available titles: www.routledge.com/Routledge-Studies-on-China-in-Transition/book-series/SE0082

45 **Elites and Governance in China**
Edited by Xiaowei Zang and Chien-Wen Kou

46 **Choosing China's Leaders**
Edited by Chien-Wen Kou and Xiaowei Zang

47 **Rural Policy Implementation in Contemporary China**
New socialist countryside
Anna L. Ahlers

48 **NGO Governance and Management in China**
Edited by Reza Hasmath and Jennifer Y. J. Hsu

49 **Dams, Migration and Authoritarianism in China**
The Local State in Yunnan
Sabrina Habich

50 **New Mentalities of Government in China**
Edited by David Bray and Elaine Jeffreys

51 **China's Cinema of Class**
Audiences and Narratives
Nicole Talmacs

52 **Economic Development in China's Northwest**
Entrepreneurship and identity along China's multi-ethnic borderlands
Joshua Bird

53 **Governing HIV in China**
Commercial Sex, Homosexuality and Rural-to-Urban Migration
Elaine Jeffreys and SU Gang

Governing HIV in China

Commercial Sex, Homosexuality and Rural-to-Urban Migration

Elaine Jeffreys and SU Gang

Routledge
Taylor & Francis Group
LONDON AND NEW YORK

First published 2018 by Routledge

2 Park Square, Milton Park, Abingdon, Oxfordshire OX14 4RN
52 Vanderbilt Avenue, New York, NY 10017

Routledge is an imprint of the Taylor & Francis Group, an informa business

First issued in paperback 2018

British Library Cataloguing-in-Publication Data
A catalogue record for this book is available from the British Library

Library of Congress Cataloging-in-Publication Data
Names: Jeffreys, Elaine, 1960– author. | Gang, Su, author.
Title: Governing HIV in China : commercial sex, homosexuality and rural-to-urban migration / Elaine Jeffreys and Su Gang.
Description: Milton Park, Abingdon, Oxon ; New York, NY : Routledge, 2018. | Series: Routledge studies on China in transition ; 53 | Includes bibliographical references and index.
Identifiers: LCCN 2017016568 | ISBN 9781138039957 (hardback) | ISBN 9781315175546 (ebook)
Subjects: LCSH: HIV infections—China—Prevention | AIDS (Disease)—China—Prevention. | China—Politics and government.
Classification: LCC RA643.86.C6 J44 2018 | DDC 614.5/9939200951—dc23
LC record available at https://lccn.loc.gov/2017016568

ISBN: 978-1-138-03995-7 (hbk)
ISBN: 978-0-367-20626-1 (pbk)

DOI: 10.4324/9781315175546

For SU Qiangchang and Cui Runhua

Contents

	List of figures	viii
	Acknowledgements	ix
	Notes on terminology and referencing	x
	Abbreviations	xi
1	Governing HIV in China: an introduction	1
2	AIDS and the sex industry: the 100 Per Cent Condom Use Program	18
3	China's condom use program and the media	36
4	Changing policies on prostitution, censorship and disease control	54
5	Health interventions focused on sex workers	74
6	Men who have sex with men	94
7	Rural-to-urban migrant labourers	117
8	Afterword: ending AIDS?	140
	References	151
	Index	184

Figures

3.1 Chinese press coverage of '*aizibing*' (AIDS) (2000–2015) 46
4.1 Chinese press coverage of '*anquantao*' (safety sheath) and '*biyuntao*' (prevent pregnancy sheath) (2000–2015) 67
6.1 'Did you bring a condom?' 'Are you wearing a condom?' 95
6.2 'Let's both get tested' 108
7.1 China's four main economic regions and developing megacities 122
7.2 Zhang's story 133

Acknowledgements

This work was supported by the Australian Research Council's Discovery Project funding scheme (DP0985709) and Future Fellowship funding scheme (FT100100238).

Governing HIV in China: Commercial Sex, Homosexuality and Rural-to-Urban Migration is composed chiefly of previously unpublished materials. However, the authors and publisher would like to thank Taylor and Francis journals for permission to reproduce parts of Elaine Jeffreys and Su Gang (2011) 'China's 100 Per Cent Condom Use Program: customising the Thai experience', *Asian Studies Review*, 35, 3: 315–33. We would also like to thank the National Center for AIDS/STD Control and Prevention for permission to reproduce Figures 6.1 and 6.2, and Niu Wenyi, Sun Zhe and Wang Chaoying from the China Association of Agricultural Science Societies for permission to reproduce Figure 7.2.

Every effort has been made to contact copyright holders for their permission to reprint material in this book. The publishers would be grateful to hear from any copyright holder who is not here acknowledged and will undertake to rectify any errors or omissions in future editions of this book.

Notes on terminology and referencing

The book uses, where possible, the preferred terminology provided in guidelines issued by the Joint United Nations Programme on HIV/AIDS (UNAIDS 2015). Although UNAIDS recommends avoiding the use of the term HIV/AIDS, the term is used when it occurs in the original version of documents, including documents produced by the World Health Organization and UNAIDS, and also when it is used in English-language translations of Chinese documents. Likewise, although UNAIDS recommends using the terms sex work, commercial sex and sex worker rather than prostitution and prostitute, the latter terms are used when referring to certain aspects of the PRC's history and laws.

The expression sexually transmissible infection (STI) is used in preference to venereal disease (VD) and sexually transmitted disease (STD) to indicate that sexual contact does not necessarily result in the contraction of an STI (Jeffreys and Huang 2009: 168). The term STD is used when referring to quotations or organizations that use such terminology, for example, the Chinese Association of STD/AIDS Prevention and Control.

Names in Chinese are usually presented as family name followed by a personal name. That practice is followed with two exceptions; the first is where a Chinese person has a non-Chinese personal name, in which case the personal name is presented before the family name; the second is where a person with a Chinese name has indicated through publication in English that they wish to be known by their personal name followed by their family name.

Abbreviations

100% CUP (100 Per Cent Condom Use Program)
AIDS (Acquired Immunodeficiency Syndrome)
CCP (Chinese Communist Party)
CCTV (China Central Television Station)
CDC (Chinese Center for Disease Control and Prevention)
CPPCC (Chinese People's Political Consultative Conference)
Global Fund (Global Fund to Fight AIDS, Tuberculosis and Malaria)
HIV (Human Immunodeficiency Virus)
LGBT (lesbian, gay, bisexual and transgender)
NCAIDS (National Center for AIDS/STD Control and Prevention)
NGO (non-governmental organization)
NHFPC (National Health and Family Planning Commission)
NPC (National People's Congress)
NPFPC (National Population and Family Planning Commission)
PRC (People's Republic of China)
PSA (public service advertisement/advertising)
STD (sexually transmitted disease)
STI (sexually transmissible infection)
UN (United Nations)
UNAIDS (Joint United Nations Programme on HIV/AIDS)
UNDP (United Nations Development Programme)
WHO (World Health Organization)
WHO/WPR (World Health Organization Regional Office for the Western Pacific)

1 Governing HIV in China

An introduction

This book explores the recent representation of the sexual behaviours of female sex workers, men who have sex with men and rural-to-urban migrant labourers as a problem for public health, and thus of government, in the People's Republic of China (PRC). It examines the pilot implementation in the early 2000s and national roll-out since the mid-2000s of health interventions designed to control the spread of sexually transmissible infection (STI) in China, especially the Human Immunodeficiency Virus (HIV) and hence Acquired Immunodeficiency Syndrome (AIDS). The term 'sexually transmissible infection' is used in preference to the expression 'sexually transmitted disease' (STD) to indicate that engaging in vaginal, oral or anal sex does not necessarily result in the contraction of an STI.

We use a genealogical method to examine the evolution of public health campaigns in China that provide information about how to use condoms to help prevent the sexual transmission of HIV, showing how particular populations of people have been identified as in need of such education, and the methods and media used to communicate that information. In the process, we trace the rapid transformation of PRC discourses and policies on AIDS, commercial sex, condoms, homosexuality and sex in general. AIDS is now a public health issue, instead of being a 'state secret', with easier access to government-subsidized rapid testing and early treatment turning the identification of HIV infection into a manageable chronic disease as opposed to a death sentence. Commercial sex is banned, but there is public debate on the question of how the sex industry might be better managed. Condoms are marketed as a personal sexual hygiene product rather than a state-provided marital contraceptive. Homosexuality, an 'invisible' practice in the PRC until the 1990s, is an increasingly visible feature of everyday life. The imperatives of AIDS-related public health communication and care have ensured that issues of sex and sexuality are matters of public discourse.

This chapter introduces the key concepts, themes and contents of *Governing HIV in China: Commercial Sex, Homosexuality and Rural-to-Urban Migration.* It first outlines the concept of 'governmentality', which focuses analytical attention on how AIDS has been problematized as an object of governance in international and national political frameworks and institutions, and through health interventions aiming to transform individual decision-making and behaviours. It then contextualizes the study by providing a short history of the emergence of STI

DOI: 10.4324/9781315175546-1

and prostitution, and, more recently, HIV and AIDS, as objects of governance and media publicity in contemporary China. Finally, it summarizes the subject matter and arguments of the remaining seven chapters.

Key concepts and themes: government, governmentality and 'making up people'

Michel Foucault (1991) coined the term 'governmentality' to describe the raison d'être and goals of modern government as concerned with 'the conduct of conduct'. Contemporary government refers to the activity of conducting others or things, and also to the ways in which one conducts oneself, 'lets oneself be conducted', 'is conducted', and the manner in which one behaves 'as an effect of a form of conduct' (Foucault 2007: 193). This way of thinking about government revises conventional understandings of the relationship between government and power by decentring 'the problem of the State'. Power is typically viewed as being concentrated in the authority and actions of a nation-state, understood as a relatively coherent and often 'predatory' political subject, which extends its authority throughout society through an apparatus of control.

The concept of governmentality draws attention to the diverse forces, knowledges and experts that are involved in efforts to regulate the lives of individuals, and the conditions within national territories, in pursuit of various goals. It suggests that government is neither operationalized nor exercised strictly through prohibitions and controls. Instead, the government of society is achieved through the (biopolitical) processes of managing and nurturing life – for example, attending to the processes of health, disease, sexuality, fertility, birth and lifespan, and their relationship to particular lifestyles (Bray and Jeffreys 2016: 2).

Foucault (1991: 93, 95) further describes governmentality as: 'the right disposition of things, arranged so as to lead to a convenient end . . . for each of the things that are to be governed'. Government thus defined is about how to guide the evolving interactions between 'people' and 'things'. This includes the relations between people and territory, wealth, resources and means of subsistence, and variables such as climate, soil, water, flora, fauna and pathogens. It also includes the changing relations between people and other 'things' such as customary ways of thinking and behaving, and the creation of new technologies and forms of expertise that may inspire or demand new ways of thinking and behaving. A governmentality framework therefore draws attention to the ways in which processes of social, economic, political and technological change can give rise to new ways of thinking about the kinds of problems that government should address, and how to resolve them, which may also involve new types of experts and expertise (Bray and Jeffreys 2016).

AIDS, for example, was only identified in the early 1980s but is now a major focus of global health governance. In 1981, the Centers for Disease Control and Prevention (CDC) of the United States of America (USA) published a report describing the unusual occurrences of opportunistic infections in five previously healthy gay men in Los Angeles (U.S. Department of Health and Human Services n.d.).

By late 1981, there were 270 reported cases of severe immune deficiency among gay men in the USA and more than 120 of those individuals had died. In September 1982, the CDC first used the term 'AIDS' to describe 'a disease at least moderately predictive of a defect in cell-mediated immunity, occurring in a person with no known case for diminished resistance to that disease' (Ibid.). By December 1982, the CDC reported a case of AIDS in an infant who had had blood transfusions; and, in January 1983, the CDC reported cases of AIDS in female sexual partners of males with AIDS.

Shortly after the discovery of HIV and the transmission routes of the virus, the World Health Organization (WHO) held its first meeting to assess the AIDS situation in October 1983, and began international surveillance resulting in the formation of a United Nations (UN) system on AIDS (Ibid.). The Global Program on AIDS was launched in 1987 to raise public awareness of AIDS, promote research, encourage the participation of non-governmental organizations (NGOs) in AIDS-related efforts, champion the rights of people living with HIV, and provide policy, technical and financial support to countries around the world. In 1996, the Joint United Nations Programme on HIV/AIDS (UNAIDS) was established to advocate for global action on the AIDS epidemic. UNAIDS now heads an international program that aims to unite the UN system, national governments, the private sector, NGOs, and people most affected by or living with HIV in innovative partnerships to achieve universal access to HIV prevention, treatment, care and support services.

The UN's current mission of ending the AIDS epidemic as a global health threat by 2030, as affirmed in the 2016 Political Declaration on HIV and AIDS, involves 'fast-tracking' national health policies to reduce the prevalence of HIV among key and vulnerable populations (United Nations General Assembly 2016). Key populations previously included sex workers, men who have sex with men and people who inject drugs using non-sterile equipment; they now also include transgender people and people in prisons or other closed settings (WHO 2014, 2015; UNAIDS 2015b: 8). These groups of people are defined as key to the epidemic's dynamics, and hence international and national responses. Key populations are viewed as facing increased risk, vulnerability and burden with respect to HIV and AIDS due to a combination of biological, socio-economic and structural factors. Yet they often have the least access to prevention and treatment services because their behaviours are stigmatized or even criminalized. Vulnerable populations such as women, migrants and mobile workers do not necessarily face the same epidemiological risk as members of key populations, but they are often vulnerable to infection because of societal pressures or social circumstances. To realize its 2030 mission, the UN aims to eliminate HIV-related discrimination, and reduce the number of people newly infected with HIV and dying from AIDS-related causes to fewer than 500,000 respectively, by 2020, which means scaling up access to information about HIV prevention, and access to rapid testing and treatment services (UNAIDS 2015b).

UNAIDS' account of key and vulnerable populations, which legitimizes and demands certain forms of national governmental action, is presented as a more or less self-evident representation of reality. This leaves out the complex and often slow processes, involving myriad professionals, government leaders, the media and so forth, that have been and are involved in identifying and presenting the conduct of persons individually and collectively, and in different locales, as a 'problem' that *has* to be governed to protect and preserve humankind. Translating that 'problem' into transnational programs of corrective intervention requires that political and organizational differences of opinion, whether fundamental or not, are addressed or brought into some kind of alignment with each other, in order to create a common language and technical measures for presenting and remedying the identified issue (Miller and Rose 2008: 14–15). In turn, the implementation of associated public health interventions is transforming aspects of national government and social mores.

Viewed from a governmentality perspective, the process of classifying certain populations as key to the AIDS epidemic and response involves what Ian Hacking (2006) describes as the 'making up of people', or the creation of 'human kinds'. As Hacking (2006) explains, processes of classifying and subsequently intervening into groups of people can create both 'moving targets' and kinds of people that in certain senses and contexts did not exist before. A classic example is homosexuality. People have probably engaged in same-sex sexual practices throughout human history. However, 'homosexuals' as a category of people only emerged in Western societies in the late nineteenth century along with the rise of new medical and legal discourses that presented same-sex desire and sex acts as aberrant and deviant, resulting in associated treatments and punishments (Foucault 1998: 43–4; see also Greenberg 1988). The contemporary discourse of gay pride, LGBT activism and attempts to find the 'gay gene' are variously marked by efforts to counter, reconfigure or resist such classifications, and to give same-sex attracted people more control over the categories into which they have been placed (Foucault 1998: 101).

Our history of AIDS-related health interventions and communication in the PRC consequently centres on three main questions. How have certain groups of people come to be classified as key to China's AIDS response, and hence as legitimate objects of public health interventions? How have these classifications affected the people that are classified? How are the effects of such classifications on people in turn changing the original classifications and altering associated fields of government?

The following sections contextualize these questions by providing a short history of the emergence of STI and prostitution, and then HIV and AIDS, as objects of governance and media attention in contemporary China.

Governing STI and prostitution in the PRC

Although there was no language to describe HIV and AIDS as a problem for global health governance before the late 1980s, that situation has clearly changed. Numerous documents issued by UNAIDS underscore the importance of representing the multiple issues associated with AIDS in ways that make them amenable to political and individual deliberation. A key technology here is the broadcast media, defined by UNAIDS as 'having tremendous reach and influence, particularly with young people who represent the future and who are the key to any successful fight against HIV/AIDS' (UNAIDS 2004: 4).

A 2004 document, 'The Media and HIV/AIDS: Making a Difference', argues that media representations have a pivotal role to play by educating listeners and viewers about the facts of the AIDS epidemic, including the availability of services, and overcoming prejudice against people living with or affected by HIV. UNAIDS (2004: 15) therefore recommends that national media incorporate AIDS storylines in existing programming, and also provide regular and entertaining public service messages that encourage discussion of how individuals can protect themselves and change their behaviour, if necessary, which may mean combating existing social norms, values and conditions. The 2015 UNAIDS Terminology Guidelines further encourage the 'considered use of appropriate language' when talking about HIV and AIDS, because 'language shapes beliefs and may influence behaviours', and therefore appropriate 'language has the power to strengthen the global response to the AIDS epidemic' (UNAIDS 2015c: 3). As this suggests, the language of 'good governance' is programmatic: it aims to transform ways of thinking and behaving to achieve specific goals.

In China, the development of an 'appropriate' language for talking about AIDS, that is, one informed by international best practice, has involved replacing in part the language of revolutionary socialism. That language turned on the historical achievements of the early communist regime in founding the PRC, and then embarking on a course of nation building and modernization. These achievements informed public discourses on the nature and causes of STI from the 1950s until the 1990s, and were reinforced through state control of the media.

Most notably, the Chinese Communist Party (CCP) claimed to have made world history in 1964, when it declared to the WHO that active venereal disease had been eradicated from mainland China. This achievement was heralded as extraordinary both at home and abroad. Apart from the fact that no other government has managed to achieve such a feat, the PRC was only founded in October 1949 and venereal disease was endemic at that time (Abrams 2001: 431; Hesketh, Ye and Zhu 2008). The testing of nearly 5,300 prostitutes in Shanghai in 1950 revealed that more than 58 per cent had syphilis (Liu Yushu 1989). A survey conducted by the Inner Mongolian government between 1950 and 1953 found that the prevalence of syphilis among members of the rural population was as high as 48 per cent (Ibid.).

The early communist regime responded to endemic venereal disease by conducting mass education and screening campaigns, providing free treatment, and also by eradicating prostitution. People identified with venereal disease were given penicillin, which was an expensive new drug at that time, especially for a poor and newly formed nation (Cohen *et al.* 1996: S225). Concomitantly, the CCP set about eradicating prostitution, which was viewed as a source of national shame and as a feudal-capitalist institution that oppressed women, and therefore had no place in a socialist society (Abrams 2001: 431; Hershatter 1997: 246; Sigley 2009: 46; Ye Ganyun 2001). This goal was accomplished by closing brothels in an overnight sweep and rounding up prostitutes for medical treatment and re-education, as was the case in Beijing in November 1949, or by gradually restricting business in brothels until they eventually closed, which was the case in Tianjin (Hershatter 1997: 304–13; Ma Weigang 1994; Mu Yumin 2003).

The establishment of socialist-style, centralized economic planning subsequently ensured that rates of STI and prostitution remained extremely low in China until after the introduction of market-based economic reforms in December 1978. Centralized planning involved the nationalization of industry and state allocation of employment. This resulted in severe restrictions on population mobility because the fledgling Party-state needed to know the identity and location of its workers (Jeffreys and Sigley 2009: 9).

The introduction of a household registration system (*hukou, huji*) in 1955, and especially after 1960, tied almost every individual to their mother's place of birth for life, and severely limited the opportunities for moving somewhere else until the 1980s. As David Goodman explains:

> Each household and all its individual members were classified according to whether they lived in an urban or rural area; and whether they had a right to buy from the public supply of grain (non-agricultural household registration) or were expected to feed themselves under all circumstances (agricultural household registration).
>
> (Goodman 2014: 35–6)

This system prevented people from relocating to another locality unless they had official permission to do so, which was extremely difficult to obtain (unless they were willing to move to a poorer, less developed area). It prevented rural residents (peasants), in particular, from relocating to the cities and accessing the welfare benefits associated with urban life. Only '329,000 rural residents were ever permitted to change to a hierarchically superior household registration before 1979' (Ibid.: 36). It also prevented impoverished rural women from relocating for the purposes of prostitution, by limiting their ability to access accommodation and food rations in urban areas.

By 1959, an estimated 90 per cent of China's urban population belonged to a work unit (*danwei*), a state-owned enterprise or institution that was meant to overcome the alienation of labour by merging life and work, and which provided all manner of welfare and services for its employees – housing, education, healthcare, policing, consumption goods and entertainment (Bray 2005). As the basic unit of urban society, each work unit became a community, providing its members with a social identity and sense of belonging, which was enhanced through engagement in collectivist political movements until the mid-1970s (Dutton 2009: 31–5). The comprehensive and politicized nature of this system enabled the early CCP to not only implement wide-ranging socio-economic reforms, but also to micro-police social attitudes and behaviours on an individual and day-to-day level.

The work-unit system contributed to the absence of visible prostitution in urban China from the late 1950s until the early 1980s by restricting both the capacity of individuals to trade sex for money or goods *and* the physical and moral spaces in which commercial sex could occur. The initial eradication of prostitution, for example, was assisted by the practice of police informing a work unit if they apprehended a man at a brothel or in the immediate vicinity of a brothel. The individual's actions would then be discussed at work-based political study meetings, thereby deterring potential brothel customers with the threat of public shaming (Ma Weigang 1994: 56). The physical venues in which individuals could engage in anonymous or private behaviours were also limited until the opening up of the commercial hospitality and service industry in the late 1980s (Jeffreys 2012b: 3).

Prostitution and STI emerged as newfound 'problems' for government in the PRC coincident with the post-1978 adoption of market-based economic reforms. The Ministry of Public Security issued a 'Notice on Resolutely Curbing Prostitution' in 1981 (*Gonganbu guanyu jianjue zhizhi maiyin huodong de tongzhi*) (Gonganbu 1981). Using the language of revolutionary socialism, it stated that the early CCP had eradicated prostitution to public acclaim. It added that prostitution had resurfaced in the reform era and was corrupting social morality and people's thinking, endangering social order and damaging China's international reputation, and hence should be targeted by police-led crackdowns. It recommended that urban-based women who had left employment in a state-run work unit to engage in prostitution as a means to earn a livelihood should be sent to institutes for reform through legal, moral and political education (Ibid.). Women who had employment but sold sexual services occasionally to earn extra income should be disciplined by their work unit. Rural women who sold sexual services in cities should be returned to their native homes and disciplined by their agricultural production unit (Ibid.). Male buyers of sex should be disciplined by their work unit. The latter three recommendations would have involved public shaming at work-based political study meetings, and highlight the dependence of early prostitution controls on socialist-era forms of labour organization and social control.

The first government announcement to address the subjects of prostitution *and* STI in the reform era was issued on 1 September 1986, the 'Notice of the State Council on Resolutely Banning Prostitution and Curbing the Spread of Sexually Transmitted Disease' (*Guowuyuan guanyu jianjue qudi maiyin huodong he zhizhi xingbing manyan de tongzhi*) (Guowuyuan 1986). It stated that prostitution and venereal disease, which had been eradicated from the PRC by 1964, had resurfaced and were spreading to the detriment of China's socialist development and international reputation, and the health of the population and future generations. It called on local governments to severely punish organizers of prostitution, and to send sellers and buyers of sex to re-education through labour, involving compulsory, self-funded health checks for STI, with the results to be submitted to public security organs, who would inform the workplaces and families of those apprehended about their actions. It also stated that previous restrictions on the dissemination of information about the resurgence of STI were henceforth cancelled so that policing, health and other government departments could start communicating information to the broader public about the causes and harm of STI (Ibid.: Article 9).

However, direct and indirect forms of censorship ensured that the state-controlled media did not discuss the resurgence of STI and prostitution in detail nor outside the parameters of Communist Party–established discourses on the issue until the 1990s. This censorship is highlighted in a document issued by the Ministry of Public Security in 1988 titled 'Minutes of the Symposium on Advancing Campaigns Against Prostitution Activities and Improving Reeducation Work' (*Jinyibu daji qudi maiyinpiaochang huodong he zuohao shourong jiaoyu gongzuo zuotanhui jiyao*) (Gonganbu 1988). The document used XXX when referring to figures about prostitution-related crimes and arrests. It concluded that public security forces could release information about 'typical, serious cases' to government departments, state-owned enterprises, educational institutions and Party-affiliated mass organizations, in order to publicize policing successes and educate them about the harm of prostitution. But it added that such information was not to be released for publication in the media (Ibid.).

Blanket censorship was redundant by the 2000s, as rates of STI soared and commercial sex became a publicly visible phenomenon. Fewer than 6,000 cases of STI were documented in the PRC in 1985; that number had risen to over 700,000 cases by 2005 (Jeffreys and Huang 2009: 152). While there are no accurate figures regarding the extent of China's underground sex industry, a report by the U.S. Department of State (2009) claims that between 1.7 and 6 million women in the PRC earn their primary income from prostitution. A further 8 to 10 million women occasionally accept money or gifts in exchange for sexual services. The common presence in urban streets of stickers and cards that advertise commercial sex attests to the widespread nature of sex work in present-day China.

Government concerns over the now publicly acknowledged existence of commercial sex and STI are linked to the new threat posed by AIDS. This is because international medical experts argue that the same behaviours and circumstances that may put people at risk for getting an STI can put them at greater risk for getting HIV (CDC Centers for Disease Control and Prevention 2015). As a consequence, the epidemiological and behaviour-change-focused language of global AIDS governance, which emphasizes management of risks, has partly displaced the abolitionist discourse of revolutionary socialism. The next section outlines this shift by offering a short history of the emergence of and changing nature of government responses to AIDS in China.

Governing AIDS in China

The spread of HIV has occurred in different and evolving patterns around the world. In the USA, AIDS was first associated with men who have sex with men living in major cities. In fact, the newly identified disease was briefly called gay-related immunodeficiency syndrome, until the presence of infection in people who had injected drugs using non-sterile injecting equipment, women who were married to bisexual men, and children who had had blood transfusions, suggested a virus that was blood-borne and sexually transmissible (Osmond 2003). In African countries, and in the context of civil war, the spread of AIDS was associated with people who injected drugs, military-associated prostitution and migrant labour (Cliff and Smallman-Raynor 2003). In Asian countries such as Thailand, it was associated with people who injected drugs and a military- and tourism-associated sex industry ('HIV in Thailand' 2011). The spread of HIV in China was initially associated with people living in ethnic minority border regions who had injected drugs using non-sterile equipment, and with commercial plasma donors from rural areas of poor central provinces (Wu, Rou and Cui 2004: 8).

China started AIDS surveillance in 1986; official notification of HIV infection became a legal requirement in 1989 (Ibid.). In 1995, the Ministry of Health established 42 national sentinel surveillance sites in 23 provinces with the support of the WHO. By 2002, the number of sites had increased to around 160, providing national surveillance across the country's 31 provincial-level administrative divisions. The number of sites rose to nearly 1,900 in 2010 (Wen *et al*. 2012: 79). New sites are established when the HIV prevalence among key populations is registered as higher than 5 per cent in a localized area (Ibid.: 80).

Drawing on national sentinel surveillance data, scholars often divide the spread of HIV in the PRC into four stages, which highlight China's changing HIV demography and evolving approaches to the governance of HIV and AIDS (Jeffreys and Yu 2015: 123; Yu 2016: 183–6). Stage One began with the identification in Beijing of the country's first AIDS case in 1985; it involved a foreign tourist. Most of the cases that were subsequently reported involved overseas Chinese and foreign residents in the PRC, and were located in cities on the eastern seaboard that had been opened to export-orientated economic development (Smith 2005: 66). AIDS was consequently viewed as an 'imported disease' and government policies focused on preventing its entry into China (Hayes 2005: 2; Wu, Rou and Cui 2004: 10–11).

The PRC's first national AIDS-related regulation, the Certain Regulations on the Monitoring and Control of AIDS, came into effect in January 1988 (State Council 1987). Article 1 stated that the regulations were 'formulated to prevent the AIDS virus from spreading into China from abroad or from occurring and becoming prevalent in China and to safeguard the health of the people' (Ibid.). Strategies based on exclusion included prohibiting or monitoring the importation of blood products into the PRC. Long-term visitors from overseas were also required to undertake physical health examinations prior to entry, which theoretically precluded the issue of visas to people who were HIV-positive (Ibid.: Article 5).

Stage Two (1989–1993) relates to the identification of HIV among people who had injected drugs using non-sterile equipment in China's western and south-western border regions, including the Xinjiang Uyghur Autonomous Region, and Yunnan Province and the Guangxi Autonomous Region (Jeffreys and Yu 2015: 124; Smith 2005: 66). These cases were linked with drug-using cultural practices among ethnic minorities (Hayes 2005: 2–3). While indicating that the spread of HIV had domestic dimensions, the association of these cases with ethnic minority populations living in rural areas meant that HIV continued to be framed as a 'peripheral' problem, or as a disease that was not associated with urban Han

Chinese. The PRC's adoption of exclusionary measures and distancing frameworks is sometimes characterized as 'the era of denial' (Yu 2016: 184).

Stage Three, starting in late 1994, is associated with commercial plasma donors and the recipients of blood transfusions in poor central provinces (Anagnost 2006: 509–29; Gu and Renwick 2008: 89–91). Henan was one of many provinces during the early 1990s where commercial companies and provincial health authorities offered rural agricultural workers money for blood. The collected blood was then pooled together and the plasma was extracted, and the remaining red blood cells from an unscreened pool were reinjected into blood sellers to speed recovery time. Such practices resulted in an estimated 500,000 HIV infections in Henan Province alone (Gittings 2001).

The dramatic rise in the number of domestic HIV infections via commercial plasma donations was accompanied by policy efforts to mitigate the spread of infection. In late 1994, China signed the Paris Declaration at the International AIDS Summit, which called on national governments to formulate AIDS prevention and treatment policies. By 1998, HIV infection had been reported in all of the PRC's 31 provinces, autonomous regions, and municipalities, with over 70 per cent of all reported cases being in the countryside (Zhang, Mao and Xia 2004: 39). International commitments and the growing number of domestic AIDS cases ensured that neither denial nor the use of exclusionary tactics constituted a viable approach to the governance of HIV in China.

Since 2001, the spread of HIV in China has followed a Stage Four pattern: the majority of new cases of infection are domestically generated and linked to sexual transmission. Sexual transmission accounted for around 33 per cent of all newly diagnosed cases of HIV infection in 2006 and more than 94 per cent in 2016 (Ministry of Health of the PRC 2012: 5–6; '654,000 living with HIV/AIDS in China' 2016). Before 2009, the majority of new cases were related to contaminated blood transfusions, mother-to-child transmission and the sharing of drug-injecting equipment. The number of infections from these transmission routes has been reduced by closing down commercial blood centres, improving antenatal services, and providing needle exchange and methadone treatment programs for people who inject drugs. The rising rate of HIV infection from sexual transmission has encouraged what Haiqing Yu (2016: 185) calls the 'sexualization' of China's AIDS response. The threat of AIDS has become linked to the sexual behaviours of people classified as members of key populations.

Also since the 2000s, the PRC's health authorities have started actively working with the UN and other international agencies, as well as with local governments, the private sector and the media, to design, implement and publicize AIDS awareness programs. These public-private collaborations initially focused on female sex workers. They have since expanded to include other key and vulnerable populations such as men who have sex with men and rural-to-urban migrant labourers.

In December 2016, the *China Daily* announced that the PRC's approach to combating HIV and AIDS had proved successful, with UNAIDS popularizing aspects of this approach in countries in Africa ('China's anti-AIDS, HIV practices successful: experts' 2016). This is a remarkable turnaround, given UNAIDS' claim that the PRC faced a 'titanic peril' in 2002 because of government neglect of AIDS (The UN Theme Group on HIV/AIDS in China 2002: 7). The country's AIDS response is still inconsistent, as demonstrated by plans to provide greater free supplies of medicines for the prevention and treatment of HIV and AIDS in the Thirteenth Five-Year Guidelines for National Economic and Social Development for 2016–2020, and in PRC's national action plan (2016–2020) for the containment and prevention of HIV/AIDS (Guowuyuan bangongting 2017; National People's Congress 2016b). The local implementation of national policies and the availability of services have varied according to degrees of decentralized government, and hence the political will, budgets and resources of local governments (Hood 2015b: 357; Huang, Y. 2013: 88–9). Improvements to China's HIV governance were also demanded at a time when the public health sector was chronically underfunded (Hood 2015b: 366). Yet the PRC's AIDS response has shifted from being funded by international agencies in the early 2000s to being domestically funded by the start of 2015 (National Health and Family Planning Commission of the PRC 2015: 12). Significant changes have also taken place in the realm of public access to information about HIV and AIDS.

Representing AIDS in China

Before 2002, China's state-controlled media was largely silent on the subject of AIDS. The PRC's Medium- and Long-Term Strategic Plan for HIV/AIDS Prevention and Control (1998–2010), issued in December 1998, stated that the media should plan to incorporate regular publicity and education about STI and AIDS by 2002 (Guowuyuan 1998: Section 4, Item 3). The issuing of this document was preceded by the establishment of two institutions in July 1998, which were renamed in 2002 as the National Center for AIDS/STD Control and Prevention (NCAIDS), under the supervision of the Chinese Center for Disease Control and Prevention (CDC). On 25 May 2001, the State Council issued the PRC's first national action plan (2001–2005) for the containment and prevention of HIV/AIDS. The action plan stipulated that the broadcast media and central and local newspapers should release news stories and public service advertisements (PSAs) about the work of AIDS education and HIV prevention at least once a week (Guowuyuan bangongting 2001: Item 3, Article 2). This led to a rapid increase in media coverage of AIDS from 2002 onwards, with China Central Television broadcasting around 230 news items on HIV and AIDS in the first 10 months of 2003 (UNAIDS 2004: 22).

The PRC government's failure to respond proactively to the policy imperatives of AIDS until more than a decade after the country's first AIDS case was identified attracted trenchant criticism from international organizations. In 2002, UNAIDS famously described the PRC's sluggish response to the work of AIDS prevention as a 'titanic peril' (The UN Theme Group on HIV/AIDS in China 2002: 7). The country's AIDS response was criticized for being 'too medical and too narrow' (Ibid.: 73). It was further criticized for failing to incorporate private sector resources and making limited use of the media, other than as a means to disseminate 'scary' AIDS stories (Ibid.).

A media content analysis of AIDS reportage between 1986 and 2002 in the *People's Daily* – the public 'voice' of the CCP and a primary conduit for official discourse in China – confirms that the topic of AIDS received minimal media coverage until after 2002 (Dong, Chang and Chen 2008). Of a total of 465 stories, only 3 were reported on the front page (Ibid.: 363–4). AIDS was generally presented as an inconsequential and non-national issue that affected foreigners and injecting drug users, with limited attention paid to prevention methods and local people affected by AIDS (Ibid.). Moreover, media stories about people living with HIV and AIDS often referred to poor and suffering Africans (Hood 2011).

While it is not difficult to find examples of sensationalist media coverage of AIDS in China (Yu 2016: 185), a comparison of AIDS stories in the *New York Times* and the *People's Daily* between January and December 2014 reveals that Chinese media coverage is broadly equivalent to that of its Western counterparts, while having a more local AIDS focus. Based on a search in the Factiva.com (global news) database, the *New York Times* ran 34 dedicated articles on AIDS in 2014, only 2 of which were featured on the front page. Some dealt with AIDS in New York and the USA, but the majority focused on AIDS in Africa. Numerous articles referred to the development of new drugs and treatment regimes, but only three mentioned the utility of condoms in preventing HIV transmission. The stories referred to women, children, sex workers, and men who have sex with men as being among the people most affected by AIDS. However, the people speaking about AIDS were mainly medical researchers, government representatives and members of private foundations and NGOs, rather than people living with HIV.

Based on a search in the China National Knowledge Infrastructure, China Core Newspapers Full-text Database, the *People's Daily* ran 29 dedicated stories about AIDS in 2014, with 3 on the front page and 1 editorial (cnki.net). Only three articles focused on AIDS in non-local contexts. Most focused on China's AIDS response and how to improve access to AIDS prevention and treatment services (19 in total), with the remainder talking about China's collaboration with the UN system, and the development of new drugs and treatments. Only two articles mentioned condoms, a front-page story on World AIDS Day and a related article on another page. Many stories referred to Chinese women, children, young adults, sex workers, and men who have sex with men as being among the groups of people most affected by AIDS, and some mentioned the need to overcome AIDS-related stigma and discrimination. While some stories were about people living with HIV, the people speaking about AIDS were mainly Chinese medical researchers, health officials and celebrity ambassadors, or international spokespersons.

As in Western societies, however, nearly 95 per cent of the Chinese population now receive information about AIDS from increasingly diversified media, which includes the Internet and social media, and AIDS storylines in television programming, films and PSAs (Hood 2011: 35–6; Li *et al.* 2009). Blogs and online diaries about HIV are readily available in which Chinese people living with HIV describe how the virus, and social discrimination, affect their lives (Hood 2015b: 366). In 2004–2006, the television soap opera *Bai Xing* (*Ordinary People*), which is about a rural village and rural development, included AIDS-related themes as a significant part of the storyline (UNAIDS 2004: 20). A government-backed film about two people living with HIV who fall in love was released in 2011. Titled *Love for Life*, the film starred major Chinese celebrities Zhang Ziyi and Aaron Kwok, and people living with HIV in supporting roles (Lee 2011).

One example of AIDS-related public service advertising based on public-private collaborations is the 2008 *Life Is Too Good* campaign, featuring celebrity actors Jackie Chan and Pu Cunxin, and soprano Peng Liyuan, the wife of President Xi Jinping ('Life is too good' 2007). The campaign, which was coordinated by the UN and the PRC's Ministry of Health through partnerships with China's media and advertising sector, provided a simple message about how to prevent the sexual transmission of HIV in the form of short video clips. In one of these videos, Jackie Chan performs on a movie set to a script that states: 'I love making movies and I love life. An action movie needs danger but life needs protecting. Sexual transmission of AIDS is on the rise; condoms help reduce the risk. Life is too good, protect yourself' (Ibid.).

As the turn to representing AIDS in entertainment media and PSAs suggests, government authorities in China are engaging in innovative public-private partnerships to halt the spread of HIV by encouraging individuals to transform their own sexual behaviours and use condoms. In 2014, China's Blued, the most popular mobile gay dating application in the world with more than 27 million users, began promoting AIDS awareness with funding from China's CDC and UNAIDS ('"Nantong" ganran aizibing zengjia tongzhi shejiao pingtai huyu baohu ziji' 2015). The dating application was launched in 2012 by Danlan.org, a gay website (bluedapp.com). A red ribbon icon within the user interface links users to 'information about the importance of correct and consistent condom and lubricant use' (UNAIDS 2015b: 85). It also 'engages users to answer questions that are intended to increase their knowledge of HIV treatment, prevention tools and care options, and it points them to locations where they can access HIV testing and counselling' (Ibid.: 86). Guidelines for health interventions among men who have sex with men issued by the CDC and NCAIDS in 2016 further recommend leveraging social networking sites such as WeChat and QQ, and other dating applications, such as Grindr, GayPark and Jack'd, to provide information about safer sex (Zhongguo jibing yufang kongzhi zhongxin, xingbing aizibing yufang kongzhi zhongxin 2016a: 60).

To offer another example, on World AIDS Day in December 2015, the CDC posted a 39-second, cartoon-style PSA video on using condoms to prevent AIDS on Ku6.com, an online video company. The Ku6 website targets youth and features news, movies, television dramas, music videos, entertainment sports and user-generated content. The PSA shows a hockey match in a major sports stadium in which the goalkeeper (a condom) enthusiastically hits back numerous balls (HIV). The PSA tagline is 'Condoms Prevent AIDS: "Sex", Be Happy and Healthy' ('Anquantao fang aizi, "xing" fu you jiankang' 2015).

Thus, the development of Chinese digital and social media is facilitating the provision of information to interested individuals about HIV prevention and treatment via the private sector. The PRC government no longer relies solely on the top-down provision or transmission of AIDS education through medicalized health campaigns. China's citizens are now being encouraged to access information about how to protect themselves from HIV infection, and therefore to govern themselves, through social networking sites and commercial lifestyle, entertainment and advertising media.

Chapter contents

The remaining chapters examine China's HIV governance by exploring the interweaving of procedures for representing AIDS and intervening upon people classified as members of key and vulnerable populations. They outline the development of public health programs designed to promote condom use and prevent the spread of HIV in the PRC. They trace the evolution of such programs from a 'covert' pilot program focused on sex workers in undisclosed locations in the early 2000s to the roll-out of a nationwide program with broadcast media publicity in 2006. They consider the origins, rationale and implementation of initiatives focused on female sex workers and look at the extension of such initiatives to include other populations identified as key to ending the AIDS epidemic in China, especially men who have sex with men and male rural-to-urban migrant labourers. In the process, they document how the PRC's evolving AIDS response has promoted new ways of 'knowing' particular sectors of the population, and different approaches to the governance of commercial sex, homosexuality and sex in general. The concluding chapter looks at some of the challenges and openings that are being presented by the PRC's commitment to UNAIDS' goal of ending the AIDS epidemic as a global health threat by 2030.

Chapter 2 examines the pilot implementation of a 100 Per Cent Condom Use Program (100% CUP) in the PRC in the early 2000s, and the subsequent adoption of national guidelines for action. The 100% CUP is a transnational health intervention that aims to prevent the sexual transmission of HIV by transforming the behaviours of people classified as sex workers. This category originally referred only to women. The 100% CUP is defined by the WHO as a collaborative programme between government authorities (health, police and Governor/Mayor's office) and all sex entertainment establishments (owners, managers and sex workers) that aims to reduce the spread of HIV and other STI by assuring that (male latex) condoms are used: '100 per cent of the time; in 100 per cent of risky sexual relations; and in 100 per cent of the sex entertainment establishments in a large geographic area such as a town, district, province or country' (World Health Organization Regional Office for the Western Pacific 2004: 5).

The chapter explains how the perceived success of the original 100% CUP in Thailand in the late 1980s was translated into a framework for government action in China that has involved ideational, political and social change. It details the introduction of five localized pilot projects during the early 2000s, followed by the evolution of a national program with central government support and enabling legislation by 2006. This development highlights the remarkable pace at which the PRC adopted an international program for government action on AIDS, once the utility of that program was accepted. Public health interventions promoting HIV prevention through condom use have since become commonplace. Such interventions are supported by new government frameworks and funding arrangements.

Chapter 3 examines the development of Chinese media coverage of the 100% CUP, demonstrating an important shift in political communication on AIDS and the sex industry. In Thailand, the 100% CUP was trialled in Ratchaburi Province with some media publicity in 1989. It was promoted nationally by mid-1992 concurrently with a national AIDS education and condom promotion campaign, which was a focus of government-led public service advertising in the mainstream media (television, radio and newspapers) (UNAIDS 2000: 25). Media publicity was viewed as integral to the success of the Thai 100% CUP and is upheld by UNAIDS (2004) as a key vehicle for promoting AIDS-related attitudinal and behavioural change in general. However, there was no accepted political basis and corollary language for talking about the goals of piloting a 100% CUP in China at the start of the new millennium.

In China, the 100% CUP was initially implemented without national media coverage because it involved then controversial issues that one health official described as akin to a 'bomb' when put together: namely, AIDS, prostitution and condoms (Zhang Li 2002). Local government authorities actively discouraged media coverage of the preliminary pilot projects in 2001–2002, fearing that media publicity would cause public panic and damage the reputation of participating regions because of the stigma attached to AIDS and commercial sex (Lixian xiangmuban 2004). The chapter consequently tracks the evolution of government responses and the role of the media – from initially keeping a low profile on the pilot projects in order to avoid raising public concerns, towards actively promoting a national 100% CUP with the support of the central government. This demanded the development of a media strategy to modify public thinking on the appropriate nature of government responses to the sex industry.

Chapter 4 examines the evolving nature of policies and laws on prostitution and STI in China, providing the historical policy background required to understand the controversial nature of implementing a national 100% CUP, and detailing the legal and social changes that the implementation of that program has brought in tow. The chapter first outlines the significant changes that have taken place with regard to the PRC's prostitution policies, and legislation linking the sex industry and STI. In the process, it explains why coercive law-enforcement strategies were viewed as the primary means to control commercial sex and the spread of HIV in China until after the turn of the century, when PRC health authorities started to collaborate with international organizations to implement pilot versions of the 100% CUP. It then traces the shift from explicit censorship of media discussion of prostitution in China during the 1980s towards permitting restricted media coverage of police campaigns against the prostitution industry in the 1990s, and eventually encouraging broad media publicity of HIV prevention measures relating to the sex industry in the late 2000s.

Finally, the chapter shows that the expansion of AIDS-related health communication has generated new Chinese-language terms for condoms and sex sellers, flowing from the reconfiguration of STI and prostitution as objects of government from the perspective of public health, and not just policing. Condoms have been rebranded as a 'safety sheath' (*anquantao*), as opposed to being primarily a contraceptive device or 'prevent pregnancy sheath' (*biyuntao*). Terms such as 'sex worker' and 'sex industry' have been translated into Chinese and used in official health documents, although they have yet to become a part of everyday speech. The PRC's adoption of international governance strategies designed to minimize the health risks associated with the sex industry has thus turned commercial sex into a matter of ongoing health management, rather than strictly policing.

Chapter 5 surveys the nature and effects of behavioural health interventions providing AIDS education and promoting condom use to sex workers. It outlines the planning instructions issued by the CDC for conducting such interventions in entertainment and leisure venues (Zhongguo jibing yufang kongzhi zhongxin 2004). It then looks at examples of AIDS education booklets for sex workers and their clients (Zhongguo jibing yufang kongzhi zhongxin n.d.; Zhongguo xingbing aizibing fangzhi xiehui and UNAIDS n.d.). Finally, it discusses public responses to the provision of AIDS education for sex workers, or what China's media dubbed 'the working-girl training classes'. Media publicity on the goals of the 100% CUP has encouraged a diversification of opinions on how the sex industry is best understood and handled. Retired Communist Party officials, lawyers, NGOs and sex workers alike have argued through the media, and in political and public venues, that the PRC's ban on commercial sex should be overturned to promote public health and sex workers' rights (Branigan 2010; Yang Zhongxu 2008; Ye Haiyan 2010; Zhou Ruijin 2006b).

The perceived successes and failures of these behavioural health interventions are routinely translated into calls for more and improved health interventions. One proclaimed success is that the percentage of female sex workers living with HIV in the PRC has remained at a relatively low level – 0.2 per cent in 2015 (UNAIDS 2016a). The perception of post-intervention success has legitimized both the original intervention and the introduction of similar programs in new locations and areas across China. Perceived problems impacting on the general effectiveness of such interventions include the continued stigma attached to sex workers; the tendency for health intervention to focus on particular groups of sex workers to the exclusion of others; and the limited attention paid until recently to other populations classified as key to the global AIDS response. These populations include men who have sex with men, male-male sex workers and male migrant labourers.

Chapter 6 explores the changing nature of public discourses on male homosexuality and the emergence of men who have sex with men as a key focus of HIV prevention training in China. It traces shifts in public representations of homosexuality, from a subject that was virtually absent from public discourse in the early years of the PRC to a topic that is now of significant interest in discussions about public health. It then outlines the expanded roles played by health authorities and community organizations in providing AIDS awareness programs for men who have sex with men. This key population was typically referred to in UN and medical documents in the abbreviated form of MSM. However, the 2015 UNAIDS

Terminology Guidelines recommend abandoning this abbreviation because it is dehumanizing (UNAIDS 2015c: 33).

The chapter also considers the changing nature of media discussions of men who have sex with men in the context of AIDS prevention and developing struggles for gay civil rights. In doing so, it shows how the act of classifying and administering human kinds as 'MSM' has had a 'looping or feedback effect' (Hacking 2002: 99). People who have been classified as MSM, and people claiming to speak on their behalf, are contesting their construction as vectors of disease and demanding anti-discrimination measures.

Chapter 7 looks at the extension of health campaigns promoting AIDS awareness and safer-sex practices to male rural-to-urban migrant labourers. It provides a short history of internal migration in the PRC, showing how urbanization and the legacy of Mao-era controls on population mobility have disadvantaged rural-born compared to urban-born residents. It explains how structural inequality, reflected in poor education, precarious employment and reduced access to local government services, may exacerbate the vulnerability of rural-born migrant workers to HIV infection. It then outlines policy developments designed to improve access to HIV prevention, testing and care services for migrant populations, before describing diverse efforts to promote AIDS awareness in migrant workplaces and communities. These efforts involve numerous ministries and government departments, Party-affiliated mass organizations, state-owned and private businesses, and volunteers.

Finally, the chapter looks at celebrity-endorsed public service advertising designed to popularize AIDS education for migrant workers and discourage social discrimination against people living with HIV. Such PSAs constitute a new way of communicating information about AIDS in China. They offer informal and entertaining educational tools that large sectors of the population can access informally through broadcast, digital and social media, rather than referring to top-down medicalized health interventions conducted in specific locations and venues. They also form a novel attempt to combat prejudice against people living with HIV in the Chinese context. At the same time, the focus on rural-to-urban migrant workers as vulnerable to HIV infection may perpetuate the association of HIV with poverty, sex work and homosexuality, and reinforce the perception that HIV is not a problem for people migrating between Chinese cities to take up higher-paid work in government and corporate sectors.

In conclusion, Chapter 8 examines the issues raised for China's HIV governance by the UNAIDS plan to end the AIDS epidemic as a global health threat by 2030. The WHO has issued guidelines to support this goal, which both consolidate information about how to conduct health interventions focused on key populations, and provide detailed instructions about how the actions of participating countries are to be monitored, evaluated and 'scored'. The chapter argues that, considered in the Chinese context, the linking of HIV to key populations can create 'moving targets' for government intervention, direct attention away from local variants and even produce 'new' kinds of people. The latter argument is illustrated with reference to the WHO's recent determination that transgender people are key to the global AIDS response.

2 AIDS and the sex industry

The 100 Per Cent Condom Use Program

This chapter examines the pilot implementation of a 100 Per Cent Condom Use Program (100% CUP) in the People's Republic of China during the early 2000s, and the subsequent adoption of national guidelines for action. The act of governing the conduct of people as individuals or groups presupposes that some aspect of their existence has been identified and presented through complex processes, involving myriad professionals, government agencies, the media, and so forth, as a 'problem' that is in need of governing to improve the commonweal (Miller and Rose 2008: 14–15). Translating such 'problems' into corrective programs of government intervention also requires that differences of opinion, whether fundamental or not, are addressed and brought into some kind of alignment with each other, in order to create a common language and technical measures for presenting and remedying the identified issue (Ibid.).

In the case of the 100% CUP – a transnational public health intervention that aims to prevent the spread of HIV by transforming the behaviours of sex workers – the program's organizing rationale is provided by the World Health Organization (WHO). The 100% CUP is defined as

> a collaborative programme between local authorities (health, police/public security and Governor/Mayor's office) and all 'sex entertainment establishments' (owners/managers and sex workers) that aims to reduce the sexual transmission of HIV and STI by assuring that [male latex] condoms are used:
>
> - 100 per cent of the time;
> - in 100 per cent of risky sexual relations; and
> - in 100 per cent of the sex entertainment establishments in a large geographic area such as a town, district, province or country.
>
> (World Health Organization Regional Office for the Western Pacific (WHO/WPR) 2004: 5)

The use of the 100 per cent figure refers to a goal rather than a numerical target. Programs that achieve a compliance rate of at least 90 per cent are viewed as successful (Ibid.: 5).

DOI: 10.4324/9781315175546-2

The 100% CUP was first piloted in Thailand during the late 1980s, and has been 'widely cited as one of the few examples of an effective national AIDS prevention program anywhere in the world' (Ainsworth, Beyrer and Soucat 2003: 13). The Thai 100% CUP is credited with increasing the rate of consistent condom use in sex establishments from around 14 per cent in the early 1990s to over 93 per cent by the late 1990s. This dramatically reduced the number of men presenting at STI clinics – around 220,000 men per year in 1988 compared to 20,000 in 1995 (Ibid.: 17). The 100% CUP is also praised for contributing to an 80 per cent drop in new HIV infections in Thailand between 1990 and 2000 (Ibid.: 22).

Thailand's 100% CUP mobilized local authorities 'to empower sex workers to refuse unprotected risky sexual practices that are a danger to their health', by normalizing condom use among sellers and buyers of sex (WHO/WPR 2004: 5). Risky sexual practices refer to those involving penetration or potential 'exposure to bodily fluids that spread disease' (Ibid.). Obtaining a commitment across a large geographical area to 100 per cent condom use in all high-risk sexual encounters on the part of sex sellers, and with the support of owners and managers of sex establishments, aimed to reduce any economic disincentive stemming from condom use by making it difficult for buyers of sex to purchase condom-free sex (Ibid.: 10).

In theory, the Thai 100% CUP did not target female sex workers but rather *focused* on them. Such women are presented in the related health literature as facing socio-economic disadvantages (poverty and poor education) that limit their knowledge of STI and capacity to negotiate for 100 per cent condom use in the context of a military- and tourism-driven sex industry ('HIV in Thailand' 2011: 6; WHO/WPR and CDC 2004: 10). Instead, the 100% CUP targeted owners and managers of sex establishments, by making them responsible for supporting outreach education projects and making condoms available onsite. Local governments provided educational materials and free condoms, and potentially penalized non-compliance by suspending operating licenses (WHO/WPR 2004: 11: United Nations Development Programme (UNDP) 2004: 18).

The efficacy of the original Thai 100% CUP was monitored by questioning men presenting at STI clinics about their condom use in 'particular establishments, and not with particular sex workers', although health examinations were arranged for sex workers (WHO/WPR 2004: 12; see also UNDP 2004: 18). It was also monitored by testing men who were conscripted into the military at the age of 21 years through a national lottery, and hence provided a nationally representative sample of young Thai men (Ainsworth, Beyrer and Soucat 2003: 14). Studies of conscripts between 1991 and 1993 revealed that more than 70 per cent had paid for sex at least once during their period of service (Reingold and Phares 2006: 157).

In China at the start of the 2000s, the adoption of a 100% CUP was complicated by the marginal attention paid to AIDS in public health communication, and a history of political opposition to the sex industry. On 1 October 1949, the Chinese Communist Party (CCP) founded the PRC. This followed the CCP's victory over the Nationalist Party after the end of World War II in 1945 and the subsequent end of the second phase of the Chinese Civil War in September 1949. As part of its nation-building program, the new regime set about eradicating the endemic prostitution industry, which was looked upon as a source of national shame (Hershatter 1997: 246; Ma Weigang 1994; Sigley 2009: 46; Zhang Jun 1999). Following a large-scale testing, treatment and education campaign, the CCP also declared to the WHO, in 1964, that China had eradicated active venereal disease, resulting in the closure of the country's venereal disease clinics (Abrams 2001: 433; Cohen *et al.* 1996: S223–9; Chen and Zhang *et al.* 2007: 132). These proclaimed achievements, whether accurate or not, made the resurgence of prostitution and STI in reform-era China a newfound problem for government.

But pilot versions of the 100% CUP were implemented in China with international funding in the early 2000s, resulting in the introduction of supportive legislation in 2006 and the nationwide roll-out of a 100% CUP (Guowuyuan 2006a, 2006c; WHO/WPR 2004). The PRC's Ministry of Health and the WHO first piloted a 100% CUP in four rural sites in different parts of China: the Huangpi area of Wuhan City and Jingcheng Township of Jingjiang City in Jiangsu Province in 2001; and Danzhou City in Hainan Province and Liyang Town, Li County, in Hunan Province in 2002 (WHO/WPR 2004: 19). The four pilots were followed by the introduction of a fifth pilot site in 2003, at Liuzhou City in the Guangxi Zhuang Autonomous Region. The fifth pilot was run by the United Nations Population Fund (UNFPA) and the National Population and Family Planning Commission of the PRC (NPFPC) (Ibid.: 6).

According to figures released by the PRC's Ministry of Health and the NPFPC, the national roll-out of such programs has been successful. Surveys of female sex workers revealed a condom use rate of nearly 88 per cent in 2012 and more than 90 per cent in 2015, which means that China has met the WHO's compliance target of 90 per cent (Ministry of Health of the PRC 2012: 8; UNAIDS 2016b: 35). The reported HIV prevalence among female sex workers has also remained relatively low at 0.3 per cent in 2012 and 0.2 per cent in 2014, compared to around 0.04 per cent for the general population during the same time period (National Health and Family Planning Commission of the PRC 2014: 5; 2015: 7, 13).

The chapter consequently first examines the implementation of a 100% CUP in Thailand and explains how this was translated into a framework for government action in other developing countries such as China. It then looks at the introduction of five localized pilot programs in the PRC, before outlining the development of a national program with central government support and enabling legislation by 2006. These developments highlight the remarkable pace at which the PRC adopted an international program for government action on AIDS, once the utility of the 100% CUP was accepted. Public health interventions promoting condom use as a means of preventing the sexual transmission of HIV have since become commonplace. Such interventions are supported by new governmental frameworks and funding arrangements involving national legislation, cooperation between multiple government agencies, domestic government funding and public-private collaborations.

The example of Thailand

The 100% CUP originated in Thailand, where it is credited with achieving significant outcomes, at least initially, in controlling the spread of STI and HIV through the nationwide promotion of safer sexual behaviours and condom use ('Thailand's new condom crusade' n.d.; UNAIDS 2000: 1–2). In Thailand, as in China, AIDS was presented at first as a 'foreigner's disease' (Ainsworth, Beyrer and Soucat 2003: 14; UNDP 2004: 7). This meant that domestic prevention policies originally were restricted chiefly to ensuring the safety of the blood supply and mandating that AIDS cases be reported.

With the establishment of Thailand's HIV sentinel surveillance system in 1989, it became clear that previous reporting systems had failed to capture the rapid spread of HIV infection among both people who had injected drugs using non-sterile injecting equipment and other sectors of the population. During 1988, the HIV prevalence among people who injected drugs in Bangkok had skyrocketed from 1 to 43 per cent (Ainsworth, Beyrer and Soucat 2003: 14; Punpanich, Ungchusak and Detels 2004: 121). Reports from the launch of a national sentinel system across 14 provinces revealed that 44 per cent of brothel-based female sex workers in Chiang Mai, a town in northern Thailand, were infected with HIV, a figure that rose to 67 per cent by 1993 (Ainsworth, Beyrer and Soucat 2003: 15; Reingold and Phares 2006: 157). In fact, between 1989 and June 1991 the reported HIV prevalence among female sex workers in Thailand rose from just over 3 per cent to more than 15 per cent (WHO/WPR 2004: 2: UNAIDS 2000: 1). A corollary survey of young Thai men, who were tested when conscripted into the military, demonstrated an increased HIV prevalence from less than 1 per cent in 1989 to 3 per cent in 1991 (Ibid.). An increased HIV prevalence was also reported among women attending antenatal clinics (Rojanapithayakorn and Hanenberg 1996: 1). In short, information derived from the expansion of the national sentinel surveillance system, and other monitoring systems, suggested that the threat of HIV transmission in Thailand stemmed not only from the behaviours of people who had injected drugs using non-sterile equipment, but also from those engaging in risky sexual behaviours.

A 1990 national survey, the Survey of Partner Relations and Risk of HIV Infection in Thailand, further indicated that commercial sex was a potential major route for HIV transmission by highlighting high levels of risky sexual behaviours in Thai society (Ainsworth, Beyrer and Soucat 2003: 15). The survey, undertaken by the Thai Red Cross and Chulalongkorn University with funding from the WHO's Global Program on AIDS, revealed that 22 per cent of Thai men aged between 15 and 49 years and 37 per cent of those aged between 20 and 24 years had paid for sex in the previous year (UNAIDS *et al.* 1998: 6). But only 38 per cent of the participants who engaged in commercial sex said that they had used condoms consistently (UNDP 2004: 11).

Thus, the results of epidemiological and behavioural surveys, and information gathered from the Thai sentinel surveillance system, suggested that preventing the spread of HIV throughout Thai society required the introduction of prevention strategies promoting safer-sex practices for sex workers and their clients. This situation encouraged the Thai government to implement a series of intervention programs in regional areas in 1991, based on the promotion of 100 per cent condom use in sex establishments (Punpanich, Ungchusak and Detels 2004: 122).

Concerned that the sex industry would play a key role in the spread of AIDS in Thailand, public health authorities had already launched a pilot 100% CUP in the Thai province of Ratchaburi in 1989. The pilot program was introduced based on the observation that male clients were reluctant to use condoms when engaging in commercial sex, and sex workers were unable to negotiate condom use effectively because of their disadvantaged economic and social position (Rojanapithayakorn W. 2006: 41–2; WHO/WPR 2004: 2). The pilot program consequently aimed to ensure that all sex workers working in sex establishments in the province adopted a 'no condom, no sex' policy, thereby making it difficult in theory for buyers of sex to purchase condom-free sex and normalizing the use of condoms in commercial sexual encounters (UNAIDS 2000: 2).

Due to the illegal status of Thailand's sex industry, owners and managers of sex establishments reportedly were afraid to distribute condoms openly in their venues, in case this was construed as evidence of organizing prostitution in the event of a police raid (Phoolcharoen 2006: 71). Public health officials therefore employed a collaborative strategy designed to garner support for the objectives of the program. They enlisted the help of local police, and owners of sex establishments and sex workers, to implement the program under the leadership of local government authorities, with all of the participants working to achieve the common goal of promoting condom use in high-risk sexual encounters (UNAIDS 2000: 2).

The implementation of the pilot 100% CUP in Ratchaburi Province demonstrated positive results in terms of recording increased condom use and declining rates of STI among female sex workers and male clients (WHO/WPR 2004: 3). Hence, in August 1991, then Prime Minister Anand Panyarachun endorsed the promotion of a nationwide 100% CUP and the program was extended to all of Thailand's provinces by mid-1992 (Rojanapithayakorn and Hanenberg 1996: 4; UNAIDS 2000: 3). At the national level, Thailand's government demonstrated its commitment to promoting the 100% CUP by holding meetings with high-level local officials. The Ministry of Public Health ensured the provision of free and high-quality condoms to sex establishments, and information about the effectiveness of condom use as a means of preventing STI was given widespread publicity in the media and through other kinds of public health education programs. At the provincial level, the 100% CUP was implemented through local public health and disease control officers, who collaborated with local police, owners of sex establishments, sex workers and members of non-governmental organizations (UNAIDS 2000: 10–12).

As with the pilot program, the national promotion of the 100% CUP in Thailand generated impressive results, at least initially. Female sex workers self-reported increased use of condoms when engaging in commercial sex, with the reported rate of condom use increasing from 25 per cent in June 1989 to 94 per cent in June 1993 (Hanenberg *et al.* 1994: 523). Pharmacists also reported to project workers that sales of antibiotics had declined during the same period, suggesting a decrease in the incidence of STI and, by implication, an increased rate of condom use (Chamratrithirong *et al.* 1999: 33–4). The successful nature of the original 100% CUP is underscored by rising rates of HIV in Thailand during the 2000s. Some researchers attribute this rise to reduced government funding for AIDS awareness programs and free condom distribution after the 1997 Asian financial crisis ('Thailand's new condom crusade' n.d.; see also Ainsworth, Beyrer and Soucat 2003: 22–4).

The apparent success of the original 100% CUP in Thailand created a framework for action in other developing countries that involves ideational, political and social change (Jeffreys and Su 2011: 318–19). First, it established the organizing rationale of the 100% CUP, which is to ensure that condoms are used in 100 per cent of commercial sexual relations, 100 per cent of the time and in 100 per cent of sex establishments in a specified large geographic area, such as a city, a province or even a country (WHO/WPR 2004: 5). Realizing this goal in Thailand demanded a pragmatic institutional response focused on the issue of public health as opposed to the moral and legal questions associated with the governmental prohibition or legalization of sex work (Ibid.: 13). Other countries are expected to adopt a similarly pragmatic approach in order to ensure the success of implementing a national 100% CUP.

Second, the success of the original Thai 100% CUP turned on the development of multi-sectoral institutional frameworks involving cooperation between international governance structures and funding bodies, national and local government authorities, the media, businesses, NGOs and non-profits, and sex establishment owners and sex workers. Implementing the Thai 100% CUP required commitment and support from multiple government departments and other organizations to identify and collaborate with people who managed and provided commercial sexual services, to ensure support for the program, and to monitor condom use in sex establishments and evaluate condom use among sex workers, clients and the general population (Ibid.: 10–11). It also demanded that inexpensive, quality condoms and clinical services were readily available and accessible in targeted areas. Implementing a 100% CUP thus requires a reconfiguration or expansion of national governing frameworks and structures.

Third, the Thai 100% CUP involved the threat of police-enforced sanctions against non-compliant sex establishments, which implied a shift in policing strategies towards managing rather than containing or ignoring the sex industry. Local police assisted with the implementation of the program by warning uncooperative owners and managers of sex establishments that future non-compliance would result in the closure of their business operations (Ibid.: 11). Although such sanctions were not imposed in practice, the threat of police action against owners who failed to support the objectives of the program distinguished the Thai 100% CUP from other condom promotion activities at the time (Chamratrithirong *et al.* 1999: 27–8; Rojanapithayakorn and Hanenberg 1996: 4; UNDP 2004: 18).

Finally, the perceived failures of the Thai 100% CUP suggested that subsequent iterations of the 100% CUP in other developing countries should be run in tandem with health campaigns promoting condom use and AIDS awareness among the broader population, which has far-reaching implications for behavioural and attitudinal change. The original Thai 100% CUP chiefly focused on 'direct sex establishments', that is, businesses that provide sexual services on site. It did not focus on 'freelance and indirect sex workers', that is, people who negotiate commercial sexual encounters on the street or through 'indirect' establishments such as massage parlours, bars and restaurants (Punpanich, Ungchusak and Detels 2004: 130; WHO/WPR 2004: 17; UNDP 2004: 3). It also focused on women who provided commercial sexual services rather than male clients, and excluded other populations of sex workers at risk of exposure to STI and HIV, for example, transgenders and men who have sex with men (WHO/WPR 2006: 8; UNDP 2004: 3).

In addition, the national implementation of the 100% CUP in Thailand did not lead to greatly increased rates of condom use in non-commercial, heterosexual relationships. A survey of HIV risk behaviours in Bangkok from 1993 to 1996 found that low condom use persisted in non-commercial sexual acts (Mills *et al.* 1997: S43–51). Nationally, the estimated levels of condom use for female sex workers when having sex with non-commercial partners, such as lovers, fiancés and male friends, varied between 32 and 73 per cent (UNAIDS 2000: 30). In terms of male clients, only 40 per cent claimed to have used condoms consistently with fiancées and girlfriends and around two-thirds with other female acquaintances (Ibid.: 32). These omissions and failures suggested that subsequent iterations of the 100% CUP in other countries should be run in conjunction with AIDS-related health campaigns focused on national populations and especially youth.

In summary, the original 100% CUP in Thailand is regarded as a positive example of an effective HIV and STI prevention strategy in a developing country, with applicability to other countries such as China. Indeed, the World Bank claimed in 2005 that seven million lives had been saved in Thailand because of large-scale HIV prevention measures introduced between 1991 and 2004 (Revenga *et al.* 2006: 25).

The example of Thailand also suggested that other countries had to meet at least four preconditions if they intended to implement a successful 100% CUP and obtain international funding to support that goal. First, effective implementation of the 100% CUP requires active and ongoing political support at both the national and local levels, although the public expression of that commitment may vary in different contexts (Rojanapithayakorn and Hanenberg 1996: 6; 'Thailand's new condom crusade' n.d.). Second, the program has to make maximum use of existing health and government infrastructures. At the same time, the effective implementation of the program requires developing and creating a new and more efficient infrastructure, in order to minimize costs and guarantee continued implementation in new geographical areas – that is, to be sustainable in the long term (UNAIDS 2000: 38–40). Third, successful implementation requires close collaboration between all of the actors involved in the roll-out of the program (Chamratrithirong *et al.* 1999: 113; UNAIDS 2000: 38–9). Finally, the program has to not only recognize the diversity of female sex workers and their clients, but also has to move beyond these groups to include men who have sex with men, and young adults and adolescents more generally (Punpanich, Ungchusak and Detels 2004: 131; UNAIDS 2000: 40).

None of these conditions was met when China started to pilot localized versions of the 100% CUP in the early 2000s.

Piloting China's 100% CUP

Unlike in many other countries, the PRC government has promoted condom use and distributed free condoms to married couples as a contraceptive device along with a national policy of family planning since 1974 (Ma Suwen 2005). The once common Chinese-language term for condoms '*biyuntao*', or 'avoid pregnancy sheath', highlights the historical link between condoms and marital contraception (Jeffreys and Huang 2009: 162). Until recently, premarital sex was actively discouraged and condoms were distributed, often free of charge, to married government employees in state-owned enterprises as a contraceptive device. In the early 2000s, the PRC government purchased an estimated 1.2 billion condoms annually, with a commercial value of between CNY 2 and CNY 20 for a 12-pack, from seven suppliers and more than 500 small manufacturers to support the goals of the one-child-per-couple family policy, which became a two-child-per-couple policy in 2016 ('What do condoms mean to the Chinese?' 2002; for a discussion of the one-child-per-couple policy, see Greenhalgh and Winckler 2005; Jeffreys and Yu 2015: 15–44).

However, health interventions focused on populations categorized by the WHO as key to the global AIDS response were rare in China before the early 2000s. The first study to test the feasibility and effectiveness of a community-based intervention for sex workers was conducted over a six-week period in 1996–1997 in 30 business establishments in southwest China, with funding from the World Bank (Wu *et al.* 2007). It focused on providing education and distributing condoms, and reported increased knowledge of HIV transmission and increased rates of condom use following the intervention (Ibid.). Ma Suwen and his colleagues describe another pilot behaviour intervention conducted in Guangzhou between March 1998 and October 1999, with support from UNAIDS and the World AIDS Foundation, where health professionals provided information about STI and condom use to nearly 1,000 sex workers. The participants subsequently reported that the use of condoms in their commercial sexual transactions had increased from 24 per cent to nearly 80 per cent (Ma and Dukers *et al.* 2002: 110). The perceived efficacy of these studies in promoting condom use suggested that broader community-based interventions were both feasible and necessary. Data from a national behaviour surveillance survey conducted in 2001 showed that female sex workers reported a low rate of condom use in commercial sexual transactions, approximately 14 per cent (State Council AIDS Working Committee Office and UN Theme Group on HIV/AIDS in China 2007: 20).

The PRC's Ministry of Health began to cooperate with the WHO in 2000 with the aim of launching four pilot projects of the 100% CUP in different parts of

China (Rojanapithayakorn 2006: 45; World Health Organization Regional Office for the Western Pacific (WHO/WPR) and the Chinese Center for Disease Control and Prevention (CDC) 2004). These pilot projects were launched without media publicity in rural county-level cities rather than in major cities, and in areas that were not associated with high rates of HIV infection. The decision to focus on rural county-level cities reflected in part the problems posed by the sheer size of China in terms of geography and population. For example, Hunan Province, one of the PRC's 31 provincial-level administrative divisions (excluding Hong Kong, Macau and Taiwan), had an estimated population of over 66 million people in the early 2000s, which was larger than the total population of Thailand (Rojanapithayakorn 2006: 45–6).

The decision to launch the pilot projects without media publicity in rural county-level cities also reflected political considerations. Project leaders actively told reporters to avoid bringing the first three pilot projects to public attention because they feared that publicity would result in public outcry and force them to abandon the pilots (Fang Meng 2002; Zhang Li 2002; Zhu Wenyi 2002). Officials were concerned that the pilot projects would attract negative public attention because people living with HIV and AIDS in China are stigmatized, and the sex industry is banned (Hood 2011; Hyde 2007; Jeffreys 2012b; Zhang 2006: 139–58). People who provide commercial sexual services (usually women) typically are also subject to social condemnation for engaging in what is viewed as an immoral and illegal income-generating activity that is adopted by poor, uncultured and structurally disadvantaged members of society (Boittin 2013: 272; Choi and Holroyd 2007: 497; Rou *et al.* 2010: II44; Xia and Yang 2005: 149).

The first site to begin piloting the 100% CUP in China was Jingcheng Township of Jingjiang City in Jiangsu Province, in March 2001. At the time, the area had a resident urban population of around 150,000 people and a migrant population of 100,000 people (Zhu Anping 2006: 13). In November 2001, Huangpi, a remote rural suburb of Wuhan City in Hubei Province, became the second site to implement a pilot 100% CUP project. Two additional sites were selected to participate in the program in mid-2002: Liyang Town in Li County, Hunan Province; and Danzhou City, a tourism hotspot, in Hainan Province (WHO/WPR and CDC 2004: 8).

Then, in July 2003, with funding from the UNFPA, a fifth pilot project of the 100% CUP was launched in Liuzhou City in the Guangxi Zhuang Autonomous Region under the guidance of the NPFPC (Ibid.: 8). Unlike the previously mentioned WHO-supported sites, Liuzhou City is a major prefecture-level, industrial city. It had an urban population of approximately one million people and a large number of registered HIV cases at that time – 600 cases in 2003 (Feng Weidong *et al.* 2006: 7). The use of non-sterile injecting equipment among people who used drugs was the main mode of HIV transmission in Liuzhou before 2003, when the first case of mother-to-child transmission was reported. This case suggested that HIV was spreading from people who injected drugs to the general population and that heterosexual transmission could become the dominant mode of transmission in China (Feng Weidong *et al.* 2006: 6–7; WHO/WPR and CDC 2004: 18–19).

Before implementing the pilot projects, project staff mapped the number of businesses associated with the provision of sexual services in each given area (WHO/WPR and CDC 2004: 13, 16, 19). All sex establishments in the PRC are indirect establishments because prostitution is a proscribed activity. Indirect establishments offer sexual services in the context of providing other services such as entertainment, food and remedial massage, with sexual activities sometimes occurring off-site. Such venues include hotels, hostels, saunas, bathhouses, beauty salons, barbershops, karaoke/dance venues, teahouses, nightclubs, and venues that provide massage services, including foot massage (Jeffreys 2012b: 4; Kong 2009: 725–6; Zheng 2009a: 55).

To map the number of indirect sex-related businesses in each area, project staff consulted with local police, health professionals, condom suppliers and owners of entertainment and leisure venues. Following the identification of target enterprises, project staff asked women working within such venues for information about their condom use, experience and knowledge of STI and HIV, the number of clients they saw on a daily basis and so on. The mapping survey also obtained information about the nature of local health services and the availability of condoms in the selected areas (WHO/WPR and CDC 2004: 177–8).

Owners and managers of entertainment and leisure venues were reluctant to cooperate with project staff at first because the sex industry is banned in China. Article 358 of the Criminal Law of the People's Republic of China (1997) forbids the third-party organization of the prostitution of others. Hence, policing authorities launch regular crackdowns against prostitution within the hospitality and service industry (Jeffreys 2012b). In fact, initial efforts at mapping entertainment and leisure venues in the pilot site of Jingjiang County in Jiangsu Province in 2001 'were complicated and delayed by a province-wide crackdown on sex work', which caused many such establishments to close temporarily or move underground (WHO/WPR and CDC 2004: 13).

Prior to 2007, police officers also often used possession of condoms as circumstantial evidence of intent to engage in prostitution. For example, the Public Security Bureau in Nanjing City released guidelines on handling cases of selling and buying sex in June 2006, which stated that condoms could be used as evidence of prostitution (Nanjing shi gonganju pukou fenju 2006). The practice became obsolete around a year after national regulations came into effect requiring entertainment and leisure venues to provide condoms and put up posters publicizing HIV prevention methods in March 2006 (Guowuyuan 2006a: Article 11 & 29; Guowuyuan 2006c: Chapter 3, Section 2, Item 1; Wang Sihai 2008). Interestingly, the New York Police Department did not overturn the practice of confiscating unused condoms as evidence of prostitution by people suspected of being sex industry workers until 2014 ('Unused condoms no longer evidence of prostitution in NYC' 2014).

First-party engagement in a voluntary prostitution transaction is not a criminal offence in China, but the police are empowered to apprehend and punish sex workers and their clients, according to a system of administrative penalties. The latter system aims to deter first-party participation in commercial sex chiefly through the imposition of fines and the social censure associated with police apprehension (Quanguo renda changwu weiyuanhui 2005; see also Tucker, Ren and Sapio 2010: 125). Given this legal context, it is unsurprising that 73 per cent of the women identified as sex workers during the WHO-supported pilot project in Li County refused to give information about their condom use habits to the project staff (WHO/WPR and CDC 2004: 16).

Project staff worked to overcome the reluctance of sex workers and owners of indirect sex establishments to participate in the pilot projects by asking local police to help with the pilot project implementation and monitoring. Police in Li County held meetings with sex workers and owners of relevant businesses and urged them to cooperate with the project staff (Lixian xiangmuban 2004). While this action may seem counterintuitive, given regular police-led crackdowns on the sex industry, local police often visit entertainment and leisure venues to check business licensing, and to apprise owners and staff of relevant laws and legislative changes that relate to their business operations (Jeffreys 2004: 2). Health professionals in the Huangpi area of Wuhan City similarly ensured that local police were involved in the design of their initial action plan (Chen and Schilling *et al.* 2008: 12). Thus, as with the example of Thailand, staff involved with the implementation of China's pilot 100% CUP projects had to initiate and develop relationships with local police, sex workers, and owners and managers of relevant businesses, to generate broader understanding of the program objectives and to gain cooperation from all relevant parties (Chen and Zhang *et al.* 2007: 12–13).

Each pilot project was governed by a leading action group containing local representatives from different government sectors, with the UNFPA-supported project in Liuzhou City being the only pilot project that involved representatives from NGOs in the leading group (WHO/WPR and CDC 2004: 23). In keeping with China's political structure, the chair of the leading group was usually a high-level local leader and member of the Communist Party, such as a mayor or deputy mayor. Officials from the Ministries of Health and Public Security were represented in all of the leading groups as playing a key role in the implementation of each pilot project. Likewise, representatives from the Ministry of Industry and Commerce were included in the leading groups because of their role in issuing business licenses. Officials from other departments were included according to local specificities and circumstances. Representatives from the Ministry of Culture were included when the selected area included a large number of karaoke/dance establishments. Representatives from the Ministry of Tourism were enlisted when the areas included hotels as places where commercial sexual activities might occur – for instance, in the WHO-supported pilot project in Hainan Province (Ibid.: 23).

Representatives of China's public security forces – the police – played an important role initially in hindering and ultimately in assisting the implementation of the five pilot projects. In the case of the first pilot project in Jingcheng Township in Jingjiang City, local police became involved in a provincial-level crackdown on prostitution in June 2001, only three months after the launch of the program (Fang Meng 2002). This action resulted in the apprehension of many owners of businesses that had cooperated with the mapping survey, on charges of facilitating prostitution. It also resulted in the apprehension of numerous sex workers. While demonstrating local government adherence to national policing directives, this action undermined the goals of the pilot project and reveals a lack of higher-level coordination between provincial-level health and policing officials. The success of the project depended on the promotion of cooperative working relations between local health officials, police officers, owners of entertainment and leisure venues, and sex workers and their clients (Ibid.; WHO/WPR and CDC 2004: 13). Ultimately, local governments and health professionals urged policing authorities to assist with the implementation of the pilot projects by temporarily halting any crackdowns on prostitution in the relevant areas (Fang Meng 2002).

Apart from assisting with compliance, local health professionals found that their work was facilitated by the provision of identity cards from local policing authorities indicating that they were working on the pilot projects in an outreach capacity, and in cooperation with public security forces (WHO/WPR and CDC 2004: 24). The provision of such cards offered legitimacy to the work of health professionals in the context of undertaking condom promotion in entertainment and leisure venues, and ensured that they would not be apprehended mistakenly as sellers and buyers of sex in the event of a police-led campaign against prostitution. Police were also asked to ensure the personal safety of condom promotion workers, the Chinese sex industry being associated with violent clients and gangs (see Hong *et al.* 2014: 1436; Zheng 2009c).

Following preliminary discussions with local sex workers, project staff produced educational materials about condoms and STI and HIV prevention, which were distributed in entertainment and leisure venues during what the press dubbed 'working-girl training classes' (*xiaojie peixunban*) (Meng Qingpu *et al.* 2004; Zhou Xiyin 2006). These materials encouraged those who engage in commercial sex to share information about STI and HIV prevention with their peers (Zhongguo jibing yufang kongzhi zhongxin n.d.-a, n.d.-b.). In addition, project staff ensured that project-affiliated clinics provided cost-free diagnosis, treatment and counselling (Chen and Schilling *et al.* 2008: 13). Such actions aimed to empower sex workers by providing them with knowledge of STI and treating them as peer educators, thereby reducing some of the stigma associated with prostitution as a perceived site of disease (Kong 2009: 737).

Owners and managers of entertainment and leisure venues were required to attend periodic meetings organized by project staff and officials from the Ministries of Public Health and Public Security (Chen and Schilling *et al.* 2008: 13). These meetings were used to promote cooperative working relations and to educate and put pressure on non-cooperative owners of relevant businesses. Additionally, proactive business owners were encouraged to act as peer educators in order to persuade other owners to cooperate with project staff (WHO/WPR and CDC 2004: 25).

Owners and managers of such venues were also required to make condoms available in their establishments. During the mapping stage of the pilot projects, project staff obtained information about the distribution of condoms in selected areas. To improve the availability of condoms in some areas, the leading group ensured that condom vending machines were placed in relevant public spaces – for example, in street locations in the case of Jingjiang City and in entertainment and leisure venues in the case of Huangpi (Fang Meng 2002; Zhang Li 2002).

The project strategy of ensuring that condoms were readily available in or near indirect sex establishments was complicated at first by the weight of Chinese law and tradition, which equated condom use with family planning. Although condoms were available for purchase in local pharmacies and supermarkets, people were unaccustomed to using coin-operated machines to purchase condoms in 'open' public spaces and in entertainment and leisure venues (Zhang Li 2002). The advertising of condoms in China's media was also banned via obscenity laws prior to July 2004, when guidelines were issued encouraging the commercial marketing of condoms to control the spread of HIV and AIDS (Rou *et al.* 2010: II41). While some condoms were provided free of charge in relevant businesses to support the pilot projects (Chen and Schilling *et al.* 2008: 13), clearly the most feasible long-term strategy, and one that has since been adopted, is to make condoms an unremarkable commodity available on site at some cost to the purchaser.

As with the example of Thailand, the pilot projects in China were deemed successful based on follow-up surveys asking sex workers about client use of condoms, tracing sources of infection from men presenting with an STI at program-affiliated STI clinics, and monitoring the rate of condom sales in local outlets (Chen and Schilling *et al.* 2008: 13; Rojanapithayakorn 2006: 48–9; WHO/WPR and CDC 2004: 25). All of the four WHO-supported projects concluded that the percentage of sex workers who reported using a condom in their last sexual encounter had reached a high of 90 per cent (WHO/WPR and CDC 2004: 20). The figures were probably exaggerated. Studies indicate that condom use surveys are unreliable. Respondents often have unclear recollections about their sexual activities and associated condom use, may not fully comprehend what they are being asked, and are inclined to answer questions in ways that present a more positive view of their behaviour (Edwards, Thomsen and Toroitich-Ruto 2005: 183–99). However, accompanying surveys emphasized the efficacy of the pilot projects by showing rapidly decreasing rates of chlamydial infection and an increase in local condom sales (WHO/WPR and CDC 2004: 20).

The apparent success of these pilot projects was soon translated into a framework for action, complete with supporting legislation, for the nationwide implementation of a 100% CUP in China.

Promoting a national 100% CUP

In July 2004, Madame Wu Yi, Vice Premier of the PRC's State Council and the Minister of Health, gave a speech at a meeting of the State Council's AIDS Working Committee that effectively endorsed the national implementation with widespread media publicity of a 100% CUP. The State Council is the highest executive organ of state power and state administration in the PRC, and is largely synonymous with the Central People's Government. The State Council AIDS Working

Committee was established in February 2004, replacing and strengthening AIDS coordinating mechanisms that had been put in place in 1996.

In this speech, Wu acknowledged the effectiveness of promoting condom use in commercial sexual encounters as part of China's AIDS response. As she put it:

> The pilot 100% CUP projects in Hubei and Hunan conducted by the Ministry of Health and the WHO have proven to be measures that have achieved significant effects in terms of reducing the incidence of STI, and preventing and controlling the spread of HIV and AIDS. The projects are worthy of expansion to other communities. Measures such as promoting condom use and installing condom vending machines and distributing condoms in public places where populations at higher risk are likely to congregate should be encouraged to cut down the sexual transmission of HIV.
>
> (Wu Yi 2004, translated by SU Gang)

Wu Yi's speech clarified the official position of the PRC government on the 100% CUP, not least by dismissing media-generated controversy about the implications of its implementation. Media reports about the fourth pilot project, while initially limited in scope, had sparked public debate and subsequently widespread media coverage because the project appeared to offer tacit support to the banned sex industry. A standard claim was that the PRC government intended to legalize prostitution because local police had supported the pilot projects rather than cracking down on prostitution (Lan Yan 2002; 'Renmin shiping: shuoshuo "100% anquantao" xiangmu' 2006).

Wu Yi (2004) rejected the general impetus of these arguments by stating that the uncontrolled spread of STI and HIV posed a major threat to the health and security of the Chinese nation, and therefore demanded immediate and direct action. She called on people to abandon their pre-existing ideas on the issue, to 'open their minds' (*jiefang sixiang*) and to 'seek truth from facts' (*shishiqiushi*), and hence to accept the reality of the situation and the necessity of the proposed response. In doing so, Wu put forward established reform-era political justifications concerning the need to change 'old' ways of thinking in order to meet the newfound problems facing present-day China. At the same time, Wu's speech highlighted a new commitment on the part of the PRC government to stressing the pragmatic necessity of first combating the spread of HIV, rather than the ethico-political necessity of first eradicating the prostitution industry.

Wu Yi's speech offered central government support for local governments to become involved in the implementation of public health interventions based on the promotion of condom use to prevent the spread of HIV. Shortly after this speech, the Ministry of Health, in conjunction with the NPFPC, the State Food and Drug Administration, the State Administration for Industry and Commerce, the State Administration of Radio Film and Television, and the General Administration of Quality Supervision, Inspection and Quarantine, released the PRC's first national guidelines on condom use and HIV prevention – the 2004 'Guidelines on

Preventing AIDS and Promoting Condom Use' (*Guanyu yufang aizibing tuiguang shiyong anquantao de shishi yijian*, hereinafter the 2004 Guidelines) (Zhonghua renmin gongheguo guojia weisheng he jihua shengyu weiyuanhui 2004). The 2004 Guidelines, unlike earlier documents advocating the promotion of condom use in 1998 and 2001, established some general strategies and responsibilities for relevant state authorities to fulfil under the coordination of the State Council's AIDS Working Committee (Guowuyuan bangongting 2001; Zhonghua renmin gongheguo guojia weisheng he jihua shengyu weiyuanhui 2004).

The 2004 Guidelines stipulated that the Ministry of Health should organize all of the nation's health authorities and institutions to disseminate information about HIV transmission and the utility of condom use in preventing infection. The Guidelines also stipulated that the Ministry of Health should supply free condoms to people living with HIV and AIDS. The NPFPC was given the responsibility of assisting the Ministry of Health in realizing these goals and organizing pilot projects relating to the social marketing of condoms. The State Food and Drug Administration was tasked with coordinating the national media to promote the use of condoms to prevent disease. It was also responsible for supervising condom manufacture and circulation to ensure the high quality of condom products (Zhonghua renmin gongheguo guojia weisheng he jihua shengyu weiyuanhui 2004).

It is worth noting that the Ministry of Public Security was not involved in the drafting of the 2004 Guidelines, even though local police were involved in the implementation of China's pilot 100% CUP projects and supported the roll-out of similar projects across the nation. This omission is based on a different kind of pragmatic rationale from that presented by Madame Wu Yi. It has enabled police to assist with the compliance aspects of the 100% CUP while retaining a commitment to the PRC's policy of banning prostitution.

But the 2004 Guidelines did promote a national action plan based on the promotion of condom use through public and community health services and commercial marketing. Although this action plan was not explicitly referred to as a '100 Per Cent Condom Use Program', the goals of the two programs are essentially the same. Hence for ease of discussion, we will refer to efforts to promote condom use in China that are based on the 2004 Guidelines and focus on key populations as China's 100% CUP.

In an effort to expand China's 100% CUP at a national level, in August 2004, the Ministry of Health and the CDC began to build professional intervention personnel teams to undertake condom promotion work (Ministry of Health 2004). These teams, known as Special Working Teams for Interventions Among High-Risk Groups (*gaoweirenqun ganyu gongzuodui*) represented a practical step towards implementing Wu Yi's speech and the condom use goals articulated in the 2004 Guidelines. They comprised between 6 and 12 members of staff at the county level, 6 at the prefecture level and 8 at the provincial level. By 2005, around 2,700 teams had been formed across the PRC (Ministry of Health, People's Republic of China, Joint United Nations Programme on HIV/AIDS and World Health Organization 2006: 8).

Two public health structures, the CDC and the NPFPC, carried the main domestic responsibility for expanding and localizing China's version of the 100% CUP. As mentioned previously, the NPFPC had conducted a pilot 100% CUP with the UNFPA in 2003, in the context of a reproductive health and family planning program (WHO/WPR and CDC 2004: 8). The advantage of involving the NPFPC, which was merged with the Ministry of Health to form the National Health and Family Planning Commission in 2013, was that it had an established organizational structure. With more than 30 years of family planning experience, it could enlist over 35,000 township-level family planning units to distribute free condoms to couples of childbearing age around the country. The NPFPC worked with several international organizations to implement AIDS prevention programs involving condom use promotion, including the WHO, UNDP, UNFPA and the Global Fund to Fight AIDS, Tuberculosis and Malaria (Zhongguo renkou yu jihua shengyu n.d.). To do so, it combined its reproductive health and AIDS prevention work (National Population and Family Planning Commission of China 2007). The CDC and NPFPC thus acted as axes to drive the implementation, localization and consequently the sustainability of the 100% CUP in China.

Following the expansion of the 100% CUP from pilot projects to a nationwide strategy with government support, the promotion of safer sexual behaviours and condom use has become a key component of China's AIDS response. On 26 February 2006, the PRC government issued the 'Regulations on AIDS Prevention and Treatment' (*Aizibing fangzhi tiaoli*) (Guowuyuan 2006a). The Regulations recognize condom use as an effective measure to control the sexual transmission of HIV, and empower health authorities to monitor condom use and supply in entertainment and leisure venues. Article 61 stipulates that condoms must be available in or near entertainment and leisure venues. It also gives policing authorities the capacity to fine operators between CNY 500 and CNY 5,000 for failure to comply, and to revoke business licenses in instances of continued non-compliance (Ibid.). The following day, the State Council promulgated China's Action Plan (2006–2010) for the Containment and Prevention of HIV/AIDS, which set targets of 70 per cent or more condom use among key populations by the end of 2007, and 90 per cent by the end of 2010 (Guowuyuan 2006c). Although these targets were subsequently deemed to be unrealistically high, China's AIDS response reports to the UN now claim to have realized those targets (UNAIDS 2016b: 35; Zou *et al.* 2012: 31).

Concluding remarks

China's AIDS Response Progress Reports to the UN for 2014 and 2015 indicate that HIV prevention strategies conducted since the early 2000s and focused on sex workers have realized positive outcomes. Surveys of female sex workers revealed a condom use rate of nearly 88 per cent in 2012 and more than 90 per cent in 2015 (Ministry of Health of the PRC 2012: 8; UNAIDS 2016b: 35). This means that China has met the WHO's 100% CUP compliance target of at least 90 per cent. The number of female sex workers living with HIV has also remained relatively low at 0.3 per cent in 2012 and 0.2 per cent in 2014 (National Health and Family Planning Commission of the PRC 2014: 5, 2015: 13).

At the same time, China's AIDS response has shifted from being almost entirely funded and directed by international organizations to being domestically managed. Prior to 2004, HIV prevention training based on condom promotion among key populations was funded and supported chiefly through international organizations, and implemented through the CDC and the NPFPC, with the support of local policing authorities. PRC government-funded interventions increased from a small number of pilot projects in 351 counties across China by 2003 and to all of the country's 2,862 county-level administrative divisions by the end of 2009 (Rou *et al.* 2010: II42). Domestic funding accounted for nearly 85 per cent of China's AIDS response by 2010 and nearly 99 per cent by 2015 (National Health and Family Planning Commission of the PRC 2015: 12).

Some public-private collaborations have been promoted in the context of this institutional shift that provide safer sex and condom use messages to the general populace, and young adults in particular. One example is the 2008 *Life Is Too Good* public service campaign, featuring celebrity actors Jackie Chan and Pu Cunxin, and soprano Peng Liyuan, the wife of President Xi Jinping ('Life is too good' 2007). The campaign was coordinated by the United Nations and the PRC's Ministry of Health through partnerships with China's media and advertising sector. It provided a simple message about how to prevent the sexual transmission of HIV in the form of short video clips directed by Ruby Yang and Thomas Lennon (2006) – the director and producer of an Oscar-winning documentary about children orphaned by AIDS in China, called *The Blood of Yingzhou District*. In one of these videos, Jackie Chan performs on a movie set to a script that states: 'I love making movies and I love life. An action movie needs danger but life needs protecting. Sexual transmission of AIDS is on the rise; condoms help reduce the risk. Life is too good, protect yourself' ('Life is too good' 2007).

However, the extension of the 100% CUP to cover new populations of sex workers is viewed as an integral yet problematic component of the PRC's evolving AIDS response. Health researchers contend that continued programs are necessitated by the high turnover of sex workers, who are typically young adults who work for a limited number of years, moving from different venues and to different places in order to maximize income-earning opportunities and evade police apprehension (Rou *et al.* 2010: II44). This situation requires ongoing outreach and funding by government departments because the number of community-based organizations working with sex workers in China is limited by government controls over the developing non-profit sector, and the illegal nature of the sex industry. For example, a 2009 survey of 340 organizations working on AIDS conducted by the China HIV/AIDS Information Network and the National Center for AIDS/STD Control and Prevention indicated that only 9 per cent worked with female sex workers (Kaufman 2012: 231; Li and Kuo *et al.* 2010: II69).

The success of health interventions focused on sex workers also turns on the extent of cooperation between health and policing authorities, and owners of sex establishments and sex workers, which is variously enhanced and undermined by police support for health interventions and crackdowns on sex establishments (Human Rights Watch 2013). Likewise, media coverage of the sometimes conflicting goals of public health and public security works to support and undermine the goals of the 100% CUP by occasionally challenging, but typically reinforcing, the social and legal marginalization of sex workers (Ibid.). Such problems are seen to require the introduction of new and improved versions of the 100% CUP in China, based on the diversification of funding and communication models, and inputs from new types of social organizations and experts.

As this suggests, the perceived failures of one mode of implementing a corrective program of governmental intervention are the perceived opportunities for the formulation of another improved or alternative program (Miller and Rose 2008: 17). In the context of China, central government endorsement of an international health program has opened the space, albeit within the constrained parameters permitted by the one-party ruling system, for a wide range of people to express different views about how the public health risks associated with the sex industry, and thus the sex industry itself, might be better governed. The next two chapters therefore look at some of the effects of implementing China's 100% CUP in terms of developing media communication and opening public debate on AIDS and the governance of commercial sex.

3 China's condom use program and the media

This chapter explores the controversy associated with the initial implementation of a 100 Per Cent Condom Use Program in the People's Republic of China, as presented in the country's state-controlled media. Although sex work in Thailand is not strictly legal, the implementation of a national 100% CUP in Thailand was accompanied by widespread media publicity about sexual health awareness and safer sex, in order to popularize knowledge of STI and HIV prevention. According to a 2004 report by the United Nations Development Programme (2004: 13–14), an estimated 90 per cent of the Thai population had heard about the goals of the program from radio and television station broadcasting. Public education and information on the program was also disseminated through print media.

Widespread publicity was viewed as integral to the success of the Thai 100% CUP, and is therefore upheld by the international AIDS governance system as an important component of implementing the 100% CUP in other parts of the world (UNDP 2004: 30). UNAIDS (2004: 4) contends that the broadcast media has 'tremendous reach and influence, particularly with young people who represent the future and who are the key to any successful fight against HIV/AIDS'. The organization recommends that national media provide regular public service messages that encourage discussion of how individuals can protect themselves and change their behaviour, if necessary, which may mean combating existing social norms, values and conditions (Ibid.: 15). The media is thus presented as a key vehicle for promoting attitudinal and behavioural change and meeting contemporary government challenges.

Yet the pilot implementation of a 100% CUP in five different sites in China during the early 2000s was conducted without any immediate national media coverage. A 2004 report by the World Health Organization Regional Office for the Western Pacific somewhat differently explains that:

> Educating 'the public' about the 100% CUP may or may not be important as this depends upon the political environment in which the programme is being organized. As it is concerned primarily with the risks associated with the often 'underground' or 'extralegal' sector of sex work, it may be prudent that the programme not be highly publicized, although the full awareness and participation of political leaders is imperative.
>
> (WHO/WPR 2004: 12)

DOI: 10.4324/9781315175546-3

In other words, obtaining the government support necessary to educate sex workers, rather than to also educate the broader public, may be viewed as the primary goal of the program in certain political contexts. In the context of China's one-party ruling system, this meant gaining the support of senior Communist Party members.

The 100% CUP was piloted in the PRC without national media coverage because it involved three then controversial issues that one health official described as akin to a 'bomb' when put together: namely, (1) AIDS (*aizibing*); (2) entertainment and leisure venues (*yulechangsuo*), that is, known venues for prostitution; and (3) condoms (*anquantao*) (Zhang Li 2002). Before 2002, AIDS was a relatively obscure topic in the Chinese media because of what many researchers describe as a national policy of neglect, or the initial failure of the PRC government to respond to the threat of HIV, based on the assumption that AIDS was a 'foreigners' disease' or something that affected nonlocal places and people (Dong, Chang and Chen 2008: 357–74; Hood 2011: 5). Businesses facilitating sexual services were the focus of anti-vice policing campaigns based on legal constructions of the prostitution industry as a social harm (Jeffreys 2012a). The State Administration for Industry and Commerce (1989), which governs the PRC's advertising industry, also banned condom advertising until the mid-2000s on the grounds that it would cause public offence. There was thus no accepted political basis and corollary language for talking about the goals of the 100% CUP in China at the start of the new millennium.

Despite these obstacles, the 100% CUP was being promoted with national media coverage by the mid-2000s. China's Action Plan (2001–2005) for the Containment and Prevention of HIV/AIDS encouraged expanded media coverage of AIDS, by stipulating that the PRC's state-controlled broadcast media, and central and local newspapers, should release news stories and public service advertisements about the work of AIDS education and HIV prevention at least once a week (Guowuyuan bangongting 2001: Item 3, Article 2). The advertising or product branding of condoms is now promoted in law. Although the sex industry is banned, media coverage of the 100% CUP has opened public debate on the nature and utility of the PRC's prostitution controls (Jeffreys 2012b: 130–46).

Analysis of media coverage of the 100% CUP thus highlights a dramatic shift in political communication on AIDS and prostitution in China and in government approaches to contemporary thought management. 'Thought management' (*sixiang guanli*) is a modern adaption of propaganda (*xuanchuan*), which is described as the 'lifeblood' of the Party-state and a key means for furthering Communist Party rule (Brady 2012: 8). Thought management refers to:

> Activities to control, guide, adjust, or develop the social or ideological relationships which influence the shaping (change or development) of people's thinking: to make their thinking conform with the dominant ideology; thereby standardizing the people's behaviour; in order to put in place a set of objectives.
>
> (Brady 2012: 2)

Putting in place the objectives of the 100% CUP in China – to transform the sexual conduct of sex industry workers and clients – demanded a media strategy to modify public thinking on the appropriate nature of government responses to the sex industry.

The chapter first examines the cautious approach that was taken by local government authorities in discouraging publicity of the first three pilot projects in the cities of Jingjiang, Wuhan and Danzhou (Fang Meng 2002; Jin Shehui 2002; WHO/WPR and CDC 2004). It then looks at the unexpected arousal of public interest that was generated by a seemingly innocuous report about the implementation of a fourth pilot project in Li County (He Gu 2002a). The report triggered a chain of mediated responses that snowballed into widespread publicity in print and online media, catapulting the 100% CUP into the public arena, and prompting government officials to adopt a media response strategy in order to allay public fears about its moral and legal ramifications (Lixian xiangmuban 2004).

Finally, the chapter examines the subsequent adoption of an open media strategy to clarify the government's position regarding its new AIDS prevention strategies, which was designed to address the issues and criticisms associated with the state-led promotion of condom use in the sex industry. Analysis of the media debate surrounding the pilot project in Li County highlights how government-promoted publicity has helped to shift the narrative of the 100% CUP away from concerns about sexual immorality and legal inconsistency, and towards one centred on the pragmatic necessity of first protecting the public health.

Piloting China's 100% CUP without media publicity

Following success in Thailand, the World Health Organization collaborated with the PRC's Ministry of Health to launch four pilot projects of the 100% CUP in China in the early 2000s (WHO/WPR and CDC 2004). The first pilot – in Jingcheng Township of Jingjiang City in Jiangsu Province in March 2001 – was launched and implemented without any media publicity. Requests from journalists to interview local health officials about the program were also turned down (Fang Meng 2002). Health officials actively avoided media publicity of the first pilot project because they were concerned that it might be construed as offering legitimacy to the existence of the banned sex industry, and therefore hinder the implementation of further programs (Ibid.).

China's second pilot project, launched in Huangpi, a remote rural suburb of Wuhan City in November 2001, was also implemented without media publicity until the middle of 2002. On 29 June 2002, *Chutian Jinbao* (hereinafter the *Golden Post*) published a short report of around 250 words titled 'The Incidence of Sexually Transmitted Infection Has Declined Sharply Following the Implementation of a Pilot Condom Use Program in Wuhan' (Jin Shehui 2002). The *Golden Post*, a subsidiary of the *Hubei Ribao* (hereinafter *Hubei Daily*), is the second most popular newspaper among residents of Wuhan with a circulation of over 400,000 copies (Wang Yong 2002: 476).

While confirming that the Huangpi pilot project was successful, the *Golden Post* report offered only limited details about the project's location and nature (Jin Shehui 2002). For example, it did not disclose exactly where the pilot project was taking place, simply noting that it was in a district of Wuhan City, the capital of Hubei Province. It also used new and scientific terminology to describe the focus population of the intervention, that is, people engaged in 'high-risk sexual relations' (*gaoweixingxingwei*) (Ibid.). This terminology, while conforming to the discursive parameters of international AIDS programs, is not a common feature of everyday language in China. A search for the number of hits for the keywords '*gaoweixingxingwei*' in the China National Knowledge Infrastructure database (CNKI) for the decade between 2000 and 2010 obtained only 12 hits (the CNKI database covers more than 10,000 academic journals and 600 newspapers in mainland China) (cnki.net). Hence, readers of the report probably would not have identified the pilot project as a program that focused on people providing commercial sexual services. Even terms that were used to describe commercial sex at the time, such as '*maiyinpiaochang*' (selling sex and buying sex from illicit prostitutes) and, more recently, '*xinggongzuo*' (sex work), were not mentioned in the report.

The Huangpi pilot project featured in a far more detailed report in the *Nanfang Zhoumo* (hereinafter the *Southern Weekend*) on 28 November 2002, shortly before the project concluded in January 2003 (Zhang Li 2002). *Southern Weekend* is a popular Guangzhou-based newspaper and a subsidiary of the Guangdong provincial Party organ, the *Nanfang Ribao* (*Southern Daily*). During the mid- to late 1990s, major Chinese newspapers began to publish weekend editions that focused on investigative journalism and current affairs, as opposed to the previously narrow focus of provincial newspapers on publishing only Communist Party–endorsed news or propaganda (Zhao 2000: 583). This shift flowed in part from market pressures. Economic reforms and the restructuring of China's media industry meant that newspapers had to publish stories that would attract readers to make a profit. The main provincial Party organs continued to fulfil the traditional 'mouthpiece' role of China's media by transmitting the concerns and policies of the CCP to the general population, while weekend subsidiaries such as *Southern Weekend* began to publish issues relating to social problems and CCP-led anti-corruption measures (Ibid.). *Southern Weekend* is now widely regarded as one of the PRC's most courageous newspapers for its bold exposure of stories relating to current affairs and social problems. However, as with many weekend subsidiaries, it tends to report on controversies occurring in other parts of the country rather than in its home province of Guangdong, in order to maintain good working relations with members of the local Party and government structures (Liebman 2005: 46).

As the *Southern Weekend* report explained, the Huangpi pilot project was implemented based on the success of AIDS prevention programs in Thailand and elsewhere, but had been trialled initially without media publicity because of its sensitive nature (Zhang Li 2002). Wei Shanbo, Head of the Disease Control Division of the Wuhan Municipal Health Department and leader of what was known in

Wuhan as the '100 Per Cent Condom Use Program in Entertainment and Leisure Venues' (*yulechangsuo 100% shiyong anquantao*), was quoted as saying that the pilot project was extremely sensitive because it involved three words that were akin to a 'bomb' when put together – entertainment venues, condoms and AIDS (Ibid.). While it was designed to limit the potential for HIV transmission from sex workers to the general population, members of the public would automatically equate the promotion of condom use in entertainment and leisure venues with sexual promiscuity and government acceptance of the sex industry. Thus, despite having the support of local policing authorities, project leaders and personnel were afraid that the pilot project would collapse at any moment because of unexpected, adverse publicity.

In fact, the Huangpi pilot project only received detailed media coverage in its home province of Hubei in April 2004 when local health officials confirmed its conclusion and successful nature. On 28 April, the *Hubei Daily* covered a story titled 'Huangpi Pilot Project Passes Evaluation, Wuhan's 100 Per Cent Condom Use Program Comes on the Stage' (Hu Man 2004). The article provided details about a press conference held by the Wuhan Municipal Health Department. During this conference, Lin Guosheng, the director of the Wuhan Municipal Health Department, announced that the WHO had approved the Huangpi pilot project and deemed it a success (Ibid.). Another article titled 'Wonderful Wuhan: Changes in 2004', published in the *Wuhan Chenbao* (*Wuhan Morning Post*) on 17 December 2004, used a more explicit subtitle when discussing significant changes in the city: namely, 'The Topic of AIDS Is Now Public' (Liu Guanju *et al.* 2004). Both articles featured an interview with Wei Shanbo, who explained why the pilot program had not been widely publicized in Wuhan City and Hubei Province. Similar to what was stated in his interview in *Southern Weekend* on 28 November 2002, Wei Shanbo emphasized that the pilot project was so sensitive that local authorities had decided that the best approach was 'only doing, not talking' (*zhi zuo bu shuo*) (Hu Man 2004; Liu Guanju *et al.* 2004; Zhang Li 2002).

As local government and health officials associated with the leadership groups later explained, the first two pilot projects in the cities of Jingjiang and Wuhan (Huangpi) were launched without media publicity because relevant local authorities were reluctant to publicize a project that might encounter objections and compromise their careers (Zhu Wenyi 2002). The work of AIDS prevention related to sex work was not implemented as a national public policy with associated supportive frameworks until after July 2004, following the introduction of the Guidelines on Preventing AIDS and Promoting Condom Use (Zhonghua renmin gongheguo guojia weisheng he jihua shengyu weiyuanhui 2004). Local officials implementing the pilot programs were apprehensive about publicizing their work prior to this because the projects potentially contravened national policy. The 100% CUP not only sought to work with members of the illegal sex industry, but also required local police to abandon the national policy of cracking down on prostitution and to temporarily cooperate with the owners, managers and workers of sex establishments to be successful. Health official Wei Shanbo told reporters that the Huangpi project could not have proceeded without the cooperation of local policing authorities and that such cooperation had taken more than six months to negotiate (Zhang Li 2002).

Local officials were also reluctant to publicize the pilot projects because of fears that the public would view their implementation as a sign of an AIDS epidemic, thereby generating public panic, endangering the local tourism industry and discouraging investment in the local economy (WHO/WPR and CDC 2004: 17; Zhang Li 2002). Similar concerns ensured that the third pilot project in Danzhou City, a tourism hotspot in Hainan Province, would also receive no media publicity.

Although the fourth pilot project, launched on 22 July 2002 in Liyang Town of Li County in Hunan Province, was initiated without major publicity, a short news report in a local newspaper called the *Xiaoxiang Chenbao* (hereinafter the *Xiaoxiang Morning Post*) on 24 July 2002 triggered widespread public debate. The report, titled 'Li County's Entertainment and Leisure Venues Put Safety First', said that condom use would be promoted in more than 100 such venues in Li County (He Gu 2002a). The report did not explicitly mention the sex industry or the subject of sex work. However, it offered a concise account of the 'who, what, when and how' of the program, stating that government authorities in Li County had established a leadership group to promote the pilot project and its implementation over a period of two years with funding of USD 30,000 from the WHO (Ibid.). The report further stated that the Li County government, together with public health and policing authorities, would monitor the level of condom use in entertainment and leisure venues. The article's reference to 'venues', 'condoms' and 'AIDS' – the three words Wei Shanbo above described as a 'bomb' – would have alerted readers to the implicit focus of the pilot project, namely, sex workers and their clients.

According to a report by the Li County 100% CUP Office, the publication of this short report on the launching of the pilot project in Li County generated unexpected and widespread debate, with the story being taken up by more than 30 media outlets as well as being hotly debated on the Internet (Lixian xiangmuban 2004). Public interest apparently forced the leadership group of the pilot project to cooperate with the media and, ultimately, to use the media as a means to publicize and raise public awareness of the goals of the 100% CUP throughout China. As a result, journalists were invited to Li County to get a first-hand experience of the pilot project, and senior government officials gave interviews to media representatives with comments in support of the pilot project and the 100% CUP (Meng Qingpu *et al.* 2004). China Central Television (CCTV), the official media outlet of the Party-state, even made a documentary about the implementation of the Li County pilot project (Lixian xiangmuban 2004).

The successful handling of media coverage of the Li County pilot project encouraged immediate rather than delayed local publicity about the fifth pilot 100% CUP, launched in Liuzhou City in the Guangxi Zhuang Autonomous Region in July 2003. The Liuzhou pilot project was organized and implemented by the United Nations Population Fund (UNFPA) under the guidance of the PRC's National Population and Family Planning Commission (NPFPC) (WHO/WPR and CDC 2004: 8). Its launch was covered by the *Nanguo Jinbao* (hereinafter the *South China Today*) in a report titled 'AIDS Is Separated From Sexual Life, Liuzhou Launches a "100 Per Cent Safety Program"', published on 1 August 2003, two days after its official launch (Meng and Long 2003). *South China Today* is a commercially orientated newspaper affiliated to the Guangxi official Party organ, the *Guangxi Ribao* (*Guangxi Daily*) conglomerate. However, the nature of the *South China Today* allows its reporters more freedom in choosing topics to publish compared to its parent outlet.

Although this report informed the local population of the launch of the Liuzhou pilot project in 2003, it simply stated that condom use was an effective means of preventing STI and the sexual transmission of HIV (Ibid.). It stated that the goal of the pilot projects was to prevent the spread of HIV from people living with HIV to their spouses and other sexual partners. But it did not mention the words prostitution, sex work or entertainment venues.

Media publicity of the 100% CUP nevertheless continued to increase across the nation, following the debate sparked by He Gu's brief report on the pilot project in Li County in July 2002.

Publicizing China's pilot projects

National media publicity of the pilot implementation of China's 100% CUP was not planned; it was triggered by general media and public interest following the publication of a short report written by He Gu (2002a) in the *Xiaoxiang Morning Post* (Lixian xiangmuban 2004). The report detailed that the pilot project was implemented under the auspices of the WHO and the PRC's Ministry of Health in Liyang Town in Li County in Hunan Province (WHO/WPR and CDC 2004). Liyang has a residential population of around 160,000 people and is a commercial centre in Li County that attracts migrant workers from local surrounding areas (Lixian xiangmuban 2004). At the time, it was estimated to have more than 650 female sex workers based in nearly 100 business settings. According to the Li County 100% CUP Office, He Gu's report on 24 July 2002 about the promotion of condom use in Liyang's entertainment and leisure venues was taken up by more than 30 media outlets, and hotly debated by Chinese netizens in blogs and other social networking forums on the Internet, over the course of two to three months (Ibid.).

In the interview, He Gu explained that he was the only journalist who had attended a meeting about the launch of the pilot project in Li County on 22 July 2002, and he did so without an official invitation (Deng Liu 2003). At that meeting, he was given some printed materials about the program, but these were promptly taken away from him and he was told not to publish any information about the pilot unless it was first checked and approved by relevant officials. While He Gu (2002b) obviously gained this approval, local officials failed to anticipate both the level of interest and furore over the underlying rationales and legality of the pilot project that his short report would attract. However, following the publication of his report, the leading group of the Li County project decided to begin cooperating with journalists and media representatives making inquiries about the program.

A second report about the Li County pilot project was published on the front page of a Hunan newspaper called the *Xiandai Xiaofei Daobao* (hereinafter the *Modern Consumer News*) on 8 August 2002 with the headline 'Is Your Sexual Behaviour Safe?' (Yang Shili *et al.* 2002: 1). The article attempted to anticipate and alleviate public concerns about the program by using subtitles such as 'Li County Is Not Severely Affected by AIDS' (*Lixian bushi aizibing zhongzaiqu*); 'Four of the Biggest Misunderstandings About the Pilot Project' (*renshishang de sida wuqu*)'; and 'Where Did the Obstructions Come From?' (*zuli laiyuan yu hechu*). Model answers to these issues and questions were provided in the explanatory text.

The report in the *Modern Consumer News* aimed to alter public perceptions on health interventions focused on sex workers and promoting condom use. It first concentrated on the 'authoritative' views on AIDS provided by Zhou Hongyan from the Li County Hygiene and Epidemic Station, and then on the need to crack down on prostitution as detailed by Jiang Fan, a police chief in Li County (Ibid.). The authors of the report described Zhou Hongyan as scholarly, or, more precisely, 'young but with a strong academic flavour' (*nianqing er yishen xuezhe wei*), and stressed the credentials of the program, calling it a genuine 'scientific research project' (*keyan xiangmu*) (Ibid.). This appeal to 'science' and 'expertise' legitimized the Li Country pilot by suggesting that it was based on ideas, practices and behaviours that might be described as modern, rational and advanced (for a discussion of the links between AIDS discourses and scientism in China, see Hood 2011: 135–74).

Zhou Hongyan explained that using condoms was the most effective and economical method to prevent HIV transmission through sexual contact. In turn, when asked whether the program entailed the legalization of prostitution, the local police chief, Jiang Fan responded with a categorical 'no', thereby extinguishing any suspicion that government policy on the sex industry had altered (Yang Shili *et al.* 2002: 1). Other non-authoritative commentators featured only at the end of the report and were depicted, unlike the now more knowledgeable readers, as being 'naive' about the issues associated with the program. For example, a young woman who worked in a bar was described as 'blushing with embarrassment' when asked for her comment on the program and an alleged sex worker told reporters that 'clients did not like to use that "thing" (*wanyier*) [a condom]' (Ibid.).

A third and lengthy article on the Li County pilot project appeared in a popular newspaper, the *Beijing Qingnianbao* (hereinafter the *Beijing Youth Daily*) in late September 2002 (He Gu 2002b). The *Beijing Youth Daily* is run by the Beijing Committee of the Chinese Communist Youth League and targets a national urban, white-collar readership, rather than a local readership. It had a daily circulation of more than 600,000 copies at the time (Duan and Zhang 2004: 738). The article was written by He Gu (2002a, 2002b), the journalist who first wrote about the Li County pilot project in the *Xiaoxiang Morning Post*. In an interview with another journalist called Deng Liu (2003), He Gu stated that he had been prompted to write the second article because of the unexpected public response to his first brief report, which had resulted in the newspaper office receiving numerous telephone calls from people asking questions about the 100% CUP.

He Gu's report in the *Beijing Youth Daily* provided detailed information on the public health and policy background of the 100% CUP and its pilot implementation in Li County. As He Gu (2002b) noted, the primary concern, reflected in the readers' reactions, was the seemingly conflicting relationship between the program and the illegal status of prostitution. While the *Modern Consumer News* article reported a local police officer's assurance that police authorities would continue to crack down on prostitution (Yang Shili *et al.* 2002: 1), He Gu (2002b) interviewed a more authoritative spokesperson to reiterate this point – Zhao Jian, a senior official from the Hunan Province Public Security Bureau. Zhao restated that promoting condom use in entertainment and leisure venues did not involve giving tacit support to the sex industry. Zhao further stated that there was no contradiction between policing authorities continuing to crack down on prostitution in entertainment and leisure venues, and health officials encouraging women who worked in such venues to insist on condom use when engaging in commercial sex. Health professionals were simply trying to reduce the risk of HIV transmission in the illegal sex industry and this would not alter or overturn policing policy (Ibid.).

To rationalize the program from a public health perspective, He Gu (2002b) interviewed Zhao Pengfei, a representative of the WHO in Beijing. As the subheading introducing this interview suggested, 'Currently, Prostitution Practices Cannot Be Eradicated Solely by Public Security Departments' (*muqian dankao gonganbumen hai buzuyi jinzhi maiyin xingwei*) (Ibid.). Zhao Pengfei listed figures on AIDS cases nationally and in Hunan Province (850,000 and 40,000, respectively), and highlighted the potential relationship between drug use, sex work and the spread of HIV. He concluded that the urgent task of preventing STI and the spread of HIV through sexual contact required the cooperation of multiple departments. The article thus demonstrates a shift in governmental practice insofar as it reiterates a point made in China's Medium- and Long-Term Strategic Plan for HIV/AIDS Prevention and Control for 1998–2010, namely, that the sex industry is unlikely to be eradicated from China in the foreseeable future, and hence the main task for government is to minimize the public health risk posed by the sex industry (Guowuyuan 1998).

He Gu's article in the *Beijing Youth Daily* further stressed that the pilot project in Li County had local government support, which was the first prerequisite used by the WHO and the PRC's Ministry of Health when selecting pilot sites (Ibid.). He emphasized local government support for the program with the subtitle 'Li County Government Openly Supports the Program' (*Lixian zhengfu gongkai zhichi xiangmu shishi*). He also noted that the program had the support of owners of local entertainment and leisure venues. This emphasis on government and business support for the pilot project would have reinforced official endorsement for the 100% CUP in Li County, and served to protect it from potential attacks by readers who might have otherwise opposed the program.

He Gu's report in the *Beijing Youth Daily* also demonstrated the different attitudes of local and provincial governments towards media coverage of the 100%

CUP. Following the release of He Gu's first report, the Hunan provincial government had overseen a policy of open media coverage on the Li County pilot. While speaking at a National AIDS Prevention Meeting in November 2005, Xu Yunzhao, the vice governor of Hunan Province, claimed that the Hunan provincial government had approved media coverage of the pilot project (Xu Yunzhao 2005). The provincial government had allowed He Gu to confirm the launch of the pilot project by permitting the publication of his article in the *Xiaoxiang Morning Post* (He Gu 2002a; Xu Yunzhao 2005). Moreover, senior members of the provincial government had mediated with Li County officials on the issues relating to media publicity of the program.

In contrast, the Huangpi local government had responded to a media report on the Huangpi pilot project by suspending the two journalists responsible because local leaders felt compromised by the details exposed in their article (Zhu Wenyi 2002). Both articles reported similar facts on the pilot programs in their respective geographical areas – Li County in Hunan Province and the Huangpi area of Wuhan City in Hubei Province. However, their publication met with two distinct reactions from provincial and local authorities.

These different responses highlight the influence of higher-level government authorities in facilitating publicity of the 100% CUP, and underscore a problem that continues to impact on the effective implementation of the PRC's AIDS policies. The decentralized governance structures and promotion of local policy autonomy that have accompanied the process of economic reform have also encouraged mixed responses to and the inconsistent enforcement of national AIDS policies (Huang 2013: 88–9). Provincial and local governments have to be incentivized and funded to execute national-level policies, which requires time spent on building interdepartmental relationships. Provincial and local governments also have considerable discretion over how funds are distributed to support social services (see Uretsky 2016: 172–206). This presents ongoing obstacles with regards to the provision of uniform and consistent access to AIDS-related information, treatment and services.

In summary, the pilot project in Li County of Hunan Province was the first of the four WHO-supported pilot projects to be promoted in the media, mainly due to the support of leaders from the provincial government. The other three projects – in Jingcheng Township of Jiangsu Province, Huangpi in Hubei Province, and Danzhou City in Hainan Province – were all conducted without major media publicity because local government leaders feared that it would attract adverse reactions from members of the public. In contrast, leaders in the Hunan provincial government evidently believed that the public would accept the 100% CUP as both a public health initiative and a manifestation of the government's commitment to 'serving the people' (*wei renmin fuwu*).

As journalist Chen Jieren (2002) explained, Li County was chosen as a site for a pilot project not because it had a high incidence of STI and AIDS, but rather because it had a 'leading and forward-thinking' government that attached great importance to this work. Such complimentary exaltation presumably reflected local government officials' request for positive reportage on the pilot and/or Chen Jieren's desire not to off-side local officials. That said, local government authorities evidently believed that different government agencies could manage the complexities of implementing a major public health intervention alongside existing practices of policing prostitution. Provincial- and county-level governments worked with the Ministry of Health and global funding bodies – the WHO and UNFPA – to pilot a public health program that demanded new forms of cooperation between different types and levels of government departments, and challenged established views on how the sex industry should be governed.

Debating the Li County pilot project in China's media

In 2002, the controversial subject of China's 100% CUP was brought into the open by widespread media coverage, with more than 30 media outlets drawing attention to the issue (Lixian xiangmuban 2004). Associated topics, such as AIDS, prostitution and safer sex, all of which were 'sensitive' although not exactly taboo subjects, were also brought into contention in that same period of time. Before 2002, AIDS was a relatively obscure topic in the Chinese media that was chiefly presented as a 'distant disease' affecting foreign or nonlocal places and people (Dong, Chang and Chen 2008: 357–74; Hood 2011: 5).

Figure 3.1 provides a graphic illustration of the increased attention paid to the subject of AIDS in Chinese newspapers since the 2000s, and especially since 2002, based on a search for the keyword '*aizibing*' (AIDS) on the China National Knowledge Infrastructure, China Core Newspapers Full-text Database between 1

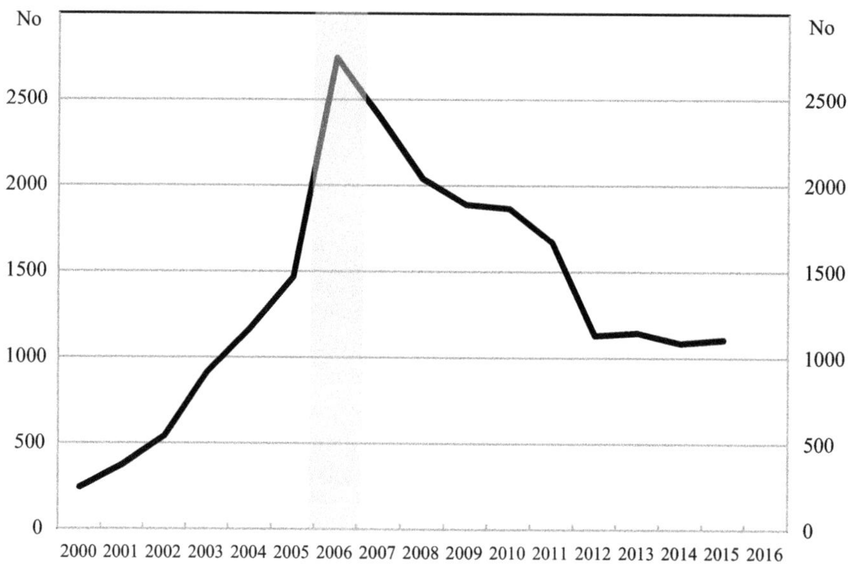

Figure 3.1 Chinese press coverage of '*aizibing*' (AIDS) (2000–2015).

Source: Compiled with data from China National Knowledge Infrastructure, China Core Newspapers Full-text Database (2000–), Beijing: Tsinghua Tongfang Knowledge Network Technology Company Ltd.

January 2000 and 31 December 2015 (cnki.net). The Chinese characters for AIDS obtained fewer than 250 hits in 2000. This figure more than doubled to reach nearly 550 hits in 2002 and peaked at more than 2,700 hits in 2006. The number of hits for the keyword AIDS in the Chinese print media has since decreased, plateauing at around 1,100 hits between 2012 and 2015. However, as in Western societies, nearly 95 per cent of the Chinese population now also receive information about AIDS from increasingly diversified media, including the Internet and social media, and AIDS storylines in television programming, films and PSAs (Hood 2011: 35–6; Li *et al.* 2009).

The rapid rise in print media coverage of AIDS-related issues between 2002 and 2006 is correlated with the issuing of specific government policies. These include the release of China's Action Plan (2001–2005) for the Containment and Prevention of HIV/AIDS and the Regulations on AIDS Prevention and Treatment in May 2001. The action plan stated that the broadcast media and central and local newspapers should release news stories and PSAs about the work of HIV and AIDS prevention at least once a week (Guowuyuan bangongting 2001: Item 3, Article 2). Article 19 of the regulations stipulated that mass media, including radio, television, press and Internet, should provide non-commercial communication on AIDS prevention and treatment (Guowuyuan 2006a).

At the start of the 2000s, government prohibitions also prevented condom manufacturers from advertising their products in the media and in public places, even though condoms had been distributed to married couples as part of the PRC's family planning policies since 1974 (Ma Suwen 2005). The State Administration for Industry and Commerce (1989), which governs the PRC's advertising industry, banned the product branding of adult goods (*xingshenghuo chanpin*), including condoms, in 1989, stating that advertisement of such products did not stand in line with Chinese social customs and morality, that is, they would cause public offence. Subsequent efforts by condom manufacturing companies throughout the 1990s to advertise their products in the media or in public places all failed (Zheng 2009b: 55). While some scholars view this failure as a sign of government repression of sex (Ibid.), it is worth noting that PSAs produced by government authorities to promote condom use suffered a similar fate. In 1998, China's inaugural condom advertisement, which was produced by a China division of the UK Jissbon Global Company and placed on 80 buses in southern Guangzhou, was removed after 33 days (Hu Wenhua 2004: B1). In 1999, a condom promotion PSA on CCTV, which was produced for World AIDS Day by the NPFPC, was cancelled after only one day (Ibid.).

In 2004, condom companies in China were first granted permission to advertise their products as part of PSAs, but not as part of product branding. In October of that year, six ministries jointly issued the Guidelines on Preventing AIDS and Promoting Condom Use, which advised that more HIV-prevention advertisements should be distributed in shopping centres, entertainment and leisure venues, ports and airports (Zhonghua renmin gongheguo guojia weisheng he jihua shengyu weiyuanhui 2004). This resulted in 40 billboards being placed in public venues and nightspots in Beijing. These advertisements promoted condom use and advised against unprotected sexual behaviours as part of World AIDS Day activities (Yu Xinming 2004: 3). According to an official from China's Center for Disease Control and Prevention, the State Administration for Industry and Commerce advertising ban on family planning products was still in force. However, condom advertisements aimed at preventing the spread of HIV were permitted, especially in the period leading up to World AIDS Day on 1 December ('China: Beijing starts promoting condom use to fight HIV/AIDS' 2004).

The 2008 Beijing Olympic Games further opened the space for condom advertising, including product branding, through association with health-related themes. In the run-up to the Beijing Games, the government-organized National Community AIDS Prevention Education Organizing Committee (*quanguo shequ yufang aizibing xuanjiao huodong zuweihui*) enrolled nearly 6,000 public places and venues in an agreement to install government-funded condom vending machines near bars, clubs, restaurants, public bathhouses and major construction sites in urban centres. These 'smart machines' broadcast AIDS prevention information during business hours. They also allowed consumers to purchase condom packs conveniently at the government-subsidized price of CNY 5 by swiping a public transit 'One Card', a card which is used to travel on buses and subways in Beijing (Wei Mingyan 2008: A12).

Some condom manufacturing companies managed to bypass restrictions on condom advertising for the purposes of product branding by advertising on subway trains, which required permission from the Subway Management Group rather than the State Administration for Industry and Commerce. For example, Durex, the world's leading condom producer, placed a television advertisement on Shanghai subway trains (Wu and Jiang 2008: A09). Following complaints about the advertisement from a mother of a 10-year-old child and other passengers, the advertisement was judged to be inappropriate by the State Administration for Industry and Commerce and taken off the subway (Ibid.). An enterprising Chinese condom manufacturer, Elasun, also devised a series of advertisements featuring condoms and sport stickmen, which reportedly went viral on the Chinese Internet (Hutcheon 2008). Durex has since exploited digital and social media to brand a range of novelty and personalized condoms, such as Chinese Valentine's Day condoms (Doland 2015).

Back in 2002, however, complaints about the implementation of the pilot project in Li County indicated that many members of the public viewed condom promotion as an unacceptable validation of immoral conduct, rather than as a personal and public health service. In his July report in the *Xiaoxiang Morning Post*, He Gu (2002a) cites a middle-aged woman who states that the implementation of the pilot project would mislead the public and that she was very worried about how it would affect her children. According to this concerned parent, condom promotion outside of marriage would increase promiscuous sexual behaviours, especially among teenagers. In a similar vein, the government-funded installation of condom vending machines as part of the pilot project in Jingcheng Township, Jiangsu Province, in March 2001, was met with resistance from concerned parents who reportedly damaged the machines deliberately (Fang Meng 2002).

As the preceding and following examples suggest, the PRC government is sometimes at the forefront of promoting positive social change rather than hindering it. Concerns about the negative impact of condom promotion on the sexual morals of China's youth even extended to university settings. In November 2004, health officials from the Beijing Haidian district government distributed condoms to students at the Peking University campus as part of their AIDS prevention activities (Zhao, Mao and Zhou 2004: A4). However, representatives from the university subsequently confiscated those condoms from students fearing that parents might view condom distribution on campus as encouraging sexual promiscuity (Ibid.).

Adding to these general concerns, several scholars indicated that the implementation of the 100% CUP potentially contravened Chinese law, especially the PRC's prostitution controls. Article 358 of the Criminal Law of the PRC (1997) stipulates sentences of between 5 and 10 years' imprisonment for anyone who organizes or forces others into prostitution. This means in theory that the running of businesses that facilitate sexual services is a criminal offence. First-party engagement in the prostitution transaction is banned according to Article 66 of the Law of the People's Republic of China on Penalties for Administration of Public Security, punishable by between 5 and 15 days' administration detention, or a fine of between CNY 500 and CNY 5,000 (Quanguo renda changweihui 2005). Prior to the introduction of that law in 2006, first-party engagement in the prostitution transaction was banned according to the 1986 Regulations of the PRC on Penalties for Administration of Public Security, which gave policing authorities the right to detain suspected offenders for investigation, for a period of up to 15 days and, in more serious cases, for a period of up to two years (Quanguo renda changweihui 1986).

The relevant laws were, and continue to be implemented through periodic police-led crackdowns on prostitution businesses and practices – an anti-vice policy known as '*saohuang dafei*' (literally, sweeping away 'the yellow' [pornography, prostitution and obscenity] and illegality). In November 2015, the Ministry of Public Security of the PRC issued a notice urging all departments to organize crackdowns on prostitution and drug-related activities in entertainment venues (Liu Ziyang 2015). In 2014, the deputy mayor and chief of police in Dongguan City in Guangdong Province was removed from his posts for dereliction of duty after a CCTV exposé showing that police raids on venues providing sexual services had failed to control the city's rampant sex industry (Zhong Xinwen 2014: 4).

Thus, the goal of the pilot projects, to encourage sex workers to insist on condom use in all commercial sexual encounters, arguably ran counter to the PRC's policy of abolishing the sex industry via police-led crackdowns. It could also have been viewed by members of the public as tantamount to accepting the existence of a sex industry or encouraging red-light districts (Zhang Li 2002). For example, although Liyang Town in Li County is only a small town, project leaders found it to have contained nearly 100 entertainment and leisure venues that may have facilitated commercial sex (He Gu 2002b). The official recognition of such a large number of businesses associated with commercial sex in a small town obviously constituted a public relations problem for local policing authorities. First and foremost, it ran the risk of being construed as a sign of the inability or unwillingness of local police to crack down on prostitution as dictated by government policy (Ren 1999: 1430). Likewise, the government-sponsored promotion of condom use among sex workers in entertainment and leisure venues might be mistakenly interpreted as a sign that the sex industry was no longer illegal (He Gu 2002b).

The contradiction implied in the provision of sexual health training by government officials to illegal sex workers was raised in a 2002 article about the pilot project in Li County, published in the *Nanfang Dushibao* (hereinafter the *Southern Metropolis Daily*). In an article titled, 'Where Does the Balance of the "Condom Project" Lie?', Han Fudong (2002) praised the pilot project as a positive and humanitarian step forward regarding the control of AIDS, but concluded that its contradictory nature would bring chaos to law enforcement. As Han explained, the government wants to prohibit prostitution while providing health protection to people who engage in prostitution. Most members of the public claim they object to prostitution as a moral offence, yet there is obviously a widespread demand for and supply of commercial sexual services. The introduction of the 100% CUP was thus bound to bring the policy of banning prostitution into question, by questioning its relevance and the commitment of policing and other government authorities to the policy.

In another report, published in the *Southern Metropolis Daily*, Tong Dahuan (2002), a famous Chinese news analyst, suggested that the implementation of the pilot project in Li County had embarrassed government authorities and hence NGOs should take over the role of implementing China's 100% CUP. Tong's argument turned on a legalistic principle: Chinese law empowers the government to ban prostitution and no regulations imply that the government should facilitate potential sexual business. Consequently, the PRC government may not have a legal mandate to implement the 100% CUP whereas NGOs might. While arguing for a more active role for NGOs in relation to AIDS prevention work, Tong (2002) also recognized that this shift might create additional problems. Most notably, precisely because of their non-governmental status, NGOs might find their capacity to implement the 100% CUP hindered by police crackdowns on prostitution practices and businesses, and those who facilitate them. The article therefore implied that preventing AIDS might require a shift from policing to managing the sex industry, and NGOs rather than government departments should do the work of minimizing the public health risk associated with the sex industry.

In refuting criticisms of the perceived contradictory nature of the Li County project, a 2002 report by Chen Jieren, in the *Zhongguo Qingnianbao* (hereinafter the *China Youth Daily*), noted that the implementation of the program marked a pragmatic and positive governmental approach to the protection of public health and civil rights. The *China Youth Daily*, run by the Communist Youth League, is a renowned national newspaper and has a daily circulation of around two million copies (All-China Youth Federation 2009). As Chen Jieren (2002) put it, people who thought the pilot project meant that government authorities in Li County had gone 'soft' on prostitution had missed the more significant objective of the 100% CUP. Given the impossibility of eradicating prostitution in the short term, it was incumbent on a responsible government to serve society by protecting the health of its citizens, and especially marginalized members of Chinese society, such as sex workers. Chen concluded that this realistic attitude did not imply government acceptance of prostitution. The continued implementation of suppression measures against prostitution reflected a balanced approach to the control of a social harm and the protection of public health.

Finally, health scholars, acting as an authoritative voice on the pilot project in Li County, actively publicized their views in support of the 100% CUP in the media. On 25 September 2002, reporters from the *China Youth Daily* interviewed Dr Wu Zunyou from the National Center for AIDS and STD Control and the CDC in Beijing (Lan Yan 2002). In that interview, Wu Zunyou stated that the introduction of a 100% CUP in Thailand and Cambodia had led to a sharp decline in the prevalence of STI and HIV (Ibid.). Wu emphasized that, although the 100% CUP focused on sellers and buyers of sex, its ultimate goal was to protect the health of the general population. Wu concluded that the implementation of the 100% CUP pilot projects did not mean that prostitution was legalized. Government authorities had implemented the pilot projects because the PRC government was the only body with the ability and responsibility to do so (Ibid.).

In summary, the pilot projects were viewed as being compromised in part by the absence of legislation that supported the promotion of AIDS education for underground sex workers. Prior to 2006, China lacked national-level regulations on AIDS prevention and control, although some regulations dealt with specific AIDS-related issues. Following requests from health officials and researchers who were associated with the 100% CUP, relevant government authorities began to draft legislation in order to facilitate public health interventions based on condom promotion (Xiao Jinliang 2008: 5; see also Duan Yuhong 2002; Ge Zongyu 2002). Consequently, a departmental rule was promulgated by six central-level ministries in 2004. This rule, called the Guidelines on Preventing AIDS and Promoting Condom Use, acknowledged that condom promotion played a useful role in HIV prevention (Zhonghua renmin gongheguo guojia weisheng he jihua shengyu weiyuanhui 2004). However, the document is best seen as a proposal, as it did not give local governments the legal right to implement condom promotion programs.

In 2006, after four years of preparation, the State Council promulgated the Regulations on AIDS Prevention and Treatment (Guowuyan 2006a). The Regulations stipulate that China's media, including television and radio stations, newspapers, magazines and the Internet are responsible for communicating knowledge about AIDS through PSAs. They also legitimize public health interventions based on condom promotion among key populations. Article 26 states that the promotion of behaviour change initiatives to help people in key populations at high risk of contracting and transmitting HIV is a major component of AIDS prevention measures (Ibid.). Given this legal mandate, versions of the 100% CUP have since been implemented throughout China.

Concluding remarks

Media publicity of the pilot project in Li County marked a significant moment in the history of political communication on AIDS prevention work in the PRC, because it opened the gates for broader media coverage of AIDS prevention programs promoting condom use. In 2004, the Guidelines on Preventing AIDS and Promoting Condom Use, which were jointly issued by the Ministry of Health and other government agencies, stated for the first time in a national policy document that promoting condom use was one of the *main tasks* of AIDS prevention (Zhonghua renmin gongheguo guojia weisheng he jihua shengyu weiyuanhui 2004). Then, in 2006, the State Council promulgated a national administrative law on HIV and AIDS, the Regulations on AIDS Prevention and Treatment (Guowuyuan 2006a). The Regulations stipulate that China's media, including television and radio stations, newspapers, magazines and the Internet, are responsible for communicating knowledge about how to prevent AIDS through PSAs.

Since 2006, media publicity on the roll-out of the 100% CUP across China has become routine rather than an unusual practice. The subject of AIDS, which was once intentionally avoided in official and mainstream media, is now widely discussed. The utility of condom use in preventing the sexual transmission of HIV is also actively promoted, and the advertising of condoms is no longer banned for offending public morality. However, commercial sex is a continued focus of legal prohibitions and associated law enforcement practices.

While media publicity associated with the 100% CUP has occurred in a more relaxed environment since 2006, the content and style of such reports often replicates the framework associated with media coverage of the pilot project in Li County. This framework aims to convince the public of the necessity for implementing the 100% CUP across China in four ways. First, expert or authoritative voices are cited to demonstrate the urgency of preventing HIV transmission in the PRC in order to protect the health and future of the nation. Second, authoritative voices are cited to demonstrate that condoms have been demonstrated to halt or slow the spread of HIV through sexual transmission, both in international best practice and based on scientific evidence. Third, the focus of the 100% CUP on entertainment and leisure venues is justified by stressing the need to focus on those most at risk. Fourth, members of the public are assured and/or reminded that the promotion of condom use within such venues does not imply any changes to the PRC's policy of banning prostitution. It simply reflects the pragmatic and necessary response of a government that is committed to protecting and serving 'the people' (see also Jeffreys 2012a).

In this way, media publicity associated with the roll-out of the 100% CUP serves to promote public confidence in China's governing authorities and to diminish the potential political controversies associated with AIDS and sex work. Such media coverage portrays the communist regime as a modern and people-centred government, as opposed to a traditional, revolutionary party. It suggests that government authorities are prepared to prioritize different goals and mobilize different moral and legal arguments when faced with a major public health problem. It further suggests that the PRC government is pragmatic and not bound to a fixed ideological position on prostitution, even as the WHO-directed focus on commercial sex as a vector of disease may reinforce the construction of prostitution as a social harm in Chinese law.

The expansion of China's 100% CUP has also encouraged significant changes to government policies and media publicity on commercial sex and condoms, as the next chapter shows.

4 Changing policies on prostitution, censorship and disease control

This chapter explores the evolving nature of policies and laws on prostitution and sexually transmissible infection in the People's Republic of China, providing the historical policy background required to understand the controversial nature of implementing a 100 Per Cent Condom Use Program, and outlining the legal and social changes that it has brought in tow. Prior to the 1990s, direct and indirect forms of censorship ensured that China's state-controlled media did not discuss the emergence of commercial sex in detail or outside the parameters of Communist Party-established discourses on the issue. In the 1980s, public discussions of prostitution chiefly focused on its harmful nature, labelling it as an 'ugly and evil social phenomenon' (*shehui chou'e xianxiang*). They also focused on the importance of eradicating the sex industry through police-led crackdowns, as per the self-proclaimed historical feat of the communist regime in the 1950s (Ma Weigang 1994; Zhang Jun 1999).

Since the mid-2000s, the implementation of health interventions providing AIDS education and promoting condom use to people who provide commercial sex via entertainment and leisure venues has helped to alter the parameters of public discussions of prostitution in China. The sex industry is still banned under Chinese law. However, questions regarding the most appropriate government response to the existence of sex workers are now publicly debated, albeit within the constrained parameters permitted by the one-party ruling system. At the same time, condom advertising is no longer banned based on obscenity laws. Instead commercial marketing is rebranding condoms as a means of promoting personal health and sexual hygiene, rather than as a marital contraceptive device.

The chapter first details the significant changes that have taken place with regard to the PRC's prostitution policies, and legislation linking the sex industry and STI. In the process, it explains why coercive law-enforcement strategies were viewed as the primary means to control commercial sex and HIV in China until after the turn of the century, when PRC health authorities started to collaborate with international organizations to implement pilot versions of the 100% CUP. It then traces the shift from explicit censorship of media discussion of prostitution in the 1980s towards permitting restricted media coverage of police-led campaigns against the prostitution industry in the 1990s, and eventually encouraging broad media publicity of HIV prevention measures relating to the sex industry in the late 2000s.

DOI: 10.4324/9781315175546-4

Finally, the chapter suggests that the introduction and expansion of AIDS-related health communication since the early 2000s has generated new terms for condoms and sex sellers, flowing from the reconfiguration of STI and prostitution as objects of government from the perspective of public health, and not just policing. Condoms have been rebranded as a 'safety sheath' (*anquantao*), as opposed to being primarily a contraceptive device or 'prevent pregnancy sheath' (*biyuntao*). Terms such as 'sex worker' and 'sex industry' have been translated into Chinese and used in official health documents, although they have yet to become a part of everyday speech. The PRC's adoption of international governance strategies designed to minimize the health risks associated with the sex industry has thus made the topic of commercial sex, and the nature of its regulation, a matter of public discourse.

China's prostitution controls

The PRC's first Criminal Law, effective 1 January 1980,[1] did not pay much attention to the subject of prostitution, reflecting the premise that prostitution was an exploitative industry that the Communist Party had eradicated from mainland China in the 1950s, and hence was a 'non-issue' in the post-1978 era of economic reform (Hershatter 1997: 331; Jeffreys 2004: 139). Article 140 proposed sentences of between 3 and 10 years' imprisonment for anyone who forced women into prostitution (Zhonghua renmin gongheguo xingfa 1979). Article 169 stipulated a maximum of five years' imprisonment, with extra provisions for more serious offences including the act of luring women into or sheltering women in prostitution for profit. In doing so, the 1979 Criminal Law banned third-party attempts to profit from the prostitution of others, but paid little attention to the activities of sex workers and their clients (Jeffreys 2004: 139).

Yet commercial sex clearly was a growing phenomenon and newfound problem for government in China, as demonstrated by the issuing of the Notice on Resolutely Curbing Prostitution by the Ministry of Public Security in 1981 (*Gonganbu guanyu jianjue zhizhi maiyin huodong de tongzhi*) (hereinafter the 1981 Notice) (Gonganbu 1981). The 1981 Notice stated that the early CCP had eradicated the prostitution industry to public acclaim. However, prostitution had resurfaced in the reform era and was corrupting social morality and people's thinking, endangering social order and damaging China's international reputation, and hence should be targeted by police-led crackdowns (Ibid.). It urged policing authorities to crack down on criminals who forced women into prostitution or who profited from the prostitution of others, including organizers of prostitution from Hong Kong and Macau. This implied that the emerging sex industry had both criminal and international dimensions.

The 1981 Notice also suggested that women who sold sexual services in the 1950s and the reform era were different. Before the PRC's founding in 1949, Chinese women were forced into prostitution by exploitative, feudal-capitalist economic relations and patriarchal customs. In contrast, some women in the reform period chose to sell sexual services because they (incorrectly) admired a 'bourgeois' and 'hedonistic' (Western) lifestyle (Ibid.). The 1981 Notice consequently separated women who sold sex into different groups – those women who were forced into prostitution by others or socio-economic hardship and therefore required support, and those who did so voluntarily from the politically incorrect standpoint of an individual desire for money and luxury.

This distinction inhered in the recommended punishments for sellers and buyers of sex. The 1981 Notice recommended that urban-based women who had left employment in a state-run work unit to engage in prostitution as a means to earn a livelihood should be sent to institutes for reform through legal, moral and political education (Ibid.). The other recommended punishments entailed public shaming at work-based political study meetings, and highlight the dependence of early prostitution controls on Mao-era forms of labour organization and social control. Yet that system was being eroded by the very conditions that had enabled the emergence of crime and a sex industry in the reform period: namely, the introduction of labour markets and hence population mobility. The 1981 Notice recommended that male buyers of sex should be disciplined by their work unit. Women who had employment but sold sexual services occasionally to earn extra income should be disciplined by their work unit. And rural women who sold sexual services in cities should be returned to their native homes and disciplined by their agricultural production unit.

In 1983, the activities of sex sellers and buyers became the indirect target of the first and most notorious of China's reform-era policing campaigns against the emerging problem of crime – the 1983 'strike hard' (*yanda*) campaign against street crime and criminal activity (Jeffreys 2012b: 9). Consensual adult prostitution was not an explicit target of this campaign. However, the activities of sellers and buyers of sex were penalized under the crime of 'hooliganism' (*liumangzui*), until this classification was deleted from the revised Criminal Law of 1997. Article 160 of the 1979 Criminal Law defined hooliganism, in the context of crowd involvement, as acts of civil disorder, including fighting (*juzhongdouou*), creating disturbances (*xunxinzishi*) and insulting women (*wurufunü*), with sentences of up to seven years' imprisonment for extreme cases (Zhonghua renmin gongheguo xingfa 1979). The category of hooliganism was nevertheless often used by the police to side-step the exact letter of the law by apprehending those who were deemed to have committed an offence against public order, but had not committed a crime according to the provisions outlined in the Criminal Law (Biddulph 1993: 341; Trevaskes 2003: 272–92). In the limited number of publications available from the early to mid-1980s about how to apply the law to the issue of prostitution, first-party engagement in commercial sex is cited as an offence that could be handled under the rubric of hooliganism (Gong Wenqiang 1984: 28–9; Li Shan 1986: 45–6).

Prostitution also featured in the 1986 Resolution of the Central Committee of the Communist Party of China on Guidelines for Building Socialist Spiritual Civilization (Zhonggong zhongyang guanyu shehuizhuyi jingshen wenming jianshe zhidao fangzhen de jueyi 1986). Deng Xiaoping (1979) – the proclaimed architect of China's economic reforms – first articulated the concept of socialist spiritual civilization in the late 1970s. It refers to the goal of upholding core socialist values, while developing a market economy, and is associated with government efforts to promote political stability and ethical-cultural development in the context of rapid economic and social change. The 1986 Resolution raised the issue of prostitution as an example of something that should be prohibited because it harmed the development of socialist democracy and the rule of law.

In keeping with this negative understanding of commercial sex, the PRC's legislature, the National People's Congress, promulgated the Regulations of the People's Republic of China on Penalties for Administration of Public Security in September 1986, effective 1 January 1987 (*Zhonghua renmin gongheguo zhian guanli chufa tiaoli*) (hereinafter the 1986 Regulations) (Quanguo renda changwu weiyuanhui 1986). Article 30 banned the acts of selling and buying sex, introducing others into prostitution and providing accommodations for prostitution. It granted policing authorities the power to detain suspected offenders for investigation for up to 15 days, and subsequently to warn offenders and force them to sign a statement acknowledging their errors. A maximum fine of CNY 5,000 was also imposed. In addition, Article 30 gave policing authorities the power to detain offenders for rehabilitative education or reform through education and labour for between six months and two years in serious cases. Until the practice was abolished in 2014, reform through education and labour referred to a controversial set of administrative measures, providing compulsory reform to those who had violated laws and regulations but had not committed a criminal offence (Green 2014). This meant that most prostitution-related offences in early reform-era China were dealt with by the police, rather than through the developing courts and criminal justice system.

These legal and ideological proscriptions combined to make commercial sex the explicit focus of a nationwide police-led campaign against the 'Six Evils' (*liuhai*) in 1989. The 'Six Evils' referred to prostitution, gambling, the manufacturing and sale of pornography, the manufacturing and sale of drugs, kidnapping and selling women, and using feudal superstition to deceive and harm people (Biddulph 2007: 136–7). This campaign heralded the start of a series of policing campaigns aimed at eradicating the 'social vices', which were viewed as contributing to the erosion of socialist values, and which had allegedly entered China along with the adoption of economic reforms and an Open Door policy.

To provide legal support for police-led campaigns against commercial sex, the National People's Congress promulgated the Decision on Strictly Forbidding the Selling and Buying of Sex in 1991 (*Quanguo renmin daibiao dahui changwu weiyuanhui guanyu yanjin maiyinpiaochang de jueding*) (hereinafter the 1991 Decision) (Quanguo renda changwu weiyuanhui 1991). This document is significant because it expanded previous rulings on prostitution and was eventually incorporated into a revised version of the Criminal Law in 1997. The provisions contained in the 1991 Decision are included in Section 8 of that Law, called Crimes of Organizing, Forcing, Luring, Sheltering or Procuring Other Persons to Engage in Prostitution.

As with the 1991 Decision, the revised Criminal Law of the PRC (1997) expanded legal punishments for organizers of forced prostitution and for those who were found to facilitate consensual prostitution via the hospitality and service industry. Article 358 stipulates sentences of between 5 and 10 years' imprisonment for anyone who organizes or forces others into prostitution. Serious crimes attract sentences of 10 or more years' imprisonment or life imprisonment. These crimes include forcing girls under the age of 14 years into prostitution; forcing several people into prostitution or an individual into repeated acts of prostitution; raping and then forcing others into prostitution; and injuring or murdering people forced into prostitution. Before 1 November 2015, serious crimes of arranging for or forcing another person to engage in prostitution could even have been meted the death penalty. That stipulation was removed from Article 358 in 2015 along with amendments that removed the death penalty from nine other crimes in the penal code (Zhang 2015).

Article 358 of the 1997 Criminal Law also stipulates sentences of not more than five years' imprisonment and a fine in ordinary cases, and between 5 and 10 years' imprisonment in more serious cases, for those who help others organize people for prostitution. Article 359 stipulates sentences of up to five years' imprisonment and a fine in ordinary cases for those who introduce and shelter other persons into prostitution. Article 361 stipulates that managers or employees who take advantage of their work unit to organize, force, introduce or shelter others into prostitution shall be sentenced based on Articles 358 and 359.

Like the 1991 Decision, the 1997 Criminal Law does not criminalize the behaviours of first-party participants in commercial sex, with the exception of clauses relating to the premeditated spread of a serious STI and sex with minors (Quanguo renda changwu weiyuanhui 1991: Article 5). Article 360 of the Criminal Law of the PRC (1997) stipulates that any person who sells or buys sex in the full knowledge that he or she is suffering from syphilis, gonorrhea, or any other serious venereal disease shall be sentenced to fixed-term imprisonment of not more than five years and shall also be fined. Before 1 November 2015, Article 360 stipulated that anyone who engaged in prostitution with a girl under the age of 14 would be sentenced to a fixed-term imprisonment of no fewer than five years. Amendments to the Criminal Law in 2015 redefined prostitution acts involving minors as rape, which is punishable by a fixed-term imprisonment of between 3 and 10 years (Zhang 2015). First-party engagement in consensual adult prostitution thus continued to be an unlawful act but not a criminal one, which policing authorities handled pursuant to the 1986 Regulations until 2006.

On 1 March 2006, three pieces of legislation came into effect that have shifted the parameters of China's prostitution controls – the Regulations on AIDS Prevention and Treatment, a revised version of the Regulations on the Management of Entertainment and Leisure Venues (*yulechangsuo guanli tiaoli*), and the Law of the People's Republic of China on Penalties for Administration of Public Security (Guowuyuan 2006a, 2006b; Quanguo renda changwu weiyuanhui 2005). The Regulations on AIDS Prevention and Treatment recognize condom use as an effective measure to control the sexual transmission of HIV, and endorse the introduction of health interventions focused on sex workers and other key populations. Article 26 states that local people's governments, and relevant departments of the people's government at the county level or above, shall take measures to promote behaviour change programs for AIDS prevention, and to help 'HIV infection vulnerable groups with high-risk behaviours change their high-risk behaviours' (*bangzhu you yi ganran aizibing bingdu weixian xingwei de renqun gaibian xingwei*) (Guowuyuan 2006a). Article 61 stipulates that condoms must be available in or near entertainment and leisure venues. It also gives policing authorities the capacity to fine operators between CNY 500 and CNY 5,000 for failure to comply, and to revoke business licenses in instances of continued non-compliance (Ibid.).

The revised Regulations on the Management of Entertainment and Leisure Venues were issued to support a nationwide crackdown on prostitution, gambling and drugs in the hospitality and service industry, which was also launched on 1 March 2006 ('China's entertainment venues' 2006). They make managers of entertainment and leisure businesses responsible for the activities occurring within them. Article 14 states that employees and patrons of such businesses must not peddle narcotics, organize others into prostitution, manufacture or distribute pornography, supply or engage in accompaniment/hostess services for profit, gamble, encourage sects and superstitions, or engage in any other illegal activity (Guowuyuan 2006b). Any venue with activities that contravene Article 14 faces closure for between three and six months and confiscation of any money or property deriving from the provision of illegal activities. Serious cases may result in the revoking of the enterprise's operating license and the responsible manager being fined between CNY 10,000 and CNY 20,000 (Ibid.: Article 42).

Articles 30 and 50 reinforce these provisions by stipulating that businesses should hang signs in prominent and visible spaces that itemize the regulations banning prostitution, gambling and drugs, and which provide a hotline complaint number to police and other relevant government departments. To minimize the potential for local police corruption and protectionism in this context, Article 31 requires managers of entertainment and leisure venues to set up regular internal checks and to notify police or relevant government departments at the county level of any illegal activities that they discover. Likewise, Articles 33 to 35 stipulate that investigating police must keep clear records of any actions or penalties that they impose on the owners, managers, staff and patrons of such venues.

However, unlike previous policing campaigns, which were accompanied by the introduction of stricter penalties for engaging in prostitution, the Law on Penalties for Administration of Public Security reduced the penalties for first-party engagement in commercial sex. Article 66 stipulates that selling and buying sex is punishable by between 10 and 15 days' administrative detention with the possible addition of a fine up to CNY 5,000; and, in less serious cases, by a maximum of five days' administrative detention or a fine of not more than CNY 500 (Quanguo renda changwu weiyuanhui 2005). It further stipulates that soliciting in entertainment and leisure venues for the purposes of prostitution is punishable by a maximum of five days' administrative detention or a fine of not more than CNY 500.

Article 67 similarly stipulates that facilitating, accommodating and introducing others into prostitution is punishable by between 10 and 15 days' administrative detention with the possible addition of a fine up to CNY 5,000; and, in less serious cases, by a maximum of five days' administrative detention or a fine of not more than CNY 500. Although these stipulations may seem harsh in that they allow for the temporary deprivation of personal freedom, they are more lenient than previous regulations, which empowered the Chinese police to detain prostitution offenders for periods of up to six months and even two years, and to fine them a maximum of CNY 5,000, with very little scope for appeal.

On 29 March 2006, the Ministry of Public Security issued the Regulations on the Procedures for Handling Administrative Cases by Public Security Organs (*gongan jiguan banli xingzheng anjian chengxu guiding*) (Zhonghua renmin gongheguo gonganbu ling: di 88 hao 2006). Among numerous other stipulations, the regulations prohibit the issuing of on-the-spot fines in prostitution cases and grant suspected offenders the right to a hearing if fined more than CNY 2,000 and the right to refuse to pay a fine if the police decline to give receipts that are not printed and issued by financial departments at the provincial level or above. A revised version of the regulations came into effect in 2013 (Zhonghua renmin gongheguo gonganbu ling: di 125 hao 2012). These stipulations have limited the scope for police corruption and abuses of power associated with the fining and handling of first-party participants in commercial sex (see Jeffreys 2010).

The issuing of revised prostitution-related regulations and laws coterminous with the Regulations on AIDS Prevention and Treatment signified a continued government commitment to banning the sex industry, while simultaneously reducing the penalities for engaging in commercial sex, and also the scope for prostitution-related police corruption and malfeasance. This situation encouraged researchers with the Chinese Center for Disease Control, and Prevention and the Global Fund to Fight AIDS, Tuberculosis and Malaria, to claim that 'prostitution is illegal but openly tolerated in China' (Chen *et al.* 2008: 11). Local police have the latitude to support or undercut the work of AIDS prevention depending on the broader political climate. On the one hand, local police often turn a 'blind-eye' to the existence of certain sex establishments and types of sex workers, and may even work with health officials to obtain the support needed to undertake AIDS education in entertainment and leisure venues. On the other hand, police from outside of local jurisdictions may conduct surprise 'raids' on entertainment and leisure venues during the course of provincial or national crackdowns on organized crime.

Controlling commercial sex and STI

The first significant regulatory document to explicitly combine the subjects of prostitution and STI in the post-1978 reform era was the Notice of the State Council on Resolutely Banning Prostitution and Curbing the Spread of Sexually Transmitted Disease, issued on 1 September 1986 (Guowuyuan 1986). The Notice stated that prostitution and STD, which had been eradicated from the PRC by 1964, had resurfaced and were spreading to the detriment of China's international reputation, the development of socialist spiritual civilization, public health and the health of future generations. It called on local governments to ban prostitution by severely punishing organizers of prostitution, investigating hotels, motels and restaurants, and sending sellers and buyers of sex to re-education through labour, involving compulsory, self-funded health checks for STI, with the results to be submitted to public security organs, who would also inform the workplaces and families of those apprehended about their actions. It further required the Ministry of Health to establish sentinel surveillance sites to monitor the extent and spread of STD.

The Notice added that then existing restrictions on public information about the resurgence of STD were henceforth cancelled so that policing, health and other relevant government departments, and Party-affiliated mass organizations, could start communicating information to the Chinese population about the harm of STD and the nature of their transmission (Ibid.: Article 9). Although statistical reports on the resurgence of STD were collated in the late 1970s, these were for internal use by leading Party members only (Zhang Junyan 1998: 118). With the issuing of the Notice, such information became available to Party-affiliated mass organizations, and especially to the Communist Youth League of China, the All-China Women's Federation and the All-China Federation of Trade Unions (Guowuyuan 1986: Article 9). Such organizations act as a medium for conveying government and party policies to the public and ensuring the effective implementation of such policies at the local level.

By 1988, the prevalence of STI in China was a publicly acknowledged problem. Representatives from the PRC's Ministry of Health and the World Health Organization held a joint workshop in Nanjing in 1988 on the prevention of STI. Information about that meeting was published in a magazine called *Liaowang* (hereinafter *Outlook*), a national news weekly affiliated with the official Xinhua News Agency (Tang Hua 1989: 20–1). This meant that the PRC government was prepared to acknowledge the existence of STI to domestic and international audiences.

Yet AIDS was viewed at this time as a primarily 'foreign import' and a product of promiscuous sexual behaviours (*xingluan xingwei*) that could be controlled through border controls and by banning prostitution. In 1987, He Jiesheng, the deputy minister of the Ministry of Health, stated in an interview with *Outlook* that AIDS would be prevented in China by preventing people with HIV from entering into the country and eradicating prostitution (Song and Chen 1987: 46). He further asserted that homosexuality and sexual promiscuity, which the WHO presented as the main factors behind the sexual transmission of HIV, were uncommon in China. The Ministry of Health thus initially assumed that banning prostitution, and detaining those apprehended as sellers and buyers of sex for compulsory health checks and legal-moral re-education, would prevent STI, including the potential spread of HIV (see Gil *et al.* 1996; Guowuyuan 1993; Tucker, Ren and Sapio 2010).

The Certain Regulations on the Monitoring and Control of AIDS, issued in January 1987, stipulated that all foreigners who had HIV or AIDS would not be permitted to enter China (State Council 1987). The regulations further stipulated that overseas visitors who were found to be infected with HIV would be deported (Articles 6 and 7). The Law of Infectious Disease Prevention and Control was issued in 1989, with further instructions about how to implement that law being issued in 1991. The law required all AIDS cases to be immediately reported to local health authorities and stated that AIDS patients must be quarantined (Wu, Rou and Cui 2004: 11). Chinese people identified as HIV-positive at the time were typically rural-to-urban migrants, and health and policing authorities would force them to return to their native homes (Ibid.). Such approaches proved to be unfeasible as the prevalence of HIV rose throughout China during the 1990s.

Thus, coercive law-enforcement strategies were viewed as the primary means to control commercial sex and the spread of HIV in the PRC until the late 1990s. This is not to say that discussions of the utility of condoms in preventing STI were completely absent from mainland China. In 1991, Zhang Ju, a scholar from the Department of Social Sciences at Xiehe University, noted in an article on the state of AIDS in China that condoms were an effective means of preventing the sexual transmission of HIV. However, as Zhang Ju (1991: 45) also noted, health authorities at the time viewed promoting condom use outside of the marital relationship as equivalent to promoting premarital and extramarital sex. As a result, health interventions based on the promotion of condom use were only trialled in a limited and sporadic nature by Chinese health professionals prior to the 2000s (Jia Manhong *et al.* 1999: 62–4).

That situation started to change with the issuing in October 1998 of China's Medium- and Long-Term Strategic Plan for HIV/AIDS Prevention and Control (1998–2010) (Guowuyuan 1998). The plan was preceded by a document released jointly by the Ministry of Health, the Publicity Department and the National Board of Education, among other government authorities, in January 1998, titled Principles for STD/AIDS Education and Prevention (Weishengbu *et al.* 1998). The document stated that AIDS was a growing and potentially major problem, as the PRC had 8,000 documented cases of people living with HIV and AIDS, but estimates projected that the number of cases could reach as high as 10 to 20 million. It called for both public education about AIDS prevention and the utility of condoms in preventing STI in general, and for preventative education focusing on the sex industry and people who injected drugs in particular. It also instructed China's media to stop publishing stories about the police using possession of condoms as evidence of engagement in commercial sex when reporting on prostitution.

The 1998 strategic plan stated that China's capacity for HIV and AIDS prevention was underdeveloped, but the PRC had a large population of internal migrants, and drug abuse and prostitution were unlikely to be completely eliminated within the foreseeable future (Guowuyuan 1998). It acknowledged that government leaders, government departments and the public had a limited understanding of the potential threat of AIDS. There was also no multi-sector coordination and community participation in prevention activities, and funding, expertise and medical services were limited. However, the strategic plan noted that the promotion of condom use had been effective in international settings and should be trialled in China. It further stated that the media should plan to incorporate regular publicity and education about STI and AIDS, but did not provide explicit instructions about how to proceed in the short term (Ibid.: Section 4, Item 3).

In July 2000, at the Thirteenth International AIDS Conference in Durban, South Africa, Deputy Health Minister Yin Daqui acknowledged in his address that the PRC government had no experience of working with key populations (Bai Jingwei 2000: 1). Shortly after, the Ministry of Health began to work with representatives from the WHO to implement pilots of the 100% CUP in China, following the example of Thailand. In 2004, the CDC issued national guidelines for conducting AIDS prevention work among women working in entertainment and leisure venues (Zhongguo jibing yufang kongzhi zhongxin 2004). These changes have gradually altered the perception that the phenomenon of prostitution is strictly a matter for policing.

Censorship and the sex industry

Prior to the 1990s, direct and indirect forms of censorship ensured that China's state-controlled media did not discuss the emergence of prostitution in detail nor outside the parameters of Party-established discourses on the issue. This censorship is highlighted in a document issued by the Ministry of Public Security in 1988 titled Minutes of the Symposium on Advancing Campaigns Against Prostitution Activities and Improving Reeducation Work (Gonganbu 1988). The document used XXX when referring to figures about prostitution-related crimes, arrests, detentions and fines. However, it concluded that the public security forces could enhance the work of 'internal' publicity and education by releasing information about 'typical, serious cases' to Party-affiliated mass organizations, government departments, state-owned enterprises and educational institutions, in order to publicize policing successes and educate people about the harm of prostitution. With the exception of cases relating to Guangdong Province, which borders Hong Kong and Macau, the document added that such information should not be released for publication in the state-run media (Ibid.).

Hence, media discussions of prostitution in the Chinese media during the early 1990s emphasized the importance of cracking down on prostitution as stipulated in legal policy, especially the 1991 Decision. For example, the magazine *Outlook* published an article in 1993 with the affirmative headline, 'China Resolves to Strike Hard Against Prostitution' (Zhou Lixian 1993). The article noted that prostitution was banned according to Chinese law, and was thus an appropriate and consistent focus of policing campaigns. It further criticized local governments for failing to take strong action against the existence of prostitution, suggesting that this problem stemmed from the erroneous understanding that prostitution was an inevitable aspect of a market-based economy, or even a potential driver of local economies (Ibid.: 18–9). This criticism, which implied the existence of alternative views on how to manage the sex industry, was directed at halting direct or indirect government profiteering from the emergent sex industry. A joint circular issued in June 1992 by the Central Committee of the CCP, the State Council and the Central Military Commission, called on all Party, government and military departments to ensure that prostitution activities were banned in the burgeoning hotel industry (Zhonggong zhongyang bangongting *et al.* 1992). The sector was basically state-owned until regulations introduced in the mid- to late 1990s stopped government departments and employees from running and protecting business operations in the hospitality industry (Jeffreys 2004: 173).

Academic writings in the early 1990s also reiterated the broad parameters of official discourses on commercial sex. This point can be illustrated with reference to an article published in the *Shenzhen University Journal* by Da Dan (1990), called 'The Problem of Prostitution: An Investigative Survey and Proposed Countermeasures'. The article reiterated arguments made in the 1986 Notice of the State Council on Resolutely Banning Prostitution and Curbing the Spread of Sexually Transmitted Disease, stating that prostitution had six very harmful aspects (*liu da weihai*) (Guowuyuan 1986). First, it harmed the social atmosphere (*baihuai shehui fengqi*) (Da Dan 1990: 95). Second, it damaged China's international reputation (*sunhai guojia shengyu*). Third, it jeopardized individual and public health through the spread of STI (*chuanbo xingbing weihai jiankang*). Fourth, it destroyed families, or more specifically, family happiness (*pohuai jiating xingfu*). Fifth, it corrupted the minds and habits of state-government employees and young people (*fushi ganbu qingshaonian*). Finally, it induced crime (*youfa fanzui*). The author, writing before the introduction of the 1991 Decision, concluded that the prostitution controls outlined in the 1979 Criminal Law and the 1986 Penalties for Administration of Public Security had failed to act as a deterrent, and proposed criminalizing the first-party selling and buying of sex (Ibid.: 96).

Da Dan's conclusion underscores the official discourse on prostitution in China during the late 1980s and early 1990s, labelling it as an ethico-political problem for public security forces to handle (Da Dan 1990). Commercial sex was portrayed as a problem in that its existence was seen to harm China's domestic and international reputation, by negatively influencing the ways in which Chinese citizens and the international community viewed the performance of the reform-era PRC leadership when compared to the proclaimed achievements of the early regime. It was constructed as a problem relating to declining socialist values insofar as it was deemed to destroy families and corrupt the minds and destroy the health of cadres and teenagers – leaders and future leaders of the nation.

Public discussions focused on commercial sex as a debilitating problem, with proposed responses suggesting the enforcement of punitive laws and ethico-political rather than health education. In many ways, this response to prostitution replicated that of the early CCP during the 1950s. However, a major difference between the responses proposed in the 1950s and in the early reform era is the attitude towards women who sold sexual services. In the 1950s, women who sold sex were categorized as victims of socio-economic exploitation who needed to be rescued by representatives of the socialist state and transformed into productive citizens (Choi 2011: 98; Ruan Qinghua 2009). In the early reform period, women who sold sex were categorized in government and academic documents in terms of social harm, and hence as victimizers of society (Da Dan 1990: 90; Gonganbu 1981; see also Zhou, J. 2006: 245).

The reconfiguration of female sex sellers in the early reform period as victimizers rather than victims of society relates in part to political considerations. Following the CCP's proclaimed success in eradicating prostitution from mainland China in the 1950s, prostitution was viewed as an ugly or decadent phenomenon that only existed in capitalist countries. Viewed from the perspective of revolutionary Chinese Marxism, there was no reason for prostitution to exist in China because the state provided resources and work. The existence of prostitution could only stem from 'incorrect' ideas possessed by people who were insufficiently politicized, which explains the original emphasis on re-educating repeat offenders and disciplining minor offenders at work-based political study meetings.

Banning the prostitution industry and adopting a negative approach to women who sold sex therefore went hand in hand until it became apparent in the late 1990s that policing authorities simply could not eradicate prostitution in the same way as the early CCP. The policing of prostitution subsequently became a focus of public debate. Demands for strict policing practices created problems throughout the 1990s and early 2000s, as campaigns against prostitution were criticized by both domestic and international commentators for encouraging policing abuses (Jeffreys 2012b: 97–100). Such campaigns were also criticized for hindering the work of AIDS prevention and compromising the rights of sex workers as Chinese citizens to legal and health protections (Tucker, Ren and Sapio 2010: 123; Xia Guomei 2009: 38).

In summary, although prostitution was associated with the spread of STI in China during the 1980s and 1990s, AIDS prevention measures focused on sex workers were limited until the late 1990s. Such measures largely involved providing medical treatment to people who presented at government-run clinics with an STI (the identities of whom were disclosed to policing authorities), and testing people who had been apprehended by policing authorities for prostitution offences, and then detained under administrative regulations for re-education or put in prison (Tucker, Ren and Sapio 2010: 123). While Chinese health professionals conducted several surveys among populations of female sex workers in the 1990s to ascertain their condom use behaviours, such activities were local and restricted in scope (Liao, He and Choi *et al.* 2006; Wu, Rou and Jia *et al.* 2007). Strategies designed to minimize the health risks associated with commercial sex were reactive rather than proactive until after the introduction of a strategic plan to prevent AIDS in 1998, which stated that prostitution would continue to exist in China for the foreseeable future and that promoting condom use could limit the sexual transmission of HIV (Guowuyuan 1998).

Rebranding condoms

The promulgation in 1998 of China's Medium- and Long-Term Strategic Plan for HIV/AIDS Prevention and Control (1998–2010) signified a national-level policy concern with growing rates of indigenous HIV infection through sexual transmission, which had implications for popular understandings of both the function of condoms and the governance of commercial sex. To begin with, health-related media reports began to discuss the effectiveness of condoms as a means to prevent the sex-related transmission of HIV. In an article called 'Ending the Silence: Meeting AIDS Head-On' (*Dapo chenmo, gongtong yingzhan aizibing*), published on 4 December 2000 in the *Guangming Daily*, Deputy Health Minister Yin Dakui spoke to journalists about the need for the media to start talking about sex and AIDS (Chen Guangman 2000). Yin stated that condoms, which he referred to as '*biyuntao*' ('avoid pregnancy sheath'), were an effective means of preventing the sexual transmission of HIV, and their use should be promoted. Here, the Chinese term for condoms, '*biyuntao*', accorded with the terminology used in the Medium- and Long-Term Strategic Plan for HIV/AIDS Prevention and Control (1998–2010) (Guowuyuan 1998).

The now popular Chinese-language term for condoms, '*anquantao*' ('safety sheath'), is a more recent invention and signifies a shift away from understandings of condoms as a contraceptive device, and towards an understanding of condoms as a personal hygiene device, and method of disease prevention. Initially, the term '*biyuntao*' was applied in official health documents not only because it was used colloquially, but also because conservative health scholars opposed the active promotion of condom use as a means of preventing disease. In 1994, Zhu Qi, a sex educator with the China Health Education Institute, published an article in the *Chinese Journal of Health Education* (*Zhongguo jiankang jiaoyu*) titled 'Preventing AIDS: [Should We Be] Promoting Condoms or Sexual Morality?' Based on a survey conducted among more than 500 students from a medical university, Zhu and his coauthors concluded that promoting condom use would encourage sexual promiscuity. They argued that promoting traditional sexual morality, which discouraged premarital sex, was a far more effective means of preventing AIDS than condom use (Zhu Qi *et al.* 1994: 30).

In the early 2000s, China's media began to use the terms 'safety sheath' (*anquantao*) and 'prevent pregnancy sheath' (*biyuntao*) simultaneously in discussions of AIDS prevention. For example, a report by the PRC's official news agency, Xinhua, on the issuing of Shanghai's first long-term HIV/AIDS plan in 2000 used the new term '*anquantao*' when referring to the effectiveness of condoms as a means of disease prevention (Qiu Yi 2000: 5), whereas a local and popular Shanghai newspaper, the *Xinmin Wanbao* (*Xinmin Evening News*), used the older term '*biyuntao*' ('Shanghai qidong <yufang yu kongzhi aizibing zhongchangqi guihua>' 2000). Xinhua's adoption of the term *anquantao* reflected a changing government attitude towards the promotion of condom use. An official document published in 2004 on promoting condom use to prevent the spread of HIV used both terms '*anquantao*' and '*biyuntao*' in its title, with '*anquantao*' being presented as the main term and '*biyuntao*' following that term in brackets to clarify its meaning (Zhonghua renmin gongheguo guojia weisheng he jihua shengyu weiyuanhui 2004).

The unfamiliarity of many Chinese citizens in the early 2000s with understandings of condoms as a means of disease prevention, rather than a contraceptive device, is demonstrated by the results of a survey on HIV transmission and condom use conducted in 2003 by the Horizon Group and the Futures Group Europe. The two groups are a human resources management consulting company and international development firm, respectively. The survey was conducted among people living in seven large and medium-sized cities, and in towns and villages in seven provinces, to ascertain the extent of local knowledge of HIV transmission and the efficacy of condoms as a means of disease prevention. It revealed that many Chinese citizens believed that condoms were used for contraception and were not aware that using a condom could help to prevent the sexual transmission of HIV ('Few people well informed about AIDS: survey' 2004).

Figure 4.1 shows the number of hits for the keywords '*anquantao*' and '*biyuntao*' in the China National Knowledge Infrastructure, China Core Newspapers Full-text Database, for the years 2000–2015. The database covers more than 600 core newspapers in mainland China (cnki.net). The data reveal that the use of the term '*biyuntao*' has remained relatively consistent, whereas the use of the term '*anquantao*' rose significantly in 2003–2004 and rose again in 2006–2007. These peaks correlate to the initial publicity about and subsequent national roll-out of China's 100% CUP, and the promulgation of the Guidelines on Preventing AIDS and Promoting Condom Use in 2004 and the Regulations on AIDS Prevention and Treatment in 2006.

As the data suggest, the idea that condoms are a means of disease prevention emerged alongside the expansion of China's 100% CUP to the national level between 2006 and 2007. The program popularized the use of the term '*anquantao*'

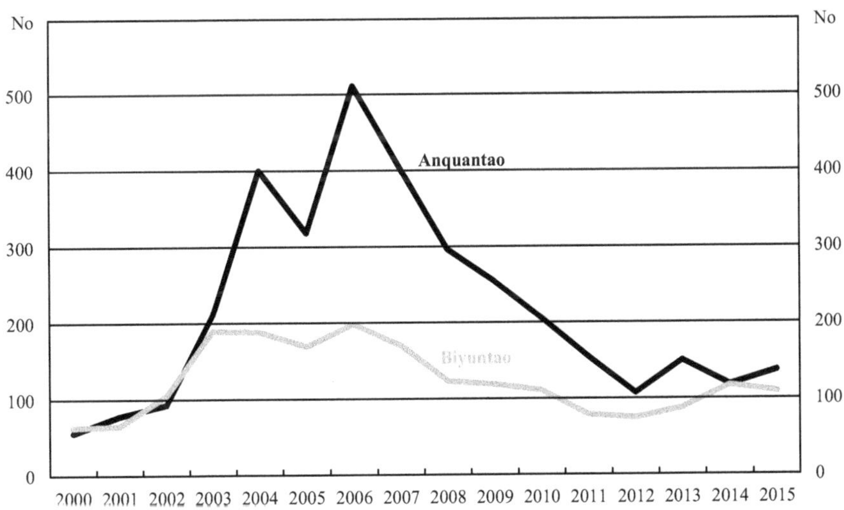

Figure 4.1 Chinese press coverage of '*anquantao*' (safety sheath) and '*biyuntao*' (prevent pregnancy sheath) (2000–2015).

Source: Compiled with data from China National Knowledge Infrastructure, China Core Newspapers Full-text Database (2000–), Beijing: Tsinghua Tongfang Knowledge Network Technology Company Ltd.

through relevant publications and advertising, helping to raise public awareness of the threat posed by unprotected sexual behaviours and the effectiveness of condom use in reducing the risk of HIV infection. Although print media coverage has since diminished, this does not indicate an absence of publicity. People in China now receive information about HIV prevention from more diversified media, including the Internet and social media, and public service advertising.

The expansion of the 100% CUP has also generated some changes in the terminology used by China's media to describe and discuss people who provide commercial sexual services.

Renaming people who sell sex

Prior to the late nineteenth century, prostitution in China sometimes referred to an elaborate set of ritualized social practices between male elites and courtesans (Hershatter 1997: 69–102). However, by the early twentieth century, prostitution had become a widespread practice. Instead of being an 'essentially luxury market', the sex trade became associated with impoverished women providing sex for money to the growing number of commercial and working-class men in Chinese cities, and with the spread of venereal disease (Ibid.: 65, 226–7).

The term '*jinü*' (prostitute) was associated in early twentieth-century China with women of low socio-economic status who had to degrade themselves to survive. Reformers seeking to replace China's imperial system with a modern system of governance often held up the existence of prostitution as a symbol of national shame, and as a social problem that needed to be resolved (Ibid.: 246; Sigley 2009: 46). This situation encouraged the newly victorious CCP to demonstrate its nation-building capacity by eradicating the prostitution industry from China during the 1950s, understood as a feudal-capitalist patriarchal institution that reflected the oppression of women (Jeffreys 2008: 234). Thus, until the 1980s, the term '*jinü*' referred to women in pre-liberation China who were forced to sell themselves to survive.

When journalists and researchers referred to the existence of prostitution in post-1978 China, they used different terms to describe women who provided commercial sex, one of which is '*xiaojie*', literally 'Miss' or 'young lady'. The term *xiaojie* became synonymous with the English expression 'working girl' due to linguistic changes and the expansion in the 1990s of the PRC's hospitality and service industry. Women working in the nascent service industry were usually addressed as *xiaojie* rather than the once ubiquitous politicized term of general address, namely, '*tongzhi*' (comrade) (Fan Xiaoling *et al.* 2004: 43). As the majority of women who were apprehended by police as prostitution offenders worked in entertainment and leisure venues, the term *xiaojie* started to be used in media reports as a means to describe women who provided commercial sex.

Many researchers now also use the term *xiaojie* to talk about female sex workers and it has become common parlance. For example, the Chinese Center for Disease Control and Prevention compiled a guidebook about HIV prevention in entertainment and leisure venues in 2004, which uses the term *xiaojie* in the title as a euphemism for female sex workers (Zhongguo jibing yufang kongzhi zhongxin 2004). While researchers often use the term *xiaojie* as a means to avoid words with more negative connotations, it has developed the negative connotation of 'prostitute/working girl', with young women who work in the hospitality and service industry often being offended if they are hailed by this term and preferring the neutral term '*fuwuyuan*' (attendant; waiter) (Wang Ningjiang 2000).

Before the implementation of China's 100% CUP pilot projects, government documents and legal documents, in particular, formally referred to women who provided commercial sex as '*maiyinnü*' or '*maiyinfunü*' (literally, women who sell sex). In Chinese, the terms '*mai*' (sell; sell out; parade; make a living by) and '*yin*' (excess; wanton; licentious) have negative connotations. Media reports about the pilot implementation of the 100% CUP showed that some health officials felt highly ambivalent about their involvement precisely because they viewed sex work negatively. For example, a medical doctor with the Li County CDC was asked how she felt about working on the 100% CUP in a documentary about the pilot project on China's Central Television Station broadcast in 2004. The doctor displayed no hesitation in saying that she was reluctant to work with female sex sellers, a group she described as 'disgusting' (*taoyan, yanwu*) (China Central Television 2004). Similarly, in interviews conducted with Chinese health officials between 2008–2010, legal scholar Margaret Boittin (2013: 259) claims that one official echoed an oft-repeated opinion when he explained to her that 'sex workers are "the lowest of the low", who "have very high rates of HIV/AIDS infection [because] they are the scum of the earth"'.

The Chinese translation of the English-language term 'sex worker' is '*xinggongzuozhe*'. This term entered the Chinese vocabulary along with media coverage of the pilot project of the 100% CUP in Li County in 2002. The use of the term in this context reflected its use in pilot project evaluations, which in keeping with international funding rules would have been couched in the required terminology. For example, although commercial sex is banned in the PRC, China's AIDS Response Reports to UNAIDS uses the preferred terminology of 'female sex worker' (National Health and Family Planning Commission of the PRC 2015).

On 8 August 2002, the *Modern Consumer News* featured an article about the pilot project which used the term '*xinggongzuozhe*'. This is not necessarily the first time that the terms 'sex worker' and 'sex workers' had been used in the PRC. Sociologist Pan Suiming (1994, 2007) used the term '*xingchanye*' (sex industry) in a 1994 publication rhetorically titled 'Does China Have a Sex Industry?' He later used the term '*xingchanye*' in a 2007 article arguing that China's sex industry had gained some degree of public acceptance, as evidenced by its widespread nature. However, the implementation of the 100% CUP in Li County brought national attention via the media to the term '*xinggongzuozhe*' as a new way of naming female sexual service providers in the context of AIDS prevention. Subsequent local and national media coverage of the pilot project in Li County referred to the term 'sex worker' (He Gu 2002b; Zhu Wenyi 2002).

This shift in terminology soon attracted responses from members of the public, as documented in media reports. A commentary published in late 2002, in a news magazine affiliated to the *Worker's Daily* (Gongren Ribao), questioned the use and accuracy of the term. As the author put it: how can you call prostitution a job? (*maiyin qineng jiao gongzuo*) (Wen Lun 2002: 20). The author objected to the use of the word '*gongzuo*' (work) to describe prostitution, understood as an illegal and immoral activity.

Scholars have similarly debated the appropriateness of different terms to describe sex sellers in China. Wang Jinling (2004: 202), a sociologist at the Zhejiang Social Science Academy, argues that the naming of prostitution and people who sell sexual services should avoid including any direct or implied moral judgment. She concludes that the key Chinese-language terms used to describe women who sell sexual services, such as '*jinü*' (prostitute), '*xiaojie*' (miss; working girl), '*maiyinnü*' (female sex seller), and '*xinggongzuozhe*' (sex worker), are inappropriate because they are gendered and incorrect from a legal perspective (Wang Jinling 2004: 202–9). They assume that the only people who sell sex are women and that the sex industry is lawful when it is not. Wang therefore recommends using the more neutral term '*shangyexing xingfuwuzhe*' (commercial sexual service provider). As this commentary suggests, the terms used to describe people who provide commercial sexual services are contested because they signify whether or not providing commercial sexual services should be considered as an ordinary form of work, and also convey different ideas about how people who buy and sell sex might be viewed by others.

The implementation of pilot projects of the 100% CUP even attracted critical commentary about the need to transform China's prostitution controls from people within the Chinese political body. In March 2003, Chen Lingfu, vice chancellor of Nanjing Normal University and a senior member of the National Committee of the Chinese People's Political Consultative Conference (CPPCC), which is a high-level political advisory body, suggested that approaches to the governance of the sex industry should be altered to assist the work of AIDS prevention ('Zhengxie weiyuan jianyi: xingjiaoyi zhong shiyong anquantao ying jianqing chufa' 2003). Chen submitted a proposal at the time of the annual meetings of the National People's Congress and the CPPCC suggesting that those people apprehended by police for engaging in prostitution, and who had condoms upon their person, should be handled in a lenient manner and given a lesser punishment. His suggestion was published in the *Southern Metropolitan Daily* and the story was taken up by media across China (Ibid.).

Chen Lingfu is the first person to our knowledge to propose at the CPPCC that the mode of governing commercial sex should be altered. His proposal also appears to have been motivated by public health concerns (Ibid.). While noting his personal objection to the existence of a sex industry, Chen argued that prostitution is widespread throughout China, despite police crackdowns, and such campaigns hinder the work of AIDS prevention. He suggested that the model of governing commercial sex based on policing, and what he described as the comprehensive management of public order (*shehui zhian guanli moshi*) should give way to an integrated management model led by health officials (Ibid.).

In Chen's view, health officials were better equipped to deal with the management of prostitution because their work with the 100% CUP encouraged sex workers to insist on condom use, and therefore protected the public health. Yet the work of health officials was complicated by the activities of police who often used possession of condoms as evidence of engagement in prostitution when apprehending suspected offenders. Chen therefore concluded that the adoption of a health-orientated style of managing commercial sex would minimize the health risks associated with the sex industry by facilitating the 100% CUP. He further concluded that the adoption of such an approach would defuse some the abuses associated with the heavy-handed policing of prostitution.

The term '*xinggongzuozhe*' has since appeared in contexts relating to other criticisms of China's prostitution controls. For example, in 2008, a well-known news magazine, the *Zhongguo Xinwen Zhoukan* (*China News Weekly*) used the term in the title of an article about crimes against female sex workers called 'Dongguan: Scar on the Face of a Female Sex Worker' (*Dongguan: yige xinggongzuozhe lianshang de daoba*) (Cheng and Chen 2008: 46–8). The article stated that female sex workers were frequent victims of violence at the hands of abusive police and clients because the illegal nature of the sex trade made it difficult for them to seek legal protections. In other words, while capitalizing on sensationalism and the readership appeal of 'prostitution' and 'crime', it also suggested that the illegality of the sex industry compromised the rights of sex workers as citizens to live safely and without fear (see Jeffreys 2009).

This is not to claim that terms such as 'sex industry' and 'sex worker' have replaced older and more pejorative terms in the Chinese media or in common speech. A search in the China National Knowledge Infrastructure, China Core Newspapers Full-text Database for the term '*xinggongzuozhe*' at various points between 2000 and 2015 received a limited number of *accurate* hits: 0 between 1 January to 31 December 2000, 2 in 2005, 11 in 2010 and 5 in 2015 (cnki.net). Although our initial search generated what appeared to be a large and increasing number of hits over time, the process of checking each and every report in specific years soon demonstrated that the majority were not explicitly related to sex work.

The Guidelines for AIDS Prevention Interventions Among Groups at High-risk Through Heterosexual Sexual Transmission, issued by the CDC and the National Center for AIDS/STD Control and Prevention in 2016, demonstrate the coexistence of new and older terminology, and neutral and negative terminology (Zhongguo jibing yufang kongzhi zhongxin, xingbing aizibing yufang kongzhi zhongxin 2016b). The Guidelines explain that such interventions are focused on female sex workers or women who provide sexual services (*nüxingxingfuwuzhe* or *nüxingfuwuzhe*). They add that different terminology is used to refer to this target population in different parts of China, such as '*maiyinfunü*' (women who sell sex), '*anchang*' (unlicensed prostitute), '*shizufunü*' (a woman who has taken a wrong step in life), and '*xiaojie*' (Miss).

The expansion of the 100% CUP since the mid-2000s has nevertheless helped to broaden the parameters of public debate on prostitution policy in China.

Commercial sex is no longer viewed as a something that can be dealt with solely by police-led crackdowns. Health interventions that promote condom use and focus on sex workers are becoming commonplace, and are supported in law and through government funding.

Concluding remarks

The promotion of condom use as a means to prevent the sexual transmission of HIV via the sex industry was accepted as an official strategy in 2004 following the completion of five 100% CUP pilot projects in different parts of China. In 2004, the Ministry of Health, together with the National Population and Family Planning Commission, promulgated a document called the Guidelines on Preventing AIDS and Promoting Condom Use, which endorses precisely this strategy (Zhonghua renmin gongheguo guojia weisheng he jihua shengyu weiyuanhui 2004). The promotion of condom use was also made into a matter of law with the promulgation of the Regulations on AIDS Prevention and Treatment in 2006 (Guowuyuan 2006a). Since then, health officials have launched a wide variety of public events promoting condom use for members of key populations, and for members of the national population in general, in keeping with shifting modes of HIV transmission.

Commercial sex became a nationwide object of public health management and not just policing when the sexual transmission of HIV became the main route of HIV transmission in China in 2007. The identification of sexual transmission as the main conduit for AIDS has followed improved testing services and the expansion of the number of national HIV sentinel surveillance sites from around 40 in 2004 to just under 160 in 2006 and nearly 1,900 in 2010 (State Council AIDS Working Committee Office and UN Theme Group on AIDS in China 2007: 6; Wen *et al.* 2012: 79). The PRC's sentinel sites now target eight groups of people: injecting drug users, female sex workers, men who have sex with men, long-distance truck drivers, male STI clinic attendees, women attending antenatal care clinics, young college students and male migrant workers. By 2016, sexual transmission accounted for more than 94 per cent of all new cases of HIV infection in the PRC, although the national HIV prevalence remains low at less than 0.06 per cent ('654,000 living with HIV/AIDS in China' 2016).

Commercial sex is still a focus of heavy-handed policing, stigma and violence in China, as the work of numerous scholars demonstrates (Anderson and Gil 1998; Boittin 2013; Choi 2011: 107, 110–13; Choi and Holroyd 2007; Gil *et al.* 1996; Hyde 2007; Jeffreys 2004, 2006, 2009, 2012b; Ren 1999; Rogers *et al.* 2002; Yu 2013; Zheng 2010). Legal acceptance of sex work is clearly also not on the government policy agenda. In February 2014, Yan Xiaokang, the deputy mayor and chief of police in Dongguan City, Guangdong Province, was removed from his posts for failing to control prostitution activities in his jurisdiction (Deng Xinjian 2014: 2). A follow-up editorial in the *People's Daily* stated that police crackdowns on the sex industry would continue for the foreseeable future because prostitution had no place in the PRC government's vision of a China as an economically developed and 'civilized' country (*wenming guojia*) (Zhong Xinwen 2014: 4). China's action plans for the containment and prevention of HIV and AIDS between 2006 and 2015 also referred to continued police crackdowns on the sex industry as part of the nation's AIDS response, as does the action plan for 2016–2020 (Guowuyuan 2006c; Guowuyuan bangongting 2012, 2017).

But the activities and publicity associated with the implementation of the 100% CUP have contributed to the diversification of debates about the sex industry, by introducing new terminology to describe people who sell sexual services, and new ideas about how the sex industry might be better managed. The next chapter explores these changes in more detail. It examines the mixed consequences of implementing a 100% CUP in China as an example of public policy that has helped to shift public, political and legal perspectives on sex workers, and other populations defined as key to the PRC's evolving AIDS response.

Note

1 During the Mao era, the formal legal system fell into disrepute as a tool of class oppression and was replaced in part by a system of administrative and Communist Party disciplinary sanctions (Starr 2001: 204–19). This system was used to police the activities of those considered to have committed social offences and political errors, but whose criminal liability was not considered sufficient to bring them before the courts.

5 Health interventions focused on sex workers

This chapter explores the nature and effects of health interventions focused on female sex workers in the People's Republic of China. The World Health Organization contends that sex workers are 'among those who are most vulnerable to HIV infection in the world today' (Amin 2005: 1). Hence the provision of effective AIDS education to sex workers is viewed as a vital component of strategies aiming to prevent the spread of HIV globally. The organizing rationale is that information about HIV and how it is transmitted can provide individuals with the knowledge needed to protect themselves and others from becoming infected with HIV, and may play an important role in reducing stigma and discrimination against people who are vulnerable to HIV infection, or living with HIV. Reducing stigma is important not only for improving the quality of life of people living with HIV, but also because stigma may encourage the spread of HIV by discouraging people from seeking testing and treatment (AVERT 2013; Meng 2012: 67).

People who sell and buy sexual services became a major focus of public health interventions in the PRC when the Regulations on AIDS Prevention and Treatment came into effect on 1 March 2006 (Guowuyuan 2006a). Article 26 states that local people's governments, and relevant departments of the people's government at the county level or above, shall take measures to promote behaviour change programs for AIDS prevention, and to help 'HIV infection vulnerable groups with high-risk behaviours change their high-risk behaviours' (*bangzhu you yi ganran aizibing bingdu weixian xingwei de renqun gaibian xingwei*) (Ibid.). Article 63 adds that 'HIV infection vulnerable groups with high-risk behaviours means people who practice the risky behaviours of engaging in commercial sex (*maiyinpiaochang*), have multiple sexual partners (*duoxingban*), inject drugs (*zhushe xidu*), or are men who have sex with men (*nanxing tongxing xingxingwei*)' (Ibid.).

The Ministry of Health of the PRC (2004, 2005) had already instructed the Chinese Center for Disease Control and Prevention in August 2004 to organize intervention teams focused on key populations at provincial, municipal, county and local levels, with trial guidelines about how to conduct those interventions being issued in mid-2005. In the case of female sex workers, the CDC issued a detailed implementation manual as early as June 2004, titled the Guidelines for AIDS and STI Prevention Work for Female Service Providers (*fuwu xiaojie*) in Entertainment and Leisure Venues (hereinafter the 2004 Guidelines) (Zhongguo jibing

DOI: 10.4324/9781315175546-5

yufang kongzhi zhongxin 2004). The promulgation of the 2006 Regulations on AIDS Prevention and Treatment facilitated the national implementation of such interventions by making them a public health priority in law. Demonstrating their ongoing nature, the CDC and the National Center for AIDS/STD Control and Prevention issued new guidelines for health interventions focused on female sex workers in 2016, titled the Guidelines for AIDS Prevention Interventions Among Groups at High-risk Through Heterosexual Sexual Transmission (hereinafter the 2016 Guidelines) (Zhongguo jibing yufang kongzhi zhongxin, xingbing aizibing yufang kongzhi zhongxin 2016b).

The chapter first examines the planning instructions for health interventions focused on female sex workers as outlined in the 2004 Guidelines, which provide an example of governmentality in action. They instruct designated experts how to act upon and address an identified ‘problem’ (the public health threat posed by individuals not using condoms during commercial sexual encounters), by transforming the conduct of governing authorities, managers of indirect sex establishments, and sex workers and their clients. The chapter then discusses examples of AIDS education booklets for sex workers and their clients, produced and distributed by the CDC and by the Chinese Association of STD/AIDS Prevention and Control, a government-organized NGO, with UNAIDS (Zhongguo jibing yufang kongzhi zhongxin n.d.; Zhongguo xingbing aizibing fangzhi xiehui and UNAIDS n.d.). It subsequently explores public responses to the provision of AIDS education for sex workers, or what China’s media described as the ‘working-girl training classes’ (*xiaojie peixunban*).

Finally, the chapter looks at public commentary by Communist Party officials, lawyers, NGOs and sex workers, regarding the need to alter the PRC’s prostitution controls in order to promote public health and sex workers’ rights. We conclude by considering the mixed consequences of implementing a 100 Per Cent Condom Use Program in China as a government intervention that has made commercial sex visible from the perspective of public health rather than policing concerns. In the process, it has helped to shift political, legal and public perspectives on sex workers, and other populations defined as key to the PRC’s evolving AIDS response.

Planning to intervene

Government-led behaviour interventions focused on women who provide commercial sex through the hospitality and service industry only became a commonplace and publicly recognized phenomenon in China after the mid-2000s. Health officials first provided AIDS-related educational materials to female sex workers in the late 1990s, but such interventions were conducted either in correctional facilities or in a limited geographical terrain (Ma and Dukers *et al.* 2002; Wu *et al.* 2007). Media reports suggest that health officials offered information and training classes to sex workers about how to prevent the sexual transmission of HIV at the First Correctional Facility in Shanghai in 1993 (Song Wei *et al.* 1995: 23). Research publications indicate that an intervention project based in entertainment and leisure venues was also conducted by staff from the CDC in Ruili City in Yunnan Province in 1997 (Jia Manhong *et al.* 1999: 62–4; Wu *et al.* 2007: S89–94). As part of this intervention, a series of cartoon-style pamphlets about AIDS awareness and sexual hygiene was used in face-to-face trainings for sex workers.

In 2004, the CDC issued a 60-page manual detailing the goals of health interventions focused on sex workers, and providing step-by-step instructions about how to organize and implement them (Zhongguo jibing yufang kongzhi zhongxin 2004). The expressed aim was to provide education to women working in entertainment and leisure venues about effective condom use, and thereby control the spread of HIV and AIDS in China, by encouraging 80 per cent of that population to insist on (male latex) condom use in all commercial sexual encounters (Ibid.: 36). To help realize this goal, the manual provided clear instructions about how to organize leadership teams to coordinate working groups and liaise with relevant people from different organizations. These included government departments, state-run and commercial media, public and private medical facilities, pharmaceutical and condom suppliers and distributors, Party-affiliated mass organizations and NGOs, and the owners, managers and employees of entertainment and leisure venues (Ibid.: 4).

Working groups were instructed to 'know' the area in which they intended to intervene by mapping the local arrangement of key 'people, places and things', and updating such maps on a yearly basis. This process involved mapping the location of all the entertainment and leisure venues that facilitated commercial sex in a specified geographical area (Ibid.: 9–11). It also involved mapping the availability of services relevant to the efficient delivery and success of the proposed intervention, such as the location of condom distributors, condom vending machines, adult goods shops, pharmacies, and public and private medical services. To do so, working groups were instructed to first liaise with members of relevant government departments (police and industry and commerce), and then to conduct personal observation and mapping exercises based on information derived from local informants – for example, taxi drivers and residents' committees. Finally, working groups were instructed to conduct in-depth interviews and focus groups with the owners, managers and women working in entertainment and leisure venues. The goal was to understand their views on the availability and accessibility of local condom supplies, and clinical services for STI and HIV counselling, testing and treatment, and how to improve service delivery and access to services.

After summarizing their findings, working groups were instructed to plan and conduct a series of pilot interventions in a limited number of venues, in order to develop an effective and financially viable intervention model for their area. This process involved piloting training classes and informational materials about the correct use of condoms to prevent STI, with the aim of obtaining feedback, and modifying the trainings and materials where necessary, and hence ensuring the success of the larger-scale delivery of such interventions. Training classes had to be run on a monthly or bimonthly basis and be quick and informative (around 30 minutes and up to a maximum of one hour in length), while also including information about how to access testing, counselling and treatments for STI and

HIV, and enabling the distribution of booklets, posters, videos and free condoms (Ibid.: 20).

The 2004 Guidelines also provided instructions on how members of the working groups, and associated CDC support services, should *conduct themselves* when conducting interventions in entertainment and leisure venues, in order to overcome obstacles to HIV testing. Members of the working groups were instructed to behave in what is generally described as a 'professional manner', indicating that this might not have been the default position adopted at that time. They were told to speak clearly and frankly to their audiences, and to demonstrate respect to those audiences by asking them open-ended questions, and listening to their responses without interrupting them. Medical personnel were instructed to overcome recognized barriers to STI and HIV testing by behaving in a courteous and helpful fashion, and demonstrating professional regard for issues of privacy and confidentiality, so that sex workers would present at testing and treatment facilities on a voluntary and regular basis in the future (Ibid.: 7). The 2004 Guidelines also recommended that local CDC branches establish more facilities for providing STI and HIV counselling, testing and treatments, but such services should be offered through particular hospital departments rather than being labelled as STI clinics, because the label might deter people from presenting for testing (Ibid.: 7).

Members of working groups were further instructed to identify sex workers, and operators of entertainment and leisure venues, with the capacity and personal communication skills required to assist the implementation of health interventions by becoming peer educators, or community-based 'experts' (Ibid.: 5–7). This process involved recognizing people with literacy skills who had influence with others, and who understood the information provided and recognized the importance of sharing that information with others. Apart from involving sex workers in health interventions, the 2004 Guidelines suggested that encouraging peer educators was necessary to overcome the problems associated with providing education about STI and AIDS to sex workers as a highly mobile (and illegal) population (Ibid.: 7). Peer educators would help to overcome this problem by visiting women working in more indirect establishments, for example, in beauty salons or on the street, to distribute free condoms and literature about safer-sex practices (Zhang, L. *et al.* 2014: 2).

Both the instructions to establish professional working relationships between health professionals and members of the sex industry, and to give members of the sex industry some responsibility for the roll-out and take-up of health interventions, *imply* a radically new approach on the part of government employees towards members of an illegal and stigmatized industry. It suggests a shift towards community-engaged service delivery, with members of key populations being trained to deliver HIV prevention and condom use promotion programs. This has not altered the top-down nature of such health interventions because the illegal nature of the sex industry and government controls over the non-profit sector mean that independent organization by sex workers, and people claiming to speak on their behalf, is limited in China. However, there has clearly been an increase in the number of NGOs working with sex workers in the intervening years. The

2016 Guidelines state that the contracting of social organizations/NGOs to access female sex workers has become an 'irreplaceable' part of such interventions since the State Council permitted government departments to contract private social services in 2013 (Zhongguo jibing yufang kongzhi zhongxin, xingbing aizibing yufang kongzhi zhongxin 2016b: 8).

Finally, and in accordance with international funding requirements, the 2004 Guidelines instructed members of local CDCs to conduct an impact assessment of such interventions and to eventually expand publicity about them to educate broader sectors of the population (Zhongguo jibing yufang kongzhi zhongxin 2004: 22–3). The interventions were funded through the Global Fund on a five-year basis, with an initial two years of funding being followed by three years of additional funding, provided such interventions had demonstrated effectiveness. The efficacy of such interventions was measured based on the capacity of the CDC to provide detailed post-intervention information about the size, characteristics, AIDS-related knowledge, and sexual attitudes and behaviours of their focus population (The Global Fund 2006). Hence the need for information that made sex workers visible as an object of public health rather than policing concerns.

Impact assessment involved the 'testing' of sex workers in entertainment and leisure venues via behavioural survey questionnaires. A sample 'impact-assessment questionnaire', which is included in the appendices to the 2004 Guidelines, states that it is an anonymous and confidential survey conducted by the CDC with the aim of improving public health services, and thanks participants for their assistance (Zhongguo jibing yufang kongzhi zhongxin 2004: 43–57). It asks respondents for demographic information about their age, ethnicity, educational level and marital status, and where they come from, that is, are they a local native or a migrant from a different county, province or country. It also 'measures' respondents' pre- and post-intervention knowledge by asking whether they have heard of 'AIDS', and, if so, from where (various media, friends, 'other' or women's health counsellors, that is, intervention teams and ancillary staff).

The questionnaire tests respondents' knowledge of HIV and AIDS and requests information about their work-related lifestyle. For example, it asks respondents whether AIDS can be cured, can you see if someone has HIV, is HIV transmitted by mosquitos or shaking hands, and can HIV be prevented by sexual monogamy, using condoms and sterile injecting equipment, or eating chicken and so forth. It asks how long individuals have been 'working' (*gan*) in entertainment and leisure venues, with options ranging from two weeks to over a year. It asks respondents whether they use condoms when they 'do it' and were they effective (did not break, slip, etc.), and if they did not use condoms, then, for what reasons (client refusal, never bought them, was not prepared, or 'other'). The questionnaire also asks female respondents about the frequency of their condom use with clients and other sexual partners, their drinking, smoking and drug use patterns, history of abortion, and whether they have a history or current symptoms of STI, and where they would choose to go to for related help (local government hospital, private clinic, pharmacy, etc.). Finally, the questionnaire asks respondents whether they have received information from intervention groups and completed a survey previously. It concludes by asking respondents whether they found the training provided interesting and useful, and whether they have any suggestions about how to improve the content and materials.

Apart from attracting additional funding by demonstrating success, the results of the impact-assessment questionnaires informed numerous research papers about the efficacy or otherwise of behaviour interventions focused on Chinese sex workers (see Rou *et al.* 2010; Ru Xiaomei *et al.* 2007). The perception of post-intervention success legitimized both the original intervention and the introduction of similar programs in new locations and areas across the country. Perceived failures generated calls for improved interventions and policy frameworks. These include calls to overcome the stigma attached to sex work, because it discourages sex workers from working with health authorities, and encourages local governments to treat health interventions focused on sex workers as a low priority in terms of the allocation of resources and funding (Rou *et al.* 2010: II44). They also include calls to end police-led crackdowns on sex work within entertainment and leisure venues, and to develop community-based support groups, which imply overturning bans on the sex industry (Ibid.).

In summary, the manual and its subsequent actualization in the form of behaviour interventions illustrate how the conduct of sex workers was presented as a problem for government in China that required corrective intervention through education about condom use, in order to prevent the spread of HIV through sexual transmission. This 'problem' was not pre-given. It was constructed on the basis of concerns articulated by the WHO, and rendered as a field that could be acted upon with funding from international AIDS organizations. However, once the 'problem' was framed in a manner that allowed dialogue between different groups – Chinese health officials, police, managers of entertainment and leisure venues, and sex workers, it also became possible to explain the nature of the 'problem' differently and even to propose different solutions, as we discuss later.

AIDS education for sex workers

This section looks at two examples of AIDS educational materials for participants in commercial sex produced by the CDC and by the Chinese Association of STD/AIDS Prevention and Control with UNAIDS. Other organizations such as the National Population and Family Planning Commission have also produced and distributed audio-visual and printed materials for sex workers and their clients about how to prevent HIV transmission. Such materials are typically produced through public-private collaborations between PRC government agencies, international development organizations, private foundations, pharmaceutical companies, and condom manufacturers. Prominent collaborators have included the China-UK HIV/AIDS Prevention and Care Project; Futures Group Europe; UNAIDS; the WHO; the Global Fund to Fight AIDS, Tuberculosis and Malaria; the Bill and Melinda Gates Foundation; and the Merck Foundation (Gåsemyr 2015: 614–20; see also Ru Xiaomei *et al.* 2007; Sun *et al.* 2010).

A booklet produced and distributed by the CDC in Qingdao City, Shandong Province, and the London Durex Company offers one example. The booklet titled *Preventing AIDS: I Have a 'Method'* [a Condom] (*Yufang aizi: wo you yi 'tao'*, hereinafter the Booklet) presents images of young attractive women wearing revealing clothing and lots of makeup, and smoking and drinking, which are presumably designed to reflect the sartorial presentation and lifestyle of their target audience. The Booklet avoids using words that stigmatize sex work, in keeping with the understanding in international discourses that effective condom use promotion requires a shift in public discourse away from moral and ideological attitudes towards sex work, and towards a more neutral public health perspective (Zhongguo jibing yufang kongzhi zhongxin n.d.). It addresses female sex workers as 'sisters' (*jiemei*), and hence as a common reading audience, rather than using negative or objectivizing terms for women who sell sexual services such as *jinü* (prostitute/whore) and *xiaojie* (working girl). The Booklet also refers to male clients as 'guests' (*keren*) rather than the Chinese-language term for male clients used in legal documents, which is 'whoremonger' or 'patron of brothels' (*piaoke*) (Ibid.: 1, 10). Media reports suggest that health officials developed these educational materials after speaking with women working in entertainment venues and incorporated the language that they used to negotiate commercial sex, for example, referring to male clients as 'guests' who want some 'fun' (*wan*) (Qiu and Wang 2006).

The Booklet provides sex workers with information about how to protect and promote their health, including basic knowledge on HIV transmission and prevention, and how to access (confidential) testing, treatment and care. It begins with a statement that warns fellow 'sisters' to be careful and pay attention to protecting one's health and preventing AIDS because having multiple sexual partners can be dangerous. It informs 'sisters' that the best way of protecting themselves from HIV, and other STI such as Hepatitis B, is to insist on condom use during every sexual encounter (Zhongguo jibing yufang kongzhi zhongxin n.d.: 1).

The text engages readers by narrating the 'story' of Xiao Hong, a female sex worker, who confides in a colleague that she feels physically uncomfortable (Ibid.: 2). Xiao Hong tells Xiao Ying, a colleague who also happens to be a peer educator, that she seldom uses condoms because she does not carry them with her. She uses pharmaceuticals to prevent pregnancy and judges the disease-associated risk of clients based on whether they look clean or not (Ibid.: 2, 7). Xiao Ying suggests that Xiao Hong may have contracted an STI and advises her to go to a local government hospital for testing and treatment (Ibid.: 4). She adds that using a condom during every sexual encounter is the best method for preventing STI and AIDS, because it is not possible to tell whether someone is HIV-positive from their appearance. Xiao Hong repeats the word 'AIDS' suggesting that she has never heard of the disease (Ibid.: 5). The Booklet subsequently explains how HIV is transmitted (via unprotected sex, mother-to-child transmission and contaminated blood transfusions) (Ibid.: 6). It then provides information about how to use condoms effectively and how to dispose of them safely (Ibid.: 9).

The Booklet also contains sections with constructive advice to women who provide sexual services about how to encourage male clients to use condoms and how to say 'if it's not on, then, it's not on' (Ibid.: 10–13). Methods include suggesting that condoms are 'fun', prevent pregnancy and may prolong pleasure. It also provides advice on what to do in the event of condom failure or breakage, which includes washing and going for government-sponsored testing and treatment (Ibid.: 15–16).

The Booklet concludes with reference to government policies that encourage people not to discriminate against people living with HIV and AIDS (Ibid.: 17). It informs readers of the services available, including free testing; free treatment for members of low-income groups, rural-to-urban migrant workers and pregnant women with HIV; free schooling for children orphaned by AIDS; and various other forms of support for people living with HIV and AIDS. The final page provides telephone numbers in major cities across the PRC for people to contact should they require more information about STI and HIV (Ibid.: 18–20).

In doing so, the Booklet conforms to the preferred models of effective AIDS communication, as advocated by international HIV and AIDS charities such as AVERT (2013), and endorsed in the CDC guidelines. It provides basic AIDS education. It attempts to appeal to an imagined community of sex workers and clients through the use of colloquial and context-specific language. It aims to reach and empower sex workers as a marginalized group by encouraging those who engage in commercial sex to share information about STI and HIV prevention among their peers. It also provides information to people living with HIV about how to access the support required to improve their quality of life, and promotes non-discriminatory attitudes towards people living with HIV and AIDS. Last but not least, the Booklet encourages proactive behaviour change by promoting safer sex and teaching people how to use and dispose of condoms, rather than only focusing on abstinence.

The promotion of proactive behaviour change is now also being supported in the PRC by ensuring that cheap and reliable quality condoms are available in recreational venues and public spaces more generally. Article 61 of the Regulations on AIDS Prevention and Treatment stipulates that condom vending machines and condoms must be available in or near entertainment and leisure venues. It gives policing authorities the capacity to fine operators between CNY 500 and CNY 5,000 for failure to comply, and to revoke business licenses in instances of continued non-compliance (Guowuyuan 2006a). Domestically produced and imported condoms of different quality and cost are readily available online and in supermarkets and convenience stores across the country, providing interested consumers with easy and anonymous access to such goods.

Other AIDS education booklets in circulation in the PRC are designed for male buyers of commercial sex. This ensures a more inclusive provision of HIV and AIDS education, and encourages everyone involved in commercial sexual encounters to be proactive about changing their behaviours and exposure to risk. One such booklet, produced by the Chinese Association of STD/AIDS Prevention and Control and UNAIDS, is titled Picturing AIDS (*Hua shuo 'aizi'*) (Zhongguo xingbing aizibing fangzhi xiehui and UNAIDS n.d.) (hereinafter Booklet 2). As with the booklet for sex workers, it provides basic education about STI and the long-term health implications of an untreated STI, how to use and dispose of condoms, and how to contact health authorities for further assistance. It also encourages peer education by encouraging readers to tell their friends about what they have read.

Booklet 2 attempts to engage an imagined community of buyers of sexual services, in this case rural-to-urban migrant workers, by relating a 'personal' narrative about Da Liu, the head of a migrant worker construction team (Ibid.). Da Liu takes a colleague out on a day off work, where they meet an attractive young woman outside a hairdressing shop – a known venue for commercial sexual services. It turns out that Da Liu and the young woman are from neighbouring villages in the rural countryside. Da Liu subsequently leaves his colleague for 'a night of fun' with the young woman. Sometime later, Da Liu tells his colleague that he is experiencing a burning sensation when urinating and has a discharge from his penis. His colleague promptly tells him to go to a public hospital, where he is diagnosed with gonorrhea.

The doctor tells Da Liu how STI and HIV are transmitted, and tells him to use condoms when he engages in sex in the future to ensure that he does not infect his wife and their future children (Ibid.). She also tells Da Liu that HIV cannot be transmitted through hugging people, shaking hands, sharing food, swimming and showering with others, using public toilets, sharing work tools, mosquito bites and so forth. She concludes by telling Da Liu how to use condoms properly and how to dispose of them safely, and how to use sterile needles and dispose of them safely.

The overall message of Booklet 2, as summarized by the images and text on the first and last page of the narrative about Da Liu, is that STI and AIDS can be prevented if people protect themselves and share their knowledge of how HIV is spread with other people that they know (Ibid.). This unity of purpose is represented on the first page through an image of Da Liu, his colleague, wife, female companion and the doctor, presented as the story's protagonists or lead actors in the narrative. They are somewhat improbably holding hands and saying: 'STI and AIDS can be prevented'. The last page shows an image of Da Liu with his arms around his wife saying 'learn how to protect yourself', and his wife saying 'tell others what you know [about STI and HIV]' (Ibid.).

Such booklets are distributed online and as part of AIDS awareness activities in entertainment and leisure venues, and other workplaces. The aim is to provide basic information about how to prevent the sexual transmission of HIV, promote condom use and encourage people who sell and buy sex to act as peer educators. Information about the purpose and nature of health interventions focused on commercial sex was also publicized, as dictated by conditions of international funding and the 2004 Guidelines.

But the provision of government-sponsored AIDS education to sex workers has proven to be both complicated and controversial in China. The next section explains why.

Publicizing health interventions focused on sex workers

On 11 October 2006, Wen Yingchun from the Harbin CDC held a training class for female sex workers on AIDS prevention and condom use (Mu and Xue 2006; Zhang Guifeng 2006; Zhou Xiyin 2006). Harbin is a major city in northern China with a population of about 10 million people. Approximately 50 women attended the class (Ibid.).

The introduction of the Regulations on AIDS Prevention and Treatment in March 2006 and China's second Action Plan (2006–2010) for the Containment and Prevention of HIV/AIDS helped to legitimize Harbin City health officials' implementation of interventions focused on sex workers, as outlined in the 2004 Guidelines. The regulations and action plan provided targets for health authorities to meet (Guowuyuan 2006a, 2006c). Most notably, the action plan stipulated that interventions designed to promote condom use among key populations should reach 90 per cent of those populations by 2010, which is the compliance rate for a 100% CUP to be deemed effective by international standards (Guowuyuan 2006c; WHO/WPR 2004: 5). These targets compelled health officials to begin working with female sex workers to demonstrate their compliance with national policy goals.

In keeping with the 2004 Guidelines, Wen and his co-workers first surveyed all the entertainment and leisure venues that facilitated commercial sex in the Harbin City area, producing a map of venue locations (Li Xiujiang 2006; Zhongguo jibing yufang kongzhi zhongxin 2004: 10). Health workers visited these venues with police officers, entertainment and leisure venues being under the jurisdiction of policing authorities (Guowuyuan 2006b). However, sex workers and the managers of venues that provided sexual services were obviously reluctant to identify themselves in such circumstances. Health workers subsequently adopted various 'unprofessional' ploys to meet their priority population, including pretending to be potential clients and/or contacting sex workers through clients (Zhang Yue 2006). The 2016 Guidelines reiterate the usefulness of such tactics in terms of enabling health authorities to access sex workers (Zhongguo jibing yufang kongzhi zhongxin, xingbing aizibing yufang kongzhi zhongxin 2016b).

After establishing contact with sex workers and the operators of entertainment and leisure venues, health workers asked the owners or managers for their permission and cooperation in running training classes to distribute materials about AIDS and condom use to sex workers. In these classes, health workers explained the basic modes of HIV transmission and showed sex workers how condoms should be used. They also provided information about where to go for confidential testing and treatment and encouraged attendees to pass on the knowledge they had acquired, and relevant information, to their friends and co-workers (Mu and Xue 2006; 'Haerbin zhiyuanzhe huizhi anchang fenbutu fangfan aizibing' 2006; Zhang Yue 2006).

Media coverage of what were dubbed the 'working-girl training classes' generated immediate debate on the implications of such government-provided training on prostitution policy. The fact that staff from the Harbin CDC had been able to invite 50 female sex workers to attend a training class raised questions about the efficacy of local police efforts to crack down on prostitution (Li Xiujiang 2006: 40–2; Mu and Xue 2006). Health officials with the Harbin CDC had drawn a map of the various recreational enterprises in Harbin City that were known to facilitate commercial sexual services. Such maps were dubbed 'working-girl maps' (*xiaojie ditu*) by bloggers and other online commentators (netizens) (Mu and Xue 2006; 'Harbin zhiyuanzhe dui tongxinglian xuanchuan fang'ai huizhi anchang fenbutu' 2006). The ability of health officials to map such enterprises and contact sex workers suggested that previous police efforts to crack down on the sex industry in Harbin City had been half-hearted or ineffective.

Representatives from the Harbin police told a reporter with the *Harbin Daily* that the provision of sexual health trainings to sex workers by health experts did not alter the policing agenda of abolishing the sex industry. They noted that the provision of such training was an important goal and indicated that the police had no plans to stop such classes. However, police representatives stated that they were not convinced that providing public and publicized classes was the most appropriate response to working with a group of people engaged in illicit activities, as it compromised the goals of policing (Zhang Yue 2006). A reporter from the *Dongfang Jinbao* (*Orient Today*) in Henan Province agreed, stating that the police should obtain information about the women who attended such classes so that they could apprehend them in the future (Zhou Xiyin 2006).

Conversely, Zhang Guifeng (2006), a freelance writer, wrote an article supporting the decision of staff from the Harbin CDC to provide 'working-girl training classes' in the *Fazhi Ribao* (*Legal Daily*). As Zhang argued, the goal of protecting public health is a government priority. Policing concerns should give way to health concerns in instances where there is a clash between the health and policing sectors.

Wang Jian, secretary of the Party Committee of the Harbin CDC, similarly told journalists that the provision of sexual health trainings to sex workers by staff from the Harbin CDC was an appropriate action that accorded with government guidelines (Li Xiujiang 2006: 40–2). Staff from the Harbin CDC had run two similar classes earlier in 2006. Although the pilot classes were deemed to be successful, they had been run without publicity to avoid negative attention (Huang 2006; Zhang Yue 2006). As Wang noted, although the Regulations on AIDS Prevention and Treatment did not outline specific types of intervention, they suggested that behaviour change interventions designed to promote condom use among key populations was a public health priority (Mu and Xue 2006). Relevant government departments not only had a responsibility to undertake such actions according to law, but also would be penalized for their failure to do so (Guowuyuan 2006a: Article 55).

The approach adopted by staff from the Harbin CDC was supported in an editorial published on 1 December 2006 for World AIDS Day in the *Nanfang Ribao* (*Southern Daily*) ('Yi xin de linian kandai aizibing fangzhi gongzuo' 2006). The *Southern Daily* is a Guangzhou-based newspaper with more than 1.1 million readers and is ranked the fourth top newspaper in China ('2011nian shijie ribao faxingliang qian100ming paihangbang' 2011). The editorial, titled 'New Thinking on the Work of AIDS Prevention', described the Harbin training class as an unusual event, but also as a positive step forward in terms of public health education ('Yi xin de linian kandai aizibing fangzhi gongzuo' 2006: A02). The editor implied that in the past it would have been unimaginable for government authorities in China to invite sex workers to voluntarily attend a government-sponsored event. However, the editor concluded that efforts to bring the underground sex industry into the open for the purposes of sexual health education benefited the whole of society from the viewpoint of public health (Ibid.).

The editor further concluded that the Harbin CDC's approach was a realistic response to the existence of commercial sex. As the editor explained, the continued existence of prostitution, despite police-led campaigns against it, indicated that commercial sex could not be eradicated from present-day China because of the country's as yet still inadequate level of socio-economic development (Ibid.). The timing of this editorial and its publication in a major national newspaper ensured positive national publicity for the provision of health-related training classes for sex workers.

Despite legal and media support, the stigma associated with sex work in China presented (and still presents) challenges for health officials who are tasked with implementing behaviour change programs based on the promotion of condom use. Female sex workers are stigmatized by negative social attitudes towards the sex industry (Choi and Holroyd 2007: 497). These attitudes are internalized by many sex workers who often defend their choices in terms of earning a livelihood, but nevertheless view themselves as engaging in work that is neither normal nor decent (Yu Jianhua 2009). Studies of female sex workers in China show that the majority do not tell their family and friends about their involvement in prostitution, and experience violence from clients and especially from stable partners (Hong *et al.* 2014: 1; Hu Xiaoyun *et al.* 2011: 44–5; Zhang, C. *et al.* 2013). Police campaigns against the sex industry augment this stigma and simultaneously make it difficult for health officials to work with sex workers who fear that public visibility will result in police apprehension (WHO/WPR and CDC 2004).

Health officials have used various tactics to overcome or reduce the reluctance of sex workers to participate in AIDS education activities. In Guangzhou, media publicity centred on the story of Ms Xu Huifang, a health official from the Guangzhou CDC, who treated a female sex worker to a meal on several occasions with the aim of building a rapport between them ('Guangzhou fang'ai renyuan jiaban piaoke jiao maiyinnü yong anquantao' 2006). Xu persuaded the woman to become a peer educator and to help health officials run AIDS prevention programs for sex workers. Other reports suggest that health workers bought gifts for sex workers and played mah-jong with them in an effort to establish trust and rapport (Meng 2013: 145).

Another strategy used by health officials in Guangzhou involved empowering sex workers as peer educators in theory by encouraging them to swear a pledge based on the 'no condom, no sex' principle of the 100% CUP (Xie

Qishan 2008: A4). Following a training class for sex workers on the utility of condom use in preventing the sexual transmission of HIV, the participating sex workers and managers of entertainment and leisure venues read aloud a public pledge written by Wan Shaoping, a medical doctor from the Sichuan Dermatology and Venereology Prevention Institute. That pledge, which took place in an entertainment venue in Huadu District, Guangzhou City, on 30 November 2008, reads as follows.

> A person's primary fortune in life is good health and good health is a precondition of happiness. We pledge to resolutely use condoms [in all commercial sexual encounters] from this day forth to ensure our personal health and happiness and that of others. (*Jiankang shi ren de diyi caifu, jiankang shi xingfu de genben baozheng, weile ziji de jiankang he xingfu, ye weile taren de jiankang he xingfu, cong jintian kaishi, women yiding yao yong anquantao, meici dou yong, jianjue shiyong!*)
>
> (Xie Qishan 2008: A4)

As with the 'working-girl training class' in Harbin, the Guangzhou pledge attracted media attention. Some netizens expressed outrage that such an event could take place. A commentary posted on Tianshannet.com.cn stated that the event contravened social norms because the women involved had admitted in public that they were sex workers – that is, participants in a 'shameful' and illicit activity (Wu Fengying 2008: A04). Others suggested that the pledge compromised the goals of policing and exposed the ineffectiveness of police efforts to crack down on the sex industry (Ibid.).

Supportive comments turned on the priority of HIV prevention. Liang Jianfang (2008) wrote in the *China Youth Daily* that the media should avoid publicizing and sensationalizing topics such as the provision of sexual health trainings to sex workers because negative publicity might hinder the goals of the 100% CUP. Mao Jianguo (2008), a blogger on the China Radio International website, said that protecting public health meant bringing the sex industry into the open, and treating it as a specific profession with professional requirements that could be managed in the same way as any other industry.

Thus, the expansion of China's 100% CUP, and associated media publicity and public awareness of its objectives, have become centred on the responsibility of health officials to undertake behaviour change programs to promote public health. In doing so, the expansion of the 100% CUP has encouraged broader discussion of sex workers' rights.

Policing versus health concerns – advocacy for the legalization of sex work

In January 2006, Zhou Ruijin (2006a), a retired senior government official and member of the Chinese Communist Party, published an article on Eastday.com, a commercial website affiliated with the Shanghai municipal government, called

'Delegates at the National People's Congress and Chinese People's Political Consultative Congress Might as Well Discuss the Underground Sex Industry' (*lianghui daibiao bufang yiyi dixia xingchanye*). The National People's Congress (NPC) is the PRC's legislature. The Chinese People's Political Consultative Conference (CPPCC) acts in theory as the 'watchdog' of the country's governance by advising the NPC on central and local government policy. Zhou's article, which was republished in a local Shanghai magazine, was controversial given his high-level Party connections and media position as a former editor for the PRC's premier state-run newspaper, the *People's Daily* (Zhou Ruijin 2006b).

Zhou Ruijin (2006a, 2006b) is the first senior Communist Party member to state in public that the sex industry in China should be *regulated* by government in the interest of public health. He noted that the country's rapidly rising rates of STI and HIV were associated with the booming sex industry, and hence commercial sex should be a focus of government management rather than policing. He deflected standard objections to the existence of prostitution in China by arguing that commercial sex is not a product of a distinct economic system, that is, capitalism or socialism. Zhou Ruijin apparently had proposed regulating the sex industry at a 1996 meeting sponsored by the Central Committee of the Publicity and Information Office of the CCP (formerly the Propaganda Department), but his suggestion would have been a matter of internal rather than public discussion at that time (Zhou Jigang 2006).

In March 2006, Chi Susheng, a lawyer from Heilongjiang Province, presented a motion to the NPC 'On Legalizing Sex Workers as Soon as Possible' (*guanyu jinzao chutai dui xingcongyezhe xingwei guifan lifa*) (Li Yunhong 2006). Chi recommended repealing Article 358 of the Criminal Law of the PRC (1997), which prohibits the third-party organization of prostitution, and amending Article 359, which prohibits the act of introducing others into prostitution, to only include acts relating to forced prostitution. She further recommended expanding Article 360, which penalizes anyone who facilitates or participates in commercial sex in the full knowledge that one or more of the participants has a serious STI. Specifically, Chi proposed the licensing of sex establishments with a system of certified health checks for sex workers, and the corollary penalizing of 'unlicensed' venues and workers (Li Yunhong 2006). Sex workers in international settings typically reject this style of legalization for subjecting sex workers to intrusive government surveillance (Jeffreys 2004: 83–91; Kilvington, Day and Ward 2001: 85–6).

Chi reportedly composed the motion after handling a case relating to the sex industry and the premeditated spread of HIV, which also heightened her awareness of violence against sex workers (Li Yunhong 2006: 7–8). In 2000, a young man living with HIV telephoned Chi to confess that he had engaged in unprotected sex with nearly 100 sex workers as an act of revenge because he believed that he had contracted HIV from a sex worker. Chi concluded that bans on the sex industry hindered the task of AIDS prevention and made sex workers vulnerable to violence, including assault, robbery, rape and murder (see also Boittin 2013: 256–7; Jeffreys 2009).

Chi's motion obtained the support of the more than 30 delegates that is required for a motion to be considered for discussion, but it was vetoed on technical grounds. Chi had drafted the motion herself, it contained too many suggestions and the deadline for framing motions for the NPC had already expired (Li Yunhong 2006: 9; Zhou and Xiong 2006). In interviews with journalists, Chi claimed that her motion had been vetoed by senior leaders because of its controversial content (Yang Zhongxu 2008). This resulted in some netizens praising her perceived courage and others ridiculing her for presenting a motion that was neither legally feasible nor morally acceptable in China. However, Chi's motion was the first attempt to raise the issue of legalizing the sex industry within the political space of the NPC.

Apart from Zhou Ruijin's and Chi Susheng's different appeals to legalize the sex industry, some China-based NGOs have used the expansion of the 100% CUP to criticize the PRC prostitution controls and appeal for sex workers' rights. In 2009, the Beijing Aizhixing Institute for Health Education compiled a Report on the Health, Legality and Human Rights of the Sex Industry and Sex Workers in China (*Zhongguo xinggongzuo yu xinggongzuozhe jiankang falü renquan baogao*). The report examined several cases of human rights abuses arising from the policing of prostitution, such as police officers depriving sex workers of the right to health by using possession of condoms as evidence of engagement in commercial sex (Beijing aizhixing jiankang jiaoyu yanjiusuo 2009: 7). The report criticized such actions for undermining the goals of the 100% CUP and violating the rights of sex workers to health (Ibid.: 8; see also Boittin 2013: 257–8; Human Rights Watch 2013).

In July 2010, Ye Haiyan, a sex blogger, sex worker and women's rights activist, held China's first street protest in support of sex workers. Ye (2010) and a small group of people walked down a busy shopping street in Wuhan City carrying red umbrellas, an international symbol of sex workers' solidarity, and held up banners calling for the legalization of sex work (*xinggongzuo hefahua*). Ye posted details and pictures of this event on her blog. The photographs indicate that only a small number of people were involved in the protest and it did not attract the attention of passers-by. However, it did attract international media coverage.

In an interview with a foreign correspondent, Ye said that the protest aimed to raise public awareness of the harm to sex workers' health caused by police crackdowns on the sex industry (Branigan 2010: 15). Ye condemned such crackdowns for putting women at risk of contracting an STI, including HIV, through fear of carrying condoms in case police authorities used possession as evidence of engagement in prostitution. Ye concluded that sex work should be legalized in China to protect the rights of sex workers to health (Ibid.; on Ye Haiyan, see Benney 2012).

Ye further stated that the protest was prompted by media coverage of women being publicly humiliated following a police crackdown on the sex industry in Dongguan City in mid-July. Related media coverage showed images of police officers leading suspected male and female offenders barefoot down a street, with leash-like restraining ropes tied around their wrists and waists (Tan Zhihong 2010; Xie and Wei 2010: A14). The images were hotly debated on the Internet as a perceived deliberate and barbaric act of public shaming. Police authorities responded that the suspects had been taken back to the 'scene of the crime' for the collection of evidence as required by law to prosecute a case. The photographs in question were a part of those procedures and had been published without permission. In other words, the images demonstrated lack of professionalism and low technology (no handcuffs and no cars). However, in response to public outrage, the Ministry of

Public Security issued a circular in late July instructing police officers to adopt professional codes of conduct when investigating prostitution-related offences, and to respect the rights of suspected offenders to dignity and reputation by not parading them in public, in particular (Gonganbu 2010; Li Hongxun 2010: A07).

In the wake of the Dongguan scandal, Liu Shaowu, Director of the Security Administration Department of the Ministry of Public Security, proposed that police officers demonstrate respect for female sex workers by changing the official terminology of *maiyinnü* (a woman who sells sex/licentiousness) to *shizunü* (a woman who has taken a wrong step in life) (Chen Ningyi 2010; Zhou Bin 2010). Liu's comments followed the release of a document titled Notice on Strengthening the Work of Educating and Rescuing Female Sex Sellers When Conducting Campaigns to Suppress Prostitution and Other Illicit and Criminal Activities (*Guanyu zai chajin maiyinpiaochang deng weifa fanzui huodong zhong jiaqiang dui maiyinnü jiaoyu wanjiu gongzuo de tongzhi*) (Zhou Bin 2010: 1). Although the document demonstrates ongoing commitment to banning the sex industry understood in negative terms, it states that women apprehended by police as suspected prostitution offenders should be treated respectfully and not humiliated in any way.

As the preceding discussion suggests, the expansion of AIDS prevention programs focused on sex workers is not the only factor contributing to a broadening of public debate on China's prostitution controls. The prevalence of commercial sexual services, despite the implementation of police-led campaigns against the sex industry, has raised questions about the merit and practicality of such controls. Abuses associated with police crackdowns have also prompted discussion of alternative modes of governing the sex industry (Jeffreys 2012b; Meng 2013).

But the public actions of people like Zhou Ruijin, Chi Susheng, Ye Haiyan, and members of the Beijing Aizhixing Institute for Health Education, have been encouraged by the implementation of AIDS prevention programs focused on sex workers. The expansion of China's 100% CUP and associated publicity has helped to open up debate in the print media, in academic circles, on the Internet and on the streets, about the most appropriate government response to commercial sex, albeit within the constrained space permitted by government censorship and associated self-censorship. Chinese law now supports the promotion of condom use among key populations as a means to prevent the sexual transmission of HIV, with police officers being told to uphold the law by refraining from using condoms as evidence of engagement in commercial sex ('Condoms no longer evidence of prostitution in China' 2007; Guowuyuan 2006c: Article 28; Wang Sihai 2008: 2). Irrespective of ongoing tensions between the policy goals of health and policing authorities, the normalization of sexual health interventions for key populations has opened up the space for a diverse array of individuals and organizations to talk about sex work and different approaches to the governance of the sex industry.

Concluding remarks

From the viewpoint of public health, the roll-out of a 100% CUP in China has been a success story in terms of increasing public awareness of HIV transmission, and slowing the spread of HIV and AIDS. The reported number of people living with HIV and AIDS in the PRC was approximately 554,000 in 2015 and 654,000 in 2016 ('654,000 living with HIV/AIDS in China' 2016; NCAIDS, NCSTD, China CDC 2015: 749). China also has a national HIV prevalence of less than 0.4 per cent, which is low compared to other developing countries, and especially given its massive population. In light of this, suggestions in the late 1990s and early 2000s that up to 15 million Chinese people would be infected with HIV by 2010 have proven to be exaggerated (The UN Theme Group on HIV/AIDS in China 2002; Weishengbu *et al.* 1998).

The national HIV prevalence among female sex workers has also remained at a relatively low level – 0.2 per cent in 2015 (UNAIDS 2016a). Data from the HIV sentinel surveillance system indicates that 94 per cent of female sex workers reporting the use of condoms with their most recent client, which exceeds the WHO's compliance target of 90 per cent (Ibid.). Health authorities claimed to have reached more than 84 per cent of female sex workers by 2015, and the 2016 Guidelines for AIDS Prevention Interventions Among Groups at High-risk Through Heterosexual Sexual Transmission advocate the continued implementation and expansion of health interventions focused on sex workers (NCAIDS, NCSTD, China CDC 2015: 749; Zhongguo jibing yufang kongzhi zhongxin, xingbing aizibing yufang kongzhi zhongxin 2016b).

Yet realizing the virtual elimination of HIV transmission through commercial sex presents evident challenges, many of which are related to the different priorities of health and policing authorities. China's two action plans for the containment and prevention of HIV and AIDS between 2006 and 2015 directed local governments to provide AIDS-related health interventions focused on sex workers (Guowuyuan 2006c; Guowuyuan bangongting 2012). But both plans also referred to police crackdowns on the sex industry as an important part of the nation's AIDS response. China's action plan for the containment and prevention of HIV and AIDS for 2016–2020 likewise states that cracking down on the sex industry is an important component of the country's AIDS response (Guowuyuan bangongting 2017).

Some studies conclude that police-led crackdowns on the sex industry heighten the vulnerability of sex workers to HIV infection in numerous ways (Boittin 2013; Meng 2013). Many sex workers do not access government-affiliated health clinics for fear that diagnosis of an STI will bring their identity and activities to the attention of authorities, including police (Jeffreys and Huang 2009: 161; Pan Jingbin *et al.* 2010: 310; Yu 2013: 359). Police crackdowns on the sex industry exacerbate the distrust felt by sex workers towards government authorities through abusive policing practices and the use of condoms as circumstantial evidence of engagement in prostitution (Boittin 2013: 259; Human Rights Watch 2013: 29; Meng 2013: 137–54). In the words of one sex worker: the 'law says it is not a problem [to carry condoms], but the police act differently' (Boittin 2013: 258). Police crackdowns also complicate health officials' access to sex workers by encouraging high levels of sex worker mobility, and the rapid turnover of small businesses, to avoid apprehension. In addition, media publicity of policing successes reinforces the social and legal marginalization of sex workers, even as it occasionally opens the space for criticisms of policing practices and associated representations (Jeffreys 2012b).

Other studies suggest that local-level relationships between police, business operators and sex workers may facilitate site-based interventions by allowing the cultivation of relatively stable relationships between health workers and operators of entertainment and leisure venues. Specifically, local police often adopt an approach based on 'non-involvement' towards health interventions – they neither interfere nor assist (Zhao Jun 2007: 343). They regularly visit entertainment and leisure venues to apprise managers and employees of business licensing and other relevant legislation, and they frequently turn a blind eye towards the existence of indirect sex establishments, either for payoffs or to maintain local economies and relationships. Interviews with women who work in such venues suggest that they are unlikely to be apprehended during the course of police crackdowns on the sex industry, because they are warned about imminent raids by venue owners and managers (Hong *et al.* 2014: 1435; Liu, M. 2011: 130–1). Venue managers are also cited as a critical link for accessing sex workers in the 2016 Guidelines (Zhongguo jibing yufang kongzhi zhongxin, xingbing aizibing yufang kongzhi zhongxin 2016b; see also Hong *et al.* 2014: 1437; Meng 2013: 144). In practice, the tacit accommodation of health interventions by local police embedded in local communities may blunt the impact of police crackdowns, which in any case are of a sporadic nature, targeted towards specific districts and generally prosecuted by officers from outside the districts in question.

Yet other studies indicate that health interventions focused on sex workers in entertainment and leisure venues are marred by low levels of professionalism. Interventions are frequently conducted in an arbitrary and coercive manner (Human Rights Watch 2013: 39–43). One CDC employee who monitors testing programs nationwide has stated that health intervention teams arrive at venues having already obtained the support of venue owners or managers who will have instructed a set number of women to attend (Boittin 2013: 260). Apart from providing AIDS education and promoting condom use, health workers will draw blood for STI and HIV testing, or send the women to a facility for testing, with the notion of consent being redundant because the women are not in a position to refuse, and may not even be informed that they are being tested for HIV (Boittin 2013: 260; Human Rights Watch 2013: 39–43).

The 2016 Guidelines reveal a different set of professional shortcomings: health interventions are often based on 'hasty' mapping procedures and chiefly focus on 'high-grade' venues with cooperative managers, and hence estimates of the HIV prevalence among certain communities of sex workers may be inaccurate (Zhongguo jibing yufang kongzhi zhongxin, xingbing aizibing yufang kongzhi zhongxin 2016b). Interventions conducted up to 2015 mainly focused on women who negotiated commercial sex through 'high- and medium-grade' nightclubs, hotels, karaoke-dance halls, and beauty and massage centres, rather than in 'low-grade' sites such as small hair and foot massage salons, hostels, cheap rental accommodations, construction sites and street-side locations. Yet the prevalence of HIV among women who work from high-grade venues is around 0.1 per cent, and such women generally insist on consistent condom use, whereas the HIV prevalence is more than 0.4 per cent among women who work from low-grade sites and they are associated with significantly lower rates of condom use. Hence, statistics regarding the overall HIV prevalence among sex workers may be misleading because interventions to date have overlooked a large population of sex workers. The 2016 Guidelines further note that commercial sex is now increasingly negotiated through social networking sites, which requires the extension of health interventions not only to more physical sites, but also to virtual meeting places (Ibid.).

The 2016 Guidelines conclude that the CDC cannot eliminate HIV transmission through commercial sex without the help of social organizations, but bans on the sex industry have ensured that such NGOs are limited in number (Ibid.; see also Kaufman 2012: 231; Li and Kuo *et al.* 2010: II69; Rou *et al.* 2010: II44). Social organizations are described as performing an indispensable role by helping intervention teams to gain access to different groups of sex workers and to overcome sex worker distrust of government officials. Interviews with sex workers indicate that they experience outreach from health officials as 'scary' and/or 'embarrassing' (Boittin 2013: 259; Hong *et al.* 2014: 1436; Human Rights Watch 2013: 43–5). Interviews with health officials similarly indicate that they found that sex workers were afraid of them (Meng 2013: 144). The 2016 Guidelines note that, although information about commercial sex in low-grade sites is obtained from men presenting at STI clinics, access to women who sell sexual services on the streets or in low-grade venues is complicated by their fear of police apprehension (Zhongguo jibing yufang kongzhi zhongxin, xingbing aizibing yufang kongzhi zhongxin 2016b).

To overcome these problems, the CDC is hiring and training members of social organizations as outreach staff and also hiring and training sex workers to work as peer educators in health interventions (Ibid.). Interventions in high-grade venues turn on the provision of information about HIV prevention, testing and treatment, either through lectures or the simple distribution of printed and audio-visual materials, and small supplies of free condoms. Interventions in low-grade venues require a more 'hands-on' approach and the extension of behavioural surveillance surveys to different communities of sex workers.

Interventions focused on low-grade sites involve gaining access to and interviewing members of covert populations for information about their age, place of birth, educational background, sexual partners and number and types of clients, history of STI, knowledge of AIDS, condom use patterns and work-related mobility. Questions on work-related mobility ask respondents whether they have moved to the investigating area to avoid police crackdowns, to find more clients or as a result of an introduction from another sex worker (*jiemei*), or for family or other reasons. Interventions in low-grade sites also involve community-based education on condom use, free condom distribution, and the promotion of rapid HIV testing and immediate take up of treatment when required.

The 2016 Guidelines have the potential to transform the governance of commercial sex in China by co-opting sex workers directly into government-led health interventions. However, this approach is counterbalanced by a recommendation that grassroots government structures – street offices and residents' committees – should be involved in the identification of low-grade sites where commercial sex is occurring, and the implementation of health interventions. In this way, health interventions become community-level affairs that remain intimately linked to local Party and governance structures.

At the same time, the focus on commercial sex in low-grade venues as a vector of disease may encourage the ongoing distancing of AIDS as a problem that affects 'other' people (Micollier 2012: 116). In the mid-2000s, the Ministry of Health of the PRC (2005) issued a document to guide health interventions among those people classified by the WHO as members of key populations. The document, titled Guidelines for Interventions Among Those at High-Risk (Trial) (*gaoweixingwei ganyu gongzuo zhidao fang'an* (*shixing*)), described female sex workers as the most at risk population in terms of contracting and transmitting HIV. It also described male rural-to-urban migrant labourers, allegedly the main clients of China's sex workers, as at high risk, but placed them at a lower level on the 'at-risk' hierarchy than women who sell sex (Ibid.). The 2016 Guidelines similarly focus on female sex workers and especially those who provide sexual services to migrant and other blue-collar workers (Zhongguo jibing yufang kongzhi zhongxin, xingbing aizibing yufang kongzhi zhongxin 2016b).

The primary emphasis on women who sell sex rather than on the men who demand their services is in part a consequence of the need to make health interventions practical or operable. As in other parts of the world, China's health authorities have found it easier to direct their attention and resources towards people who provide sexual services in a relatively regular fashion via site-based locations, rather than on the comparatively more transient population of male clients who are generally unwilling to admit that they pay for sex in the first place. But the result is that AIDS is presented as a disease that is associated with an 'underclass' of poor, young women who sell sexual services to men from low income groups. This remains the case even though sex workers constitute a diverse group of women, as demonstrated by the 2016 Guidelines' reference to high- and low-grade sites for commercial sex. Moreover, numerous studies show that married men with professional employment and money (entrepreneurs, managers and government officials) are routine patrons of venues that facilitate commercial sex (Chen *et al.* 2008: 14; Pan Suiming 2002: 19; Uretsky 2008: 801–14, 2016: 3–4; Zheng 2009a).

The next two chapters look at the two populations of men who are considered as key to China's AIDS response – men who have sex with men and male rural-to-urban migrant labourers.

6 Men who have sex with men

This chapter examines changing discourses on homosexuality and the emergence of men who have sex with men as a key focus of AIDS prevention programs in the People's Republic of China. In late 2011, a Chinese netizen posted an image online of a poster-style public service advertisement promoting safer homosexual sex, adding that s/he was surprised to have seen the poster on a community noticeboard in Beijing (Xu 2011: 20). Such notice-boards can be found in most urban residential compounds and are used to display government and local community information. The poster contained a close-up head-to-shoulder shot of two young and shirtless Chinese men, each playfully holding out a packaged condom to the other (see Figure 6.1). The poster poses two questions, both reading '*dai le ma?*', using the Chinese homonyms of *'dai'* (literally, 'to bring' and 'to wear') to ask: 'did you bring a condom' and 'are you wearing a condom?'

The netizen expressed surprise to see a PSA promoting safer homosexual sex, stating: 'I never thought government offices would print such posters, as homosexuality seems taboo in China' (Xu 2011: 20). S/he thought it was 'good' to see HIV prevention messages for homosexual men, but wondered how 'elderly' people would react. In other words, the netizen implied that some local residents might find the subject matter distasteful and was surprised that government authorities had taken the bold initiative of making safer-sex messages for homosexual men publicly available. The subsequent reporting of the posting in print media underscores its topical nature (Wei Mingyan 2011: A12; Xu 2011: 20).

As this example demonstrates, men who have sex with men have become a focus of public health campaigns designed to prevent the sexual transmission of HIV in China. The available literature mostly refers to this population in the abbreviated form of 'MSM' (Chen *et al.* 2012; Fan 2014; Huang *et al.* 2012; UNAIDS 2009a; Xiong *et al.* 2010). However, recent terminology guidelines issued by UNAIDS (2015c: 33) recommend abandoning this abbreviation because it is dehumanizing.

Globally, men who have sex with men are identified as the population most at risk of contracting and transmitting HIV, 'particularly in countries with concentrated epidemics' (McDaid and Hart 2010: 311). In 2010, 63 per cent of all new infection cases in the USA were related to sexual transmission among men ('HIV in the United States' 2015). Studies suggest that some men engage in unprotected anal sex with other men, even though they are aware of HIV prevention messages,

DOI: 10.4324/9781315175546-6

because they view condoms as unerotic and unreliable (Joint United Nations Programme on HIV/AIDS and World Health Organization 2009; Peterson and DiClemente 2000: 204). Sexual risk management approaches such as 'serosorting' and 'strategic positioning' are reportedly increasing, even though their efficacy in terms of preventing the sexual transmission of HIV remains unclear (McDaid and Hart 2010: 311). 'Serosorting' is when a person chooses 'a sexual partner known to be of the same HIV serostatus, often to engage in unprotected sex, in order to

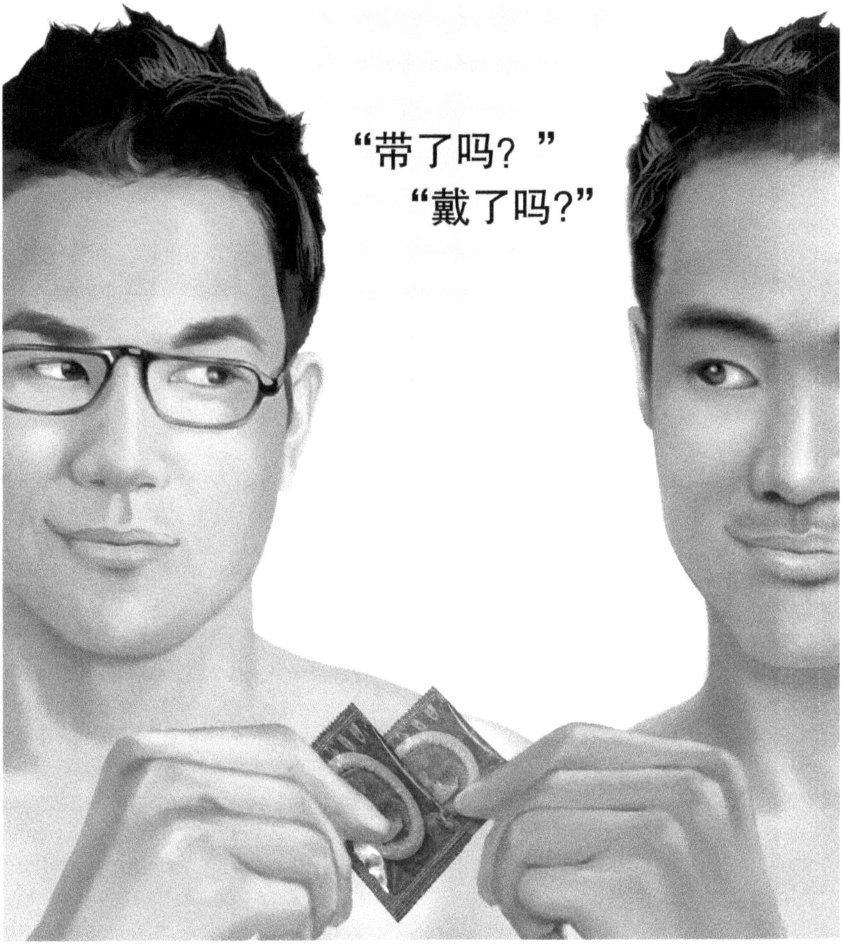

Figure 6.1 'Did you bring a condom?' 'Are you wearing a condom?'.

Source: National Center for AIDS/STD Control and Prevention, China CDC (2010) 'Xing'ai zhongxin guanyu yinfa "nannanxingxingweirenqun aizibing xingbing fangzhi xuanchuan cailiao" de han' [NCAIDS: on the issuing of AIDS prevention promotional materials for men who have sex with men], 21 December. Online. Available: http://ncaids.chinacdc.cn/fzdt/zxdt/201012/t20101221_1519120.htm (accessed 23 January 2017); reproduced with permission.

reduce the risk of acquiring or transmitting HIV' ('Serosorting and strategic positioning' n.d.). 'Strategic positioning' refers to the practice whereby a person living with HIV chooses to take the receptive position during unprotected anal sex with a partner believed to be HIV-negative, based on the assumption that it less likely for HIV to be transmitted from a receptive partner.

In China, men who have sex with men have been recently identified as both a key population and as the population most at risk of contracting and transmitting HIV. In 2002, they accounted for only 0.2 per cent of all new HIV infection cases recorded in the PRC (approximately 57 people). That figure rose to over 7 per cent in 2005 (approximately 5,110 people), peaked at 32 per cent in 2009 (approximately 15,600 people), and reached nearly 27 per cent in 2015 (approximately 3,200 people) (Guo, Li and Stanton 2011: 521; Ministry of Health, People's Republic of China, Joint United Nations Programme on HIV/AIDS and World Health Organization 2012; NCAIDS, NCSTD, China CDC 2015: 749). The documented HIV prevalence among men who have sex with men was 8 per cent at the start of 2015, which is considerably higher than the HIV prevalence among other key populations: 6 per cent among injecting drug users and 0.2 per cent among female sex workers (National Health and Family Planning Commission of the People's Republic of China 2015: 6, 13). Hence the PRC's action plan for the containment and prevention of HIV and AIDS for 2016–2020 recommends focusing on men who have sex with men, especially given the recent proliferation of gay dating applications on social media (Guowuyuan bangongting 2017).

The dramatic rise in HIV prevalence among Chinese men who have sex with men is a reflection, in part, of the expansion of sentinel surveillance, behaviour interventions and diagnostic testing. In 2002, there was only one HIV sentinel surveillance site that focused on such men (Chow *et al.* 2014: 4). That figure rose to 17 sites in 2009. By 2011, there were 108 sites across all of mainland China's administrative divisions, with the exception of the Tibet Autonomous Region (Ibid.; see also Wen *et al.* 2012: 79).

PRC health authorities began issuing guidelines and implementation plans for conducting AIDS prevention programs focused on men who have sex with men in the late 2000s. The Chinese Center for Disease Control and Prevention (CDC) and the National Center for AIDS/STD Control and Prevention (NCAIDS) issued the Guidelines for Interventions Into AIDS-Related High-Risk Behaviours Among Men Who Have Sex With Men in late 2007 (*Nannanxingxingweirenqun aizibing gaoweixingwei ganyu gongzuo zhinan*), whereas guidelines for interventions focused on female sex workers were issued in mid-2004 (Zhongguo jibing yufang kongzhi zhongxin 2004; Zhongguo jibing yufang kongzhi zhongxin, xingbing aizibing yufang kongzhi zhongxin 2007). In March 2008, the Ministry of Health released a document titled AIDS Prevention Pilot Program for Men Who Have Sex With Men (*Nannanxingxingwei aizibing fangzhi shidian gongzuo fang'an*) (Weishengbu 2008). It indicated that health authorities intended to conduct pilot projects in 61 cities across the country between 2008 and early 2009, based on the promotion of safer sex through condom use, and developing HIV testing, AIDS diagnosis and medical care facilities (Weishengbu 2008). UNAIDS (2009a) described this project, which included plans for 21,000 men to be HIV tested in order to establish a clearer statistical baseline for infection rates, as 'the first of its kind in Asia' and 'the largest such study undertaken anywhere in the world'. Demonstrating the ongoing nature of such interventions, in 2016, the CDC and NCAIDS issued the Guidelines for Interventions to Prevent AIDS Among Men Who Have Sex With Men (*Nannanxingxingwei renqun yufang aizibing ganyu gongzuo zhinan*) (hereinafter the 2016 Guidelines) (Zhongguo jibing yufang kongzhi zhongxin, xingbing aizibing yufang kongzhi zhongxin 2016a).

The chapter first provides a short history of homosexuality in the PRC, in order to explain why men who have sex with men are a recent focus of public health interventions. It examines shifts in PRC discourses on homosexuality, from a subject that was virtually absent from Mao-era discussions, to a practice that was subsequently categorized as a form of mental disorder, and to more recent discussions of homosexuality in terms of public health concerns and sexual identity and personhood. It then outlines the emerging roles played by health authorities and non-governmental organizations/social organizations in providing AIDS prevention programs for men who have sex with men.[1]

Finally, the chapter examines the changing nature of media discussions of homosexuality in the context of AIDS prevention and developing struggles for equal rights. In doing so, we show how the act of classifying and administering human kinds as MSM has had a 'looping or feedback effect' (Hacking 2002: 99). People who have been classified as MSM, and people claiming to speak on their behalf, are contesting the construction of men who have sex with men as vectors of disease, and demanding anti-discrimination measures.

The emergence of homosexuality in the PRC

Being openly 'gay' and living a gay lifestyle is a recent and minority phenomenon in mainland China; although there are no laws banning consensual homosexual sex, there are no protective laws relating to sexual orientation, and there are limited spaces for homosexual organization and representation. Beijing and Shanghai have gay bars and a gay scene, and gay pride events have been held every year since 2009 in Shanghai, typically in the form of art exhibitions and film screenings rather than a street march (Bao 2012; weblink http://www.shpride.com/?lang=en). Gay websites and queer-themed information and films with translocal and transcultural dimensions are also increasing in number (Jeffreys and Yu 2015: 81–9). But data from the PRC's 2010 Census indicates that less than 2 per cent of women and men aged 40 years and over had never married, which suggests many gays remain 'closeted' (Ibid.: 15). Homosexuality also features in the mainstream media chiefly in connection with AIDS.

In *Tongzhi: Politics of Same-Sex Eroticism in Chinese Societies*, Wah-Shan Chou (2000: 27) argues that, strictly speaking, there were no 'homosexuals', 'bisexuals' or even 'heterosexuals' in China until the late nineteenth or even early twentieth century. The classification of people as homosexual is also a relatively recent phenomenon in Western societies (Greenberg 1988). While certain sectors of both populations obviously engaged in same-sex sexual practices historically, Chou's point is that traditional Chinese society was not divided according to a homo-hetero binary, and same-sex eroticism was not associated with a particular form of personality or identity. Instead, it was organized around class hierarchies and different levels of responsibilities to family and kinship networks. This meant that same-sex eroticism among men was tolerated to the extent that it did not interfere with the obligation to marry and have children in order to continue the male family line.

After the founding of the PRC in 1949, homosexuality became an 'invisible' sexual practice flowing from the reorganization of social space to meet the needs of centralized economic planning, and the early regime's promotion of free choice, monogamous heterosexual marriage. Nationalization of industry and curtailment of the monetary economy meant that the Party-state provided citizen-workers with employment, housing and the necessities of everyday life, which had the corollary effect of restricting the space for same-sex behaviours by limiting the kinds of venues in which individuals could engage in anonymous or private behaviours (Jeffreys 2012b: 3). The promotion of free choice, monogamous marriage aimed to improve the position of Chinese women by letting them choose their own spouses, and stopping traditional practices such as mercenary marriages and concubinage. However, as Harriet Evans (1995: 370) explains, the promotion of free choice, heterosexual marriage also ensured that representations of homosexuality in terms of sexual identity 'were all but totally absent' from the 1950s discourse on human sexuality and sexual practices. Until the mid-1990s, the few Chinese references that acknowledged the existence of homosexuality in the Mao era (1949–1976) were largely retrospective and condemned homosexuality as a physical and psychological perversion (*biantai*), and even as a crime, based on legal views that were accepted in the 1980s (Ibid.).

Although there are no specific laws prohibiting consensual adult homosexuality in the PRC, constraints were placed on the activities of male homosexuals throughout the Maoist and early post-1978 reform period (Li 2006: 82). A 1956 ruling by the Supreme Court indicated that sodomy (*jijianzui*) was a crime when it related to non-consensual and violent homosexual acts, and sex with minors (Ibid.: 83). Another ruling in 1957 suggested that homosexual acts between consenting adults were not criminal because there were no laws against such behaviours (Chow *et al.* 2014: 4). However, the emphasis on monogamous marriage and reproduction meant that homosexuality was viewed as an aberrant form of behaviour. Local cadres often handled cases of homosexuality, brought to their attention through complaints by other people, in a moralistic and arbitrary manner, resulting in some homosexuals being detained for committing 'political errors' (Li 2006: 83).

By the 1980s, the importation of aspects of Western medical science into the PRC meant that homosexuality came to be defined in terms of sexual dysfunction and mental disorder. Homosexuality was defined as a psychosexual disorder in a 1981 text published by the Chinese Society of Psychiatry, which was used as a clinical guide for diagnosing mental disorders (Yang Desen 1989: 10–12). That text was retrospectively titled the first Chinese Classification of Mental Disorders (CCMD-1) in 1989, when it was replaced by the official 'second' Chinese Classification of Mental Disorders (CCMD-2 1989) (Jia Yicheng 1995). The description of homosexuality in terms of mental disorder was not removed from the Chinese Classification of Mental Disorders until it was revised again in 2001 (CCMD-3) (Chinese Society of Psychiatry 2001; Zhu Yu 2001: 5). It is worth noting that the World Health Organization (1992) only removed homosexuality from its classification of mental and behaviour disorders at the Forty-Third World Health Assembly in May 1990, with a new International Classification of Diseases coming into effect in member states in 1994. Hence, the PRC's scientific redefinition of homosexuality flowed from the eventual adoption of international standards.

Academic and media discussions of homosexuality in the early reform period expanded on negative clinical constructions of homosexuality by describing same-sex eroticism as a 'foreign import'. In the late 1980s, He Zhaoxiong (1989) from the Guangxi Social Science Academy published an article in a magazine called *Daode yu Wenming* (*Morality and Civilization*) titled 'The Unacceptable Aspects of Homosexuality in China'. He described homosexuality as an 'unhealthy' (*bu jiankang*) product of the introduction of 'Western modes of thinking' (*xifang sichao*). Medical doctors such as Wu Jieping (1987), who was renowned for treating Premier Zhou Enlai, also publicly reinforced anti-homosexuality attitudes. Although Wu advocated for sex education in schools, that education was meant to teach Chinese youth 'correct' sexual behaviours to aid the building of socialist spiritual civilization and combat the invasion of 'decadent bourgeois ideology'. Homosexuality was included in the latter category by default, with Wu Jieping describing homosexuality as an abnormal but preventable behaviour in an interview with China Central Television Station (CCTV) in November 2003 ('Zhongyangdianshitai dajia lanmu' 2005).

However, some psychologists attempted to reframe homosexuality as an issue relating to stigmatization. In the early 1990s, Lu Longguang and his colleagues reviewed 1,000 clinical cases of male homosexuality collected at the Nanjing Institute of Neurology and Psychiatry between 1981 and 1991 (Lu *et al.* 1992). They concluded that social pressure had forced these men to seek medical advice because the majority displayed no abnormal psychology. In the late 1990s, Wang Naixin (1998) published an article in *Jingshen Weisheng Tongxun* (Communication in Mental Health), questioning whether homosexuality should be considered as a psychological disorder or as a minority sexual practice.

Some sociological and medical studies published in the 1990s advocated greater social tolerance of homosexuality. Li Yinhe and Wang Xiaobo (1992, 1998) wrote a book called *Tamen de Shijie* (Their World) based on interviews with men who have sex with men, which was later revised and reprinted as *Tongxinglian ya Wenhua* (*The Sub-Culture of Homosexuality*). In *Tongxing'ai* (*Same-Sex Love*), Zhang Beichuan (1994), a medical practitioner, suggested that same-sex relations are part of a normal range of human relationships. In 1998, he founded a magazine called *Pengyou Tongxun* (*Friend Exchange*), which covered stories about the lives of Chinese men who have sex with men, AIDS awareness initiatives and relevant international news (Zhang Beichuan *et al.* 2001). By 2004, the magazine's circulation figures had reached 10,000 copies per issue; publication ceased in 2010 when external funding from the Ford Foundation ended (Wu Rihan, Cao and Yang 2010).

New terminology for homosexuals and homosexuality began to emerge in the late 1990s as gay bars, beats and gay websites became a feature of life in major Chinese cities (Bao 2012; Jeffreys and Yu 2015: 75–88). The most common terms to describe people who are erotically attracted to people of the same sex are '*tongxinglian*' (literally, 'same-sex love') and '*tongzhi*' (comrade). The term '*tongzhi*', which came to China from the former Soviet Union, originally embodied the revolutionary ideals of comradeship and was used by people as a common form of address during the Mao era (Chou 2000: 1). Following the introduction of economic reforms, the term fell out of fashion. It was appropriated in 1989 as a euphemism for homosexuality by organizers of a gay film festival in Hong Kong (Wong 2005: 769). The Chinese word '*tong*' means 'same/with' and '*zhi*' means 'goal', 'spirit' or 'orientation', and hence '*tongzhi*' was redefined as 'homosexual' in the context of struggles to affirm homosexual identity (Chou 2001: 27). By the 1990s, *tongzhi* had become the default term used for homosexuals and homosexual identity-based politics in Hong Kong and Taiwan, and it became common parlance in the PRC in the 2000s (Chou 2000: 95). The English term 'gay' is also used by Chinese self-identified homosexuals who openly engage in a 'gay' lifestyle and struggles for gay rights (Sun, Farrer and Choi 2006: 5).

In December 2004, the Ministry of Health issued the first official estimate of China's male homosexual population to the world as part of World AIDS Day activities – an estimated 5 to 10 million people. That estimate was raised upward to reach between 10 and 20 million people in 2007 (State Council AIDS Working Committee Office and UN Theme Group on AIDS in China 2004, 2007). The public nature of these announcements by government authorities illustrates the growing visibility of homosexuality in the PRC and the linking of male homosexuality with health concerns.

From 'invisible man' to 'public health problem'

Homosexuality has become a visible phenomenon in the PRC at the same time as men who have sex with men have been identified as key to the country's evolving AIDS response. This is unlike the situation in developed Western societies, where the existence of gay communities forged around campaigning activities and lifestyle politics preceded the AIDS epidemic (Miller and Rose 2008: 93). In Western societies, national governments prioritized research and policies on HIV and AIDS largely in response to the political activism of such communities, and at a time when a HIV diagnosis was a death sentence rather than a chronic disease that can be managed with prompt medical care.

Although studies conducted in China during the early 2000s highlighted the need for AIDS prevention programs focused on men who have sex with men, such men were difficult to identify and contact as a community of self-identified individuals who engage in same-sex sexual practices (Wong *et al.* 2008: 171). Many such men are married. Public spaces such as gay bars and clubs that might foster a sense of homosexual community, and enable access to relevant communities, were also limited in number and heavily policed until recently, with the exception perhaps of gay expatriate bars in metrocities. The social 'invisibility' of homosexuality hindered the collection of the kinds of data that are used to legitimize and expand public health interventions (Fan 2014: 86; Wei *et al.* 2014: 372).

Unlike commercial sex, homosexuality is not an object of prohibitory laws in the PRC, and hence the invisibility of homosexuality prior to the 2000s largely stemmed from social prejudice. The Criminal Law of the PRC (1997) contains no provisions relating to consensual, adult homosexual acts. Between 1984 and 1997, non-consensual or violent anal sex, and anal sex involving adult men with minors, were treated as crimes under the category of sodomy (*jijianzui*), based on a 1984 ruling by the Supreme People's Court and Supreme People's Procuratorate on how to handle cases of hooliganism (*liumangzui*) (Zuigao renmin fayuan, zuigao renmin jianchayuan 1984).

The Supreme Court's 1984 ruling referred to crimes of 'hooliganism' and 'other hooligan activities' (*qita liumang huodong*). 'Hooliganism' was defined in terms of fighting, looting, sexually harassing women and causing public disturbance. 'Other hooligan activities' referred to offences involving rape, group sex, the dissemination of pornography, and the not-for-profit luring or sheltering of women in prostitution. It also included seducing male adolescents and foreigners, the sodomy of children, the forced sodomy of juveniles and violent and non-consensual anal sex involving adults. However, the category of 'hooliganism' was often used as an umbrella term for any act deemed by the police as causing public disturbance until it was deleted from the Criminal Law in 1997 (Wan 2001: 53–4; Zhang Lü 1997: 40; see also Guo Xiaofei 2007). To the extent that police targeted homosexuals, they tended to police public spaces that men were known to frequent to find sexual partners, such as public toilet blocks and parks (Li 2006: 86–7).

Homosexual organization was also constrained by policing controls in the early 1990s, as the case of activist Wan Yanhai shows. A medical doctor, Wan Yanhai (2001) worked for the China Health Education Institute (*Zhongguo jiankang jiaoyu yanjiusuo*), a sub-organization of the Ministry of Health, from 1988 to 1994. Part of his work involved promoting health education, including AIDS awareness among men. During this time, Wan established the first telephone hotline providing information on AIDS in China, conducted a survey on homosexual men and HIV-risk-related behaviour, appeared on local and national radio programs to talk about AIDS, and organized outreach projects to provide AIDS education on the streets and in public parks. In late 1992, Wan (2001: 60) established a salon called 'Men's World' (*nanren de shijie*), a health promotion group for men who have sex with men, which held a Valentine's Day celebration in February 1993.

While encouraging similar gatherings in other cities, Wan Yanhai's salon was closed down shortly after the Valentine's Day event by the Ministry of Health, allegedly because of public complaints (Gonganbu 1993: Wan 2001: 60). The

Ministry of Public Security issued a notice about the closure of the salon titled Notice on the Closure of the 'Men's World' Homosexual Culture Salon (*Guanyu qudi tongxinglian wenhua shalong 'nanren de shijie' de qingkuang tongbao*) (Gonganbu 1993). The Notice stated that: 'homosexual activities were spreading in some districts and this trend had met with strong opposition from members of the public'. Police had therefore closed down the salon at the request of the Ministry of Health. The Notice rejected Wan Yanhai's contention that homosexuality was normal, stating instead that homosexuality was a perverse form of human behaviour that violated public morality, corrupted social values, destroyed family harmony, encouraged criminality, endangered public security and contributed to the spread of STI and AIDS. While noting that such gatherings did not constitute a form of hooliganism, it concluded that local public security bureaus should promptly investigate gatherings like the Men's World, which they could close as 'unlawful assemblies' (Ibid.). Wan Yanhai (2001: 61, 2014) claims that he was then transferred away from his work in Beijing to a posting in Kunming and eventually was obliged to resign, as the result of efforts by the Ministry of Health to stop his activism.

Public reaction was reportedly even responsible for the temporary closing in 2009 of a gay bar in Yunnan Province (Li Yingqing 2009; Sexton 2009). Zhang Jianbo, a medical practitioner with the Dali Number 2 People's Hospital had opened a bar where men could socialize and receive safer-sex education (Liu Juan 2009). The bar was funded by the health department of the Dali local government, the Global Fund, and the Barry and Martins Trust. It opened on a trial basis in November 2009 and was meant to be launched officially on World AIDS Day in December (Li Yingqing 2009). However, widespread coverage by CCTV and other major media outlets halted the launch, by deterring customers and the volunteers who were to provide AIDS prevention trainings from coming to the bar. Volunteers avoided the bar because they had been shunned or ridiculed by family and friends when the nature of their work was revealed. Media photographs of people in the bar also made potential customers, especially married ones, nervous that their sexual preferences would be made public (Sexton 2009).

Attempts by NGOs to work with men who have sex with men in China are also complicated by government controls over the non-profit sector. In April 2004, Madame Wu Yi, the vice premier and Minister of Health, implied that China's AIDS response required government authorities to work with NGOs in a speech that she gave to a meeting of the State Council's AIDS Working Committee, by referring to non-specified social 'partners', 'forces' and 'sectors'. In Wu's words:

> We should mobilize all the partners in the society to participate in the fight against HIV/AIDS. We need to improve our policies and strategies to build a better environment for all the forces in the society to participate in the response, and try our best to facilitate the involvement of all sectors.
>
> (Wu Yi cited by the State Council AIDS Working Committee Office and UN Theme Group on AIDS in China 2004: 13).

Wu Yi (2004) further proposed that government authorities should use publicity and education (*xuanchuan jiaoyu*) to guide all actors in the work of HIV prevention.

However, the PRC's first Charity Law only came into effect in September 2016, followed by the Law on the Management of Overseas Non-governmental Organizations' Activities Within Mainland China in January 2017 (National People's Congress 2016a, 2016c). Some restrictions on NGO registration were eased in 2011 to encourage the development of a domestic non-profit sector, and subsequently to allow government departments to contract private social services, as is common practice in Western societies (Guowuyuan bangongting 2013). Previously, NGOs had to find a government agency that was willing to act as a supervisory body before they could be legally registered as a non-profit organization. This restricted the independent development of the NGO sector because only a few government agencies were willing to supervise community-level organizations. Concomitantly, registered organizations had to have government backing, which meant that they were either fully or partially endorsed by their sponsoring government affiliation, and hence had to work within its operating frameworks (Kaufman 2011: S1220). Small organizations often bypassed these restrictions by simply not applying for official registration and working at a localized level (Li and Kuo *et al.* 2010: II66).

An early example of a successful NGO working on HIV prevention is the 99575 Beijing Tongzhi Hotline, founded in March 1997 (99575 Beijing tongzhi rexian 2005). In 2002, the hotline became the Beijing Gender Health Education Institute, the first registered social organization in mainland China to undertake HIV prevention work among both male and female homosexuals (Chow *et al.* 2014: 5). Another example is the Chengdu Gay Community Care Organization, founded in 2002 (Li and Kuo *et al.* 2010: II68). Also in the early 2000s, NCAIDS convened various seminars on homosexuality and AIDS which were attended by members of Friend Exchange and the Beijing Tongzhi Hotline, resulting in the development of AIDS-related volunteering programs (Zhang and Chu 2005: 858–64; Zheng Lingqiao 2000a, 2000b). In the mid-2000s, the Beijing Gender Health Education Institute (2005) conducted HIV prevention training for men who have sex with men through venues frequented by homosexuals, help hotlines and other activities, and published a compilation about its methodological approach, initiatives and findings. Such activities are regarded as a milestone in terms of advancing communication between homosexuals, health authorities and researchers (Zhang and Chu 2005: 858–64).

Although bans on the sex industry have prevented many NGOs from working with sex workers, the number of organizations working on AIDS awareness programs for men has gradually increased. Of the more than 300 organizations listed in the 2006–2007 China HIV/AIDS Directory, fewer than 100 focused on men who have sex with men (Fan 2014: 89). A 2009 survey of 340 organizations conducted by the China HIV/AIDS Information Network and NCAIDS indicated that 36 per cent of worked with men who have sex with men, 27 per cent worked with people living with HIV, and only 9 per cent worked with female sex workers

(Kaufman 2012: 231; Li and Kuo *et al.* 2010: II69). A directory published in 2010 suggested that 50 per cent of around 360 organizations worked with homosexual men (Li and Kuo *et al.* 2010: II68).

Many of these NGOs have developed links between local governments, health authorities, researchers and homosexual communities, by conducting outreach and AIDS education programs, typically with international funding (Chow *et al.* 2014: 6; Li and Kuo *et al.* 2010: II67; Zhang and Chu 2005: 858–64). Some of this international funding is no longer available. For example, funding from the Global Fund to China, which was largely administered through local government agencies or government-organized NGOs, ended in 2013. Many domestic AIDS-related NGOs now have to bid for funding from PRC government authorities, which means their sustainability is dependent on local government preferences (Hildebrandt 2012: 853; Li and Kuo *et al.* 2010: II67). Such organizations survive by being '"loud about AIDS but quiet about other issues" in order to enjoy the most political space' (Hildebrandt 2012: 853).

Along with these developments, there has been a proliferation of surveys aiming to identify the range and risks of the sexual behaviours of 'MSM' (Chen *et al.* 2012; Huang *et al.* 2012). Such studies typically conclude that men who have sex with men are a key population because homosexual practices are widespread throughout urban and rural China; moreover, such men are often married or have concurrent female partners, but the majority have not been tested for HIV and do not use condoms (Wang *et al.* 2015). For example, a 2013 survey of around 1,100 men who have sex with men notes that nearly 46 per cent reported bisexual behaviours, but only 27 per cent reported consistent condom use with female partners (Tao *et al.* 2013: 524). Surveys of men who have sex with men conducted by the Ministry of Health in 2009 and in 2011 indicate that nearly 70 per cent had had sex with multiple partners during the preceding six months, but only 40 per cent had used condoms consistently, and less than 45 per cent used had condoms when having sex with their regular partners (Bai Jianfeng 2009; Ministry of Health, People's Republic of China, Joint United Nations Programme on HIV/AIDS and World Health Organization 2012). A 2015 review of the available literature concludes that approximately 30 per cent of mainland Chinese men who have sex with men have concurrent female partners, with some studies revealing that around 77 per cent have unprotected sex with primary female partners (Wang *et al.* 2015: 126–7).

Male sex workers, including self-identified homosexual, bisexual and heterosexual men, have emerged as a new feature of public health concerns and research in this context (Chow *et al.* 2012; He *et al.* 2007; Liu *et al.* 2009; Tao *et al.* 2010; Wong *et al.* 2008). Male sex workers are typically young men from small towns or rural areas of China who have migrated to urban centres looking for work and enhanced socio-economic opportunities (Jeffreys and Yu 2015: 103; Kong 2016: 1). Although some of these men offer sexual services to women, the majority provide services to other men. Men who provide commercial sexual services to women are called '*shaoye*' (young masters) or '*yazi*' (literally 'ducks'). The term 'ducks' is a play in the Chinese language on the colloquial term for prostitute '*jinü*', with the abbreviated word '*ji*' (prostitute) being a homophone for the word '*ji*' (chicken) (Jeffreys and Yu 2015: 104). Men who provide commercial sex to men are called '*yazi*' (ducks) and '*haizi*' (children), or 'money boys' and 'MBs' based on the adoption of English-language expressions. These men are stigmatized because of their means of earning a living and because they often come from poor rural communities (Kong 2012: 286). Additionally, they are sometimes condemned by members of China's homosexual community for being 'improper gay men' who undermine the perceived purity of same-sex love (Kong 2012: 286, 2016: 8–12; Rofel 2010: 425–6).

Researchers suggest that male sex workers are potentially a key population in HIV transmission through homosexual contact with male clients and heterosexual contact with female lovers and wives. Studies indicate that 28 per cent of male sex workers and nearly 51 per cent of men who have sex with men have never tested for HIV, even though the PRC government provides free-of-charge voluntary HIV counselling and testing, and 76 per cent of male sex workers and other men who have had sex with men also have had sex with women (Huang *et al.* 2012: 858, 864). A survey of male sex workers conducted in the northeastern province of Shandong, suggests that nearly 37 per cent of over 100 participants self-identified as bisexual (Tao *et al.* 2010: 361). Likewise, a survey of 56 male sex workers conducted in the southern city of Shenzhen revealed that 43 per cent had female sexual partners (Liu *et al.* 2009: 657). At the same time, localized surveys indicate a high prevalence of HIV among male sex workers. A study of nearly 90 male sex workers in Tianjin, a city near Beijing, revealed a HIV prevalence of nearly 7 per cent (Liu Zhongquan *et al.* 2009).

In short, the identification of men who have sex with men as key to China AIDS response has led to a growing body of research and an increase in the number of organizations focused on such men. The next section examines some of the AIDS education materials that have been created for this key population. It also explores some of the controversies associated with health interventions to promote AIDS awareness and HIV testing among men who have sex with men.

AIDS prevention focused on men who have sex with men

Since the late-2000s, city-level branches of the CDC have organized large-scale public health interventions with the aim of providing men who have sex with men with information about HIV prevention, testing and treatment services. Supported by the Global Fund, many of these branches contracted social organizations that had full-time staff and volunteers to access a specified number of men in bars, bathhouses and other venues, within a specified period of time, to provide AIDS education and rapid HIV testing with the test results being forwarded to the CDC (Fan 2014). Social organizations, while limited in number, typically find it easier to access men who have sex with men than CDC officials (Chow *et al.* 2014: 6). Many such men distrust government authorities and fear that involvement with public health authorities will result in their families and employers becoming aware of their sexual behaviours (Fan 2014: 91; Wang *et al.* 2015: 136). Hence, it has become common practice for the CDC to contract social organizations to provide HIV prevention programs, and rapid testing and treatment services, for men who have sex with men (Zhongguo jibing yufang kongzhi zhongxin, xingbing aizibing yufang kongzhi zhongxin 2016a).

To support such initiatives, the Beijing CDC produced a number of booklets on AIDS awareness for men who have sex with men (Beijingshi jibing yufang kongzhi zhongxin n.d.-a, n.d.-b, n.d.-c). The booklets, which are available as printed and online texts, were distributed during health interventions in venues frequented by men who have sex with men, and through the websites and dating applications of homosexual organizations such as Danlan.org and the *tongzhi* working group in Hezhou City, Guangxi Zhuang Autonomous Region (http://blog.sina.com.cn/hetong2010). Similar resources are stored on a dedicated site on the NCAIDS website (http://ncaids.chinacdc.cn/zsk/mbrq/zdgwrq/msm/).

One booklet relates six cautionary tales about cases of unprotected sex resulting in HIV infection, in order to overcome the popular belief among people who occasionally engage in unprotected sexual behaviours that they are not at risk (Beijingshi jibing yufang kongzhi zhongxin n.d.-a). The findings of surveys and interviews indicate that many men do not use condoms when having sex with regular male partners because they trust their partners and believe that condom use undermines the 'loving' nature of the relationship, or interferes with sexual desire (Chapman 2009; Li and Lau *et al.* 2010). Hence the basic message of the booklet is that men who have sex with men can reduce their risk of contracting and transmitting HIV by being monogamous, using condoms in all sexual encounters and being tested for HIV.

Of the booklet's six cautionary tales, five are stories of HIV infection resulting from a failure to use condoms with a regular partner. The protagonist incorrectly assumes that his 'untested' partner is 'disease-free' and will not have unprotected sex with other men (see also Wei *et al.* 2014: 373). The remaining story warns against wrongly assuming that HIV only targets certain classes of people, by explaining how a high-status member of society – a higher-degree research candidate – was diagnosed with HIV after engaging in unprotected sex during a one-night stand with a casual partner.

The booklet concludes with a common list of reasons for inconsistent condom use obtained from a survey of nearly 1,300 men, which the 'informed' reader now knows are unhelpful in terms of disease prevention (Beijingshi jibing yufang kongzhi zhongxin n.d.-a). These reasons include: 'I know my partner really well' (32 per cent); 'my partner is a person of high quality and has never had an STI' (13 per cent); 'we did not have condoms at the time' (11 per cent); 'my partner feels uncomfortable using condoms' (11 per cent); 'I feel uncomfortable using condoms' (10 per cent); and 'my partner has recently tested negative for HIV' (8 per cent).

Another booklet encourages men who have sex with men to receive HIV testing, using bold type to reassure the potential reader that their personal information will be kept strictly confidential and will not be revealed to family members or work colleagues (*nin de gerenxinxi jianghui yange baomi buhui yingxiang nin de jiaren yijigongzuo*) (Beijingshi jibing yufang kongzhi zhongxin n.d.-b). Previously, health authorities were obliged to notify public security departments of positive test results for STI. The results of such tests were often revealed to other perceived relevant members of the community for follow-up testing and other reasons. This meant that many people were reluctant to undergo testing in the first place (Detels *et al.* 2003: 803; Wei *et al.* 2014: 374; Xia and Yang 2005: 153).

Apart from issuing booklets, the CDC has produced HIV prevention posters that are available online for government and social organizations to print and disseminate in public spaces. Local government authorities were instructed to place these posters in diverse public spaces, including on residential-community noticeboards and at public transport stops. The posters present condom use and HIV testing as an independent decision between two caring and 'aware' individuals, rather than being the outcome of information provided by medical experts to the 'inexpert' (see Figures 6.1 and 6.2).

The CDC has also contracted social organizations to conduct AIDS-awareness projects in diverse venues frequented by men who have sex with men, including bathhouses and clubs (National Center for AIDS/STD Control and Prevention 2007). In Western societies, men who frequent bathhouses to find sexual partners are viewed as especially at risk of contracting HIV through sexual transmission, and this is potentially also the case in China (Binson *et al.* 2001; Downing 2010: 7). A study of around 220 men who frequented a bathhouse in Hangzhou City in 2011 revealed a HIV prevalence of nearly 16 per cent (Ni Zhimin *et al.* 2011). This is much higher than the rate of less than 6 per cent recorded among men who frequent bars and parks looking for sexual partners, or who meet partners through the Internet, according to a study of more than 2,200 men who have sex with men in Jiangsu Province between 2008 and 2009 (Yan Hongjing *et al.* 2010: 1251; see also Chow *et al.* 2014: 2).

The Beijing Aizhixing Institute for Health Education and a Wuhan-based NGO attribute the higher prevalence of HIV among men who frequent bathhouses to spatial and social reasons (Beijing aizhixing jiankang jiaoyu yanjiusuo he Wuhan xinyuan 2009). The spatial and gender-segregated arrangements of bathhouses, many of which contain small private rooms with dim lighting, provide opportunities for negotiating and engaging in casual sex. At the same time, many of the men who frequent bathhouses are older and married. They may neither identify themselves as homosexual nor wish to be identified as such by others, and therefore may believe that they are not at risk or may not have come into contact with AIDS education materials.

Health interventions focus on 'clubs' (*huisuo*) as another place where men negotiate and engage in casual sex with other men, often through commercial sex. Some clubs have male 'technicians' (*jishi*) who provide massage services in theory, but sexual services in practice. Hence the term '*jishi*' has become a synonym for 'money boy'. Money boys working in clubs are viewed as a priority population for HIV prevention because many of these men have heterosexual relationships (Wong *et al.* 2008: 171, 173). Health interventions conducted in such venues offer the CDC access to groups of men who might otherwise remain

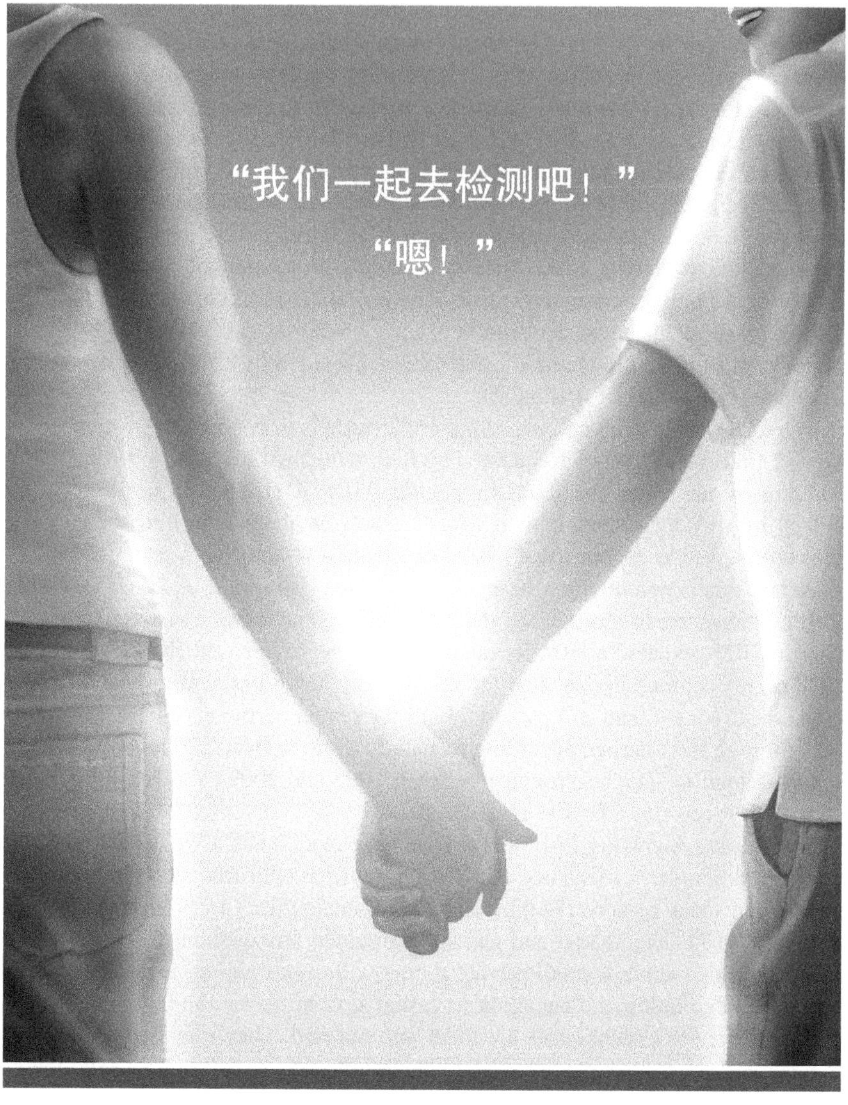

Figure 6.2 ‘Let’s both get tested’.

Source: National Center for AIDS/STD Control and Prevention, China CDC (2010) ‘Xing’ai zhongxin guanyu yinfa “nannanxingxingweirenqun aizibing xingbing fangzhi xuanchuan cailiao” de han’ [NCAIDS: on the issuing of ‘AIDS prevention promotional materials for men who have sex with men’], 21 December. Online. Available: http://ncaids.chinacdc.cn/fzdt/zxdt/201012/t20101221_1519120.htm (accessed 7 February 2017); reproduced with permission.

'hidden' because of the marginalized social position of men who have sex with men, and the illegality of sex work (Chow *et al.* 2014: 6).

But the CDC's practice of using social organizations to expand health interventions focused on men who have sex with men has met with mixed responses. As Elsa Fan (2014: 90) explains, one organization was paid CNY 25,000 per six months (approximately USD 4,000) directly from government budgets by their local CDC in return for organizing one training workshop a month, to reach a total of 2,000 men who have sex with men, and testing 400 men in the same period. This practice is expanding because it is more efficient. Social organizations are able to access greater numbers of men and persuade more men to be tested than CDC officials. It is also an income-earner for social organizations.

Many social organizations focus on men who have sex with men because they yield higher test results for new infections than other key populations. As a leader of one organization told Fan:

> Initially our project targeted three populations: [sex workers, injecting drug users and men who have sex with men]. In most of the program cities, however, there were minimal to no new infections found among [sex workers and injecting drug users]. Among MSM, though, we were finding a lot of new infections; we had spent a lot of money for these two groups [sex workers and injecting drug users] with no results to show for it, while we spent less money on MSM and yielded more results. So we decided to reallocate the funding to MSM because it was much more financially efficient.
>
> (cited in Fan 2014: 19)

Newspaper reports further suggest that some organizations used funding from the Bill and Melinda Gates Foundation to provide financial recompense to people presenting for testing, resulting in some individuals presenting for testing on multiple occasions (Jacobs 2009).

Fan (2014: 95) concludes that the CDC's practice of contracting AIDS prevention work to social organizations is both saving lives and stigmatizing men who have sex with men. It is saving lives by providing particular groups of men with information about HIV transmission and prevention, and access to testing and medical treatment. At the same time, the act of making men who have sex with men 'visible' for the purposes of accelerated HIV testing is marginalizing them as a new and perceived major conduit of AIDS in China (Ibid.).

Yet the CDC's turn to private service providers and commercial models is also transforming the top-down model of providing AIDS education through medicalized health campaigns, and reaching broader and young audiences. In 2014, China's CDC and UNAIDS funded Blued (www.bluedapp.com), a dating application launched by the gay website, Danlan.org, to promote AIDS awareness for men who have sex with men ('"Nantong" ganran aizibing zengjia tongzhi shejiao pingtai huyu baohu ziji' 2015). A red ribbon icon within the Blued user interface links users to information about correct condom and lubricant use, and encourages them to answer questions intended to raise their knowledge of HIV prevention, testing and care options (UNAIDS 2015b: 85–6). Guidelines for health interventions among men who have sex with men issued by the CDC and NCAIDS in 2016 further recommend leveraging social networking sites such as WeChat and QQ, and dating applications such as Blued, Grindr, GayPark and Jack'd, to provide information about safer sex and to facilitate online bookings for HIV testing and the communication of test results (Zhongguo jibing yufang kongzhi zhongxin, xingbing aizibing yufang kongzhi zhongxin 2016a: 60). As this suggests, Chinese men are increasingly encouraged to access information about how to protect themselves from HIV and AIDS, and hence to govern themselves, through the indirect means of social networking, and commercial lifestyle, entertainment and advertising media.

The expanding and altered nature of such health interventions is demonstrated by the 2016 Guidelines for Interventions to Prevent AIDS Among Men Who Have Sex With Men, issued by the CDC and NCAIDS (Ibid.). The 2016 Guidelines outline behavioural survey and interview questions for health authorities and NGOs to 'map' the social and sexual practices of men who have sex with men (Ibid: 36–7). Respondents are asked basic demographic information (age, education background, occupation and marital status), and whether they have migrated to the city in which they are living, and if so, for what reason. They are asked whether they self-identify as a homosexual/comrade (*tongzhi*), how many other like-minded men they know in the city, how many homosexuals in their estimation live in the city in total, what kinds of different homosexual groups and activities exist in the city, and whether members of those groups are distinguished by differences in age, education, and preferred meeting places and activities. Respondents are also asked whether they frequent homosexual venues, and whether they communicate with men who have sex with men who do not frequent such venues, and if so, how. They are then asked to mark the location and provide a name for each meeting place that they frequent on a city map, and to indicate the general age, educational background and occupation of the people who frequent such spaces, and to estimate the proportion of patrons that are heterosexual, not local city residents and money boys.

Apart from mapping the physical spaces for homosexual sociality in a given city, the 2016 Guidelines aim to map the virtual spaces for men to meet men. Respondents are asked whether they surf the Internet and 'comrade' websites, and, if so, which sites they frequent, and whether other men in the same city frequent the same sites. They are also asked whether they use dating applications and live dating sites, and, if so, to explain how often they use them and for what reasons, and what they talk about with other men on such sites. Respondents are then asked to comment on the statement that 'some people believe that using dating software promotes AIDS'.

The survey and interview questions ask respondents to describe either their own sexual relationships and practices, or those of their 'comrades', and whether they use condoms and recreational drugs. Respondents are asked whether they or their 'comrades' have female partners and casual or long-term sexual relationships with other men. They are asked in what circumstances they or their 'comrades' use and do use condoms and why. They are also asked whether they or their 'comrades' use methamphetamine and other stimulants, and if so, how often, and whether they have heard of people having any adverse reactions to the use of such drugs.

Finally, the survey and interview questions ask respondents to comment on the prevalence of STI and HIV among their circle of 'comrades', and to explain how the provision of information about disease prevention, testing and treatment might be improved. Respondents are asked whether they know anyone with a history of an STI or living with HIV, and whether the people in question saw a medical doctor, contacted the CDC and received medical treatment. They are also asked whether HIV and syphilis testing is a common experience for 'comrades', and how might 'comrades' be encouraged to undertake regular testing. Last but not least, respondents are asked for their views and ideas on the nature and placement of AIDS and drug awareness publicity for men who have sex with men in the city in which they live, and how such public service advertising might be improved.

The stated aim of this social mapping exercise is to equip more men with the knowledge required both to protect themselves from contracting HIV, and to access HIV testing and care services. Information derived from such surveys could perhaps also be used to inform the location-based policing of recreational drugs and commercial sex. However, the use of social networking sites and dating applications to provide information about AIDS, and the introduction of survey questions asking where men would like to see AIDS-related communication and in what forms, demonstrates new interest in diverse communities of homosexuals as both stakeholders in health campaigns and niche markets for public service and other forms of advertising.

As the next section explains, the linking of AIDS with men who have sex with men has drawn public attention to a previously 'invisible' group of people and accentuated the stigmatization of homosexuality. But it has also opened the discursive space for self-identified homosexuals, and people speaking on their behalf, to contest negative constructions of homosexuality and to demand anti-discrimination measures.

Contesting constructions of homosexuality and AIDS

Positive presentations of homosexuality were virtually absent from China's state-run media until recently. In the words of sociologist Li Yinhe:

> I remember about 20 years ago, in the *People's Daily*, homosexuality, prostitution, and drugs were all supposedly linked to social evils. . . . even 10 years ago . . . everybody was convinced that no one was gay, and so they had never met someone who purported to be homosexual.
>
> (Li Yinhe cited in Schreurs 2015)

Before the mid-1990s, the few articles that were published on homosexuality and AIDS defined homosexuality as a problem relating to deviancy and the introduction of 'decadent' Western mores, and prescribed heterosexuality as the cure. In 1996, a popular journal called *Shuwu* (*Book House*) published an article with the title 'AIDS: The Bitter Fruit of Homosexuality – The Background Culture of Human Disease' (Yu Fenggao 1996: 20–4). Following a brief history of homosexuality in China and in Western societies, the author recounted tales of famous homosexuals who had died of AIDS, including the Russian ballet dancer Rudolf Nureyev, the American actor Rock Hudson, and the French intellectual Michel Foucault. The author concluded that AIDS is the 'bitter fruit' of homosexuality because male homosexuals are likely to have multiple partners and unprotected anal sex, putting them at risk of contracting HIV (Ibid.).

In the 2000s, China's media started to provide news coverage and opinion pieces about AIDS in support of national policies, which variously pathologized and attempted to normalize homosexuality. In August 2000, the official newspaper of the Ministry of Health, *Jiankangbao* (*Health News*), featured an article suggesting that AIDS was 'rampant' (*sinüe*) among China's homosexual population (Zheng Lingqiao 2000a: 1). It further suggested that this was contributing to the spread of HIV among the broader population because many such men were married with children. The article concluded that AIDS awareness programs had to target men who have sex with men presented as vectors of disease (Ibid.).

On 15 April 2001, Xinhua News Agency reported that the Chinese Classification of Mental Disorders Third Revision had removed the diagnostic criteria suggesting that homosexuality referred to a form of mental illness, which encouraged broader media coverage of homosexuality as part of everyday life (Zhu Yu 2001: 5). Shortly after World AIDS Day in 2003, the *Xinhua Daily* published an article stating that public attitudes towards homosexuality had become more relaxed (*kuansong*), while noting that a growing number of married men were presenting at mental health clinics for treatment for homosexual desires (Liu Yuqin 2003: 5). The article informed readers with reference to the new psychiatric standard that homosexuality is not a mental health condition. However, it added that newfound social tolerance of homosexuality was creating problems for some families because many same-sex attracted men were husbands and fathers (Ibid.).

The first 'official counting' of the PRC's homosexual population occurred on World AIDS Day in December 2004, when a press release by the Ministry of Health stated that an estimated 5 to 10 million male homosexuals were living in mainland China (Lü Fuming 2004). The press release linked homosexuality and AIDS by noting that the HIV prevalence among men who have sex with men was second only to the prevalence among people who had injected drugs using non-sterile equipment. It further noted that homosexuals are normal members of a sexual minority rather than people with mental health problems. Thus the task posed for relevant authorities and society in general is to 'understand' and 'support' members of this sexual minority in ways best calculated to reduce the spread of HIV (Ibid.). A day later, CCTV broadcast a current affairs show on homosexuality and AIDS called *Acknowledgement Is Better Than Avoidance* ('Huibi buru zhengshi' 2004). These actions signalled a more open attitude towards homosexuality on the part of China's mainstream media to facilitate public health objectives.

In August 2005, CCTV aired a 40-minute documentary on homosexuality and AIDS awareness called *In the Name of Life* ('Yi shengming de mingyi' 2005). The program's host, Chai Jing, said that HIV was spreading from key populations to the general population. But rather than focusing on the marital arrangements of many such men, she interviewed a man living with HIV who talked about his homosexual lifestyle, and another two men who held hands and talked about how they had met and fallen in love. The documentary also showed scenes from a bathhouse frequented by men looking for male sexual partners. The bathhouse was closed down by police shortly afterwards, allegedly in response to pressure from outraged local residents (Wang Wei 2005). However, the CCTV documentary is generally viewed as marking a milestone in terms of media involvement in generating public awareness of homosexuality, and it was clearly influenced by the AIDS awareness actions initiated by the Ministry of Health in 2004 (Ibid.).

Also in 2005, China's media began to report on activism in support of equality for homosexuals, including the right to health and to marry. Sociologist Li Yinhe (2015) has unsuccessfully lobbied delegates at the PRC's top political advisory body, the National Committee of the Chinese People's Political Consultative Conference (CPPCC), to consider a proposal on legalizing same-sex marriage on multiple occasions between 2003 and 2016. Her proposal states that legalizing same-sex marriage will revive China's traditional cultural acceptance of same-sex eroticism, build the PRC's international reputation as a promoter rather than violator of human rights, and reduce the spread of HIV through sexual transmission. Although Li's proposal has not obtained the support required to be discussed formally at the CPPCC to date, legal scholar Yang Hongtai endorsed her actions in a 2005 article in the *Minzhu yu Fazhi Shibao* (*Democracy and Law Times*), a newspaper affiliated with the China Law Society (Chen Zhuo 2005: 2). Yang stated that: 'Homosexual love should be legitimate. Homosexuality is not a disease' (Ibid.). He even drafted a Regulation on Same-Sex Marriage (*Tongxing'aizhe hunyin tiaoli caoan*) to express his support for her proposal.

Gay activists also went public in 2005, with issues of same-sex marriage and HIV prevention being linked in related media discussions. On 23 October, approximately 100 people gathered on a beach in Shenzhen holding rainbow flags, a symbol of gay pride that originated in the USA. The protestors declared that homosexuals have the human right to live a happy and normal life, and hence to marry (Ren, Liu and Ran 2005: 5). A participant in the Shenzhen action told journalists that struggles for gay rights were in their infancy, and it was therefore unlikely that same-sex marriage would be legalized soon. However, the aim of the protest was to demand the reduction of discriminatory attitudes (*paichi taidu*) towards homosexuals (Ibid.).

In a subsequent editorial for the *Procuratorial Daily*, legal scholar Fu Dalin (2005: 6) stated that the Shenzhen beach protest was China's first open gay rights event, and claimed it had been triggered by the negative effects of government-led AIDS prevention initiatives. According to Fu, these initiatives had not only opened a marginal social group to public scrutiny, but also in some respects deepened social hostility towards homosexuals by associating them with AIDS. Fu concluded that the protest demonstrated that the PRC government needed to introduce anti-discriminatory measures to protect this vulnerable group in the context of a rapidly changing society.

Researchers somewhat differently note that discrimination against homosexuals creates additional problems for the work of HIV prevention. In a master's thesis on homosexual communities in Changsha City in Hunan Province, Yu Yong (2006: 56) argues that some self-identified homosexual men marry women to avoid social discrimination and to have a permanent relationship, viewing relationships with men as unstable because of the marginalized nature of homosexuality (see also Huang *et al.* 2012: 869; Wang *et al.* 2015: 130–1). Health workers argue that social discrimination makes many homosexuals reluctant to undergo HIV testing, with men who have sex with men accounting for only 2 per cent of people presenting for voluntary testing in 2008 (Xiong Ran *et al.* 2010: 251; see also Wei *et al.* 2014). Other studies contend that social discrimination is reflected in the project-driven and unsustainable nature of health interventions promoting safer sex and condom use, which are driven by health authorities rather than homosexual communities (Jiang Hua *et al.* 2009: 501; see also Fan 2014).

Senior government officials appear to have accepted that effective HIV prevention requires anti-discriminatory measures and assistance from NGOs, at least to some extent. In 2010, the Minister of Health, Chen Zhu, visited a NGO that works on HIV prevention with men who have sex with men, while investigating the state of AIDS prevention work in Nanning City, Guangxi Zhuang Autonomous Region (Tian and Wang 2010). During that visit, which was filmed by accompanying journalists, Chen acknowledged that HIV prevention work among such men was inadequate. He further noted that official support for anti-discrimination measures was necessary to improve the work of HIV prevention (Ibid.).

Reaction to actress and practising Christian Lü Liping's 2011 claim that homosexuality is sinful (*zui*) on Sina Weibo – the so-called Twitter of the East – suggests some degree of public support for anti-discrimination measures (Wang Tingting 2011: D03). Numerous intellectuals promptly criticized Lü for promoting outdated and discriminatory views, noting that young people, in particular, increasingly view sexual orientation as a private matter and a human right (Wu Dan 2011a, 2011b). Lü was criticized on a CCTV program called *24 Hours* (*24 Xiaoshi*) for using her public profile to promote discrimination rather than encouraging her fans to respect the rights of homosexuals (Chen Wen 2011: B2). The *21 Shiji Jingji Baodao* (*21st Century Business Herald*) concluded that criticisms of Lü's comments demonstrated growing social tolerance of homosexuality because, in the early 2000s, no one would have imagined that homosexuality could be so openly discussed in the media (Zhou Biao 2011: 2).

Recent activism indicates that lesbian, gay, bisexual, transgender and intersex (LGBTI) people may be marginalized in China, but they are no longer invisible or voiceless. In what the media described as the largest coordinated LGBTI effort in the PRC's history, over 190 LGBTI organizations released a joint letter condemning violence based on sexual orientation, after a gunman killed 49 people in a gay nightclub in the USA in June 2016 (Bai 2016). The letter added that Chinese LGBTI people are subject to unacceptable violence and discrimination, as evidenced by schoolyard bullying of LGBTI youth and the existence of 'gay conversion therapy'. This collective action followed a series of landmark cases presented to the Chinese courts by LGBTI activists in 2015–2016, which aimed to attract media publicity and raise public awareness of LGBTI issues by demanding legal protections, including the right to marry and an end to the existence of homophobic textbooks, censorship of gay-themed films and workplace discrimination. Hence, there is now a nascent but active LGBTI community in the PRC, which may also encourage more diverse actions on sexual health issues by self-identified homosexuals and domestic LGBTI organizations.

Concluding remarks

The classification of human kinds as 'MSM' has had varied effects in terms of public health initiatives and discourses on homosexuality. On the one hand, men who have sex with men are now identified as the population in China that is most at risk of contracting and transmitting HIV, flowing from expanded research, sentinel surveillance, diagnostic capacity and incentives to get tested. This is helping to save lives by prompting the scaling up of testing and the provision of treatments to those who need them (Fan 2014: 95). On the other hand, the medicalization of men who have sex with men as vectors of a stigmatized disease contributes to negative representations of homosexuals and homosexuality.

At the same time, behavioural surveys of men who have sex with men highlight the diverse nature of such men and the need to overcome the obstacles presented by social discrimination for understanding their sexual attitudes and practices (Li and Lau *et al.* 2010: 1485). Although the latter suggestion is intended to facilitate the more effective administration of AIDS prevention programs, it implies that homosexuality should be normalized. Indeed, many studies now draw on interviews with Chinese men to suggest that HIV prevention would be enhanced by the governmental act of promoting gay venues with legal protections, legalizing same-sex marriage, and presenting both homosexuals and people living with HIV as positive role models in mass media (Chen *et al.* 2012: 6; Shang *et al.* 2012: 577). This means making LGBTI people and lifestyles a part of everyday life.

The act of classifying and administering human kinds as 'MSM' has thus had a looping or feedback effect. Some people who self-identify as homosexual, and some people who work with men who have sex with men, are contesting the negative construction of MSM as vectors of disease, and demanding legal protections and anti-discrimination measures. The extension of AIDS awareness campaigns to men in general is an integral component of strategies aiming to raise public awareness of AIDS, and reduce the stigma attached to people living with HIV and AIDS. Hence the next chapter focuses on AIDS prevention programs for male members of China's massive rural-to-urban migrant population.

Note

1 The term non-governmental organization (NGO) refers to different types of social organizations in the Chinese context. These include registered non-profit and charitable organizations associated with state-owned and private businesses, and registered and unregistered community-based organizations. They also include non-profits associated with mass organizations and other associations that are closely affiliated with the Party-state system, and have established national networks. The latter are sometimes called 'government-organized non-governmental organizations' or GONGOs in the English-language literature. For ease of discussion, we use the terms NGOs and social organizations interchangeably.

7 Rural-to-urban migrant labourers

This chapter examines the development of public health campaigns promoting AIDS awareness and safer-sex practices to male, rural-to-urban migrant labourers in the People's Republic of China. People migrating within China are categorized as a 'focal' rather than 'key' population in terms of AIDS prevention, and male migrants are a recent focus of the HIV sentinel surveillance system and associated behavioural surveys. The website of the National Center for AIDS/STD Control and Prevention (NCAIDS), which is managed by the Chinese Center for Disease Control and Prevention, lists AIDS-related educational resources created for four categories of people. These are: (1) 'high-risk groups' (*gaoweirenqun*), that is, 'key populations', comprising people who inject drugs, men who have sex with men, 'women who sell unlawful sexual services' (*anchang*) and 'other' (*qita*); (2) 'focal populations' (*zhongdianrenqun*), comprising internal migrants (*liudongrenkou*) and students; (3) 'the general population' (*dazhongrenqun*); and (4) 'people living with HIV and AIDS' (*ganranzhe/bingren*) (NCAIDS n.d.). Five HIV sentinel surveillance sites focused on male migrant workers were established in 2009 (Wen *et al.* 2012: 79). That figure increased to 87 sites in 2010, which indicates that male migrants have become a significant feature of the cumulative number of reported HIV and AIDS cases in the regions where the sites are located (Ibid.: 80).

Internal migration, resulting from the post-1978 opening-up of the PRC's labour market and associated rapid urbanization, is viewed as a potential driver of the spread of HIV through sexual transmission (Hong *et al.* 2006; Rou *et al.* 2010: II43; Zhuang *et al.* 2012: 1). Data from the National Bureau of Statistics of China (2015) indicates that the number of internal migrants stood at nearly 274 million people in 2014. Migration within China thus represented nearly 37 per cent of internal migration worldwide in 2015 (740 million people) and was greater than the entirety of worldwide international migration (244 million people) (International Organization for Migration, Global Migration Data Analysis Center 2016). Such population mobility will continue along with increased rates of urbanization and consumption as part of the PRC's Thirteenth Five-Year Guidelines for National Economic and Social Development for 2016–2020 (National People's Congress 2016b).

According to UNAIDS (2001: 2), migrants comprise two groups of people who are 'more vulnerable to HIV/AIDS than are populations that do not move'. The

DOI: 10.4324/9781315175546-7

first group is 'mobile people', that is, 'those who move from one place to another, temporarily, seasonally or permanently for a host of voluntary or involuntary reasons', for example, truck drivers, transport workers, construction workers, business people and sex workers. The second group is 'migrants', that is, people who take up residence in another country and who therefore remain in a place away from home for an extended period of time (Ibid.: 3).

Migration in the Chinese context predominantly takes the form of internal rural-to-urban labour mobility, rather than cross-border migration, and is marked by the legacies of Mao-era social controls. The introduction of a household registration system in 1955 prevented population mobility and divided China's population into urban- and rural-born residents, with ongoing consequences (Chan and Zhang 1999; Cheng and Selden 1994; Xu 2009). Rural-born migrants are generally viewed as 'outsiders' (*wailairenkou*), and as sources of 'contamination' and 'crime', by the urban residents and governing authorities of the cities in which they have relocated for work (Liu 2005; Solinger 1999a; Xu 2009; Zhang 2001). Negative media coverage of rural-to-urban migrants as people of low 'quality' (*suzhi*) reinforced such prejudice, especially during the 1980s and 1990s (Tse 2016: 581). Rural-born migrants are also often unable to obtain permanent residency permits in their host cities, and are subsequently denied local social services such as education and healthcare, making them 'second-class citizens' (Xu 2009; Wong 2011).

The terms 'migrant' and 'migration' in the Chinese context therefore generally refer to transient internal population mobility, and especially to people with a rural household registration who work in Chinese cities but who do not possess the documentation required to be considered permanent residents of those cities. Yet some people may remain in their host cities for extended periods, and sometimes even permanently. Others may have been born in a city but have migrant parents with rural household registration (Gransow 2012: 1; Tse 2016: 583).

Although the documented HIV prevalence among China's internal migrant population is only 0.075 per cent, research and media reports highlight the potential for rural-born migrants to contribute to the nationwide spread of HIV (Ministry of Health, People's Republic of China, Joint United Nations Programme on HIV/AIDS and World Health Organization 2010). Migrant workers accounted for over 74 per cent of new HIV infections recorded in Beijing between 1985 and 2010, and nearly 43 per cent of new HIV infections recorded in Guangdong Province in 2010 (Guangdong Province Health Department 2010; Wei Chenxue 2010: 2). A 2009 report in a Hubei-based newspaper, the *Changjiang Ribao* (*Changjiang Daily*), suggested that the number of HIV infections in the farming area of Chongyang County had risen from 15 to 72 cases between 2006 and 2008 (Li Qing 2009). The article noted that 'outside workers' (*waichudagongzhe*) or 'farmer-workers' (*nongmingong*) had returned to their rural homes to visit family members during Chinese holidays and agricultural planting/harvesting seasons, or because they had been unable to find work during the Global Financial Crisis and China's accompanying economic slowdown (Ibid.). These men had subsequently infected their spouses with HIV, which they had unknowingly contracted after engaging in unprotected sex with urban-based sexual partners, including sex workers (see also Zhuang *et al.* 2012: 1). In such accounts, the threat of AIDS is linked to the mobility of rural- rather than urban-born citizens.

Rural-to-urban migrant workers are viewed as vulnerable to HIV infection because they often experience financial and psychological difficulties relating to precarious employment, and separation from their homes and families (Wu Junqing 2010: 415; Yang, Derlega and Luo 2007: 283). Studies aimed at 'knowing' the sexual behaviours of male migrants, especially men working in construction sites, factories and markets, suggest that they are young and sexually active, but either have a limited understanding of HIV and its causes, or else seldom use condoms consistently (He *et al.* 2013: 84; Pan *et al.* 2013: 3; Zhuang *et al.* 2012: 5). Compounding these problems, many migrant workers are reportedly unwilling to be tested for HIV because of financial concerns, lack of knowledge of the availability of free and confidential testing and treatment services, and fear of social and workplace discrimination should they test positive ('China launches AIDS prevention among migrant workers' 2007; Wang *et al.* 2010: 902).

The chapter first provides a short history of internal migration in the PRC, showing how urbanization and the legacy of Mao-era social controls have disadvantaged rural- compared to urban-born citizens. It explains how structural inequality, reflected in poor education, precarious employment and reduced access to local government services, may exacerbate the vulnerability of rural-born migrant workers to HIV infection. It then outlines policy developments designed to improve access to HIV prevention, testing and care services for migrant populations, before describing diverse efforts to promote AIDS awareness in migrant workplaces and communities. These efforts involve numerous ministries and government departments, Party-affiliated mass organizations, state-owned and private businesses, and volunteers.

Finally, the chapter looks at celebrity-endorsed public service advertising (PSAs) designed to popularize AIDS education for migrant workers and discourage social discrimination against people living with HIV. Such PSAs are a new way of communicating information about AIDS in China. They offer informal and entertaining educational tools that large sectors of the population can access informally through broadcast, digital and social media, rather than referring to top-down medicalized health interventions conducted in specific locations and venues. They are also a novel attempt to combat prejudice against people living with HIV in the Chinese context. At the same time, the focus on rural-to-urban migrant workers as vulnerable to HIV infection may encourage the continued association of and allocation of blame for AIDS with marginalized groups of people.

Population mobility in the PRC

Migration is viewed as a major factor contributing to the spread of HIV both internationally and within national borders, not because migration causes HIV but rather because migration contributes to HIV-related vulnerabilities (UNAIDS 2001: 2).

Unlike other infectious diseases, HIV does not necessarily follow population flows. Migrants' vulnerability to HIV infection stems from their often low socio-economic position and associated circumstances. For example, people living in sub-Sahara Africa accounted for 46 per cent of new HIV infection cases reported globally in 2015, with young women between 15 and 24 years of age being disproportionately affected (AVERT 2016). This highlights the importance of addressing the economic and social factors that make particular groups of people vulnerable to HIV infection, rather than focusing strictly on individuals and their risk-taking behaviours.

Population mobility is a relatively recent phenomenon in the PRC and predominantly takes the form of rural-to-urban labour migration. During the 1950s and until the early 1980s, the Chinese Communist Party restricted population mobility to meet the requirements of socialist centralized planning. Nationalization of industry and state control over the distribution of labour and resources meant that the Party-state needed to know the identity and location of its workers (Jeffreys and Sigley 2009: 9). The introduction of the Regulations on Household Registration of the PRC in 1958 tied rural citizens to agricultural collectives and their place of birth, and it tied urban citizens to state-run work units and ultimately their place of birth (Goodman 2014: 35–6). With the corollary curbing of the monetary economy, people became fixed to their place of birth/work because they were unable to access food rations and the means of obtaining a livelihood in other areas (Gransow 2012: 2; Rush 2011: 33). People could only move for work with government approval, which was difficult to obtain being dependent on quotas determined by national economic and development plans (Yang and Xia 2008: 323). China's population was thus geographically 'fixed', with residents of major cities typically receiving better access to education, employment and welfare opportunities than their rural counterparts. This situation exacerbated an already existing rural-urban divide, even though the CCP was theoretically committed to overcoming such a division (Chan and Zhang 1999: 841–2).

The PRC's population only started to 'move' after the introduction of market-based economic reforms in December 1978. The reforms, irrespective of whether they were motivated by government or popular support, led to the dismantling of rural agricultural cooperatives (Perkins 1994). In rural areas, land was re-allocated to individual households. Households could determine which crops to grow, and had an incentive to grow extra crops because they could freely dispose of surplus production over and above national and collective quotas. In many areas the result was more efficient and profitable agricultural enterprises. Millions of rural people also found themselves without work and with the newfound capacity to move to other parts of the country to engage in different forms of labour (Yang and Xia 2008: 323). The corollary, gradual dismantling of the work-unit system, and opening-up of urban labour and housing markets created new opportunities for rural-born people to work and live in cities. Surplus labourers in rural areas subsequently moved to developing cities, contributing to China's urban development and export-oriented industrialization (Fan 2003: 28; Rush 2011: 29; Xu 2009: 41).

The PRC is currently divided into four economic regions – the eastern, north-eastern, central and western regions – based on the Eleventh Five-Year Guidelines for National Economic and Social Development (2006–2010) (Zhonghua renmin gongheguo guomin jingji he shehui fazhan di shiyi ge wunian guihua gangyao 2006). It was previously divided into the eastern, central and western regions, based on the Seventh Five-Year Plan (Fan 1995: 425). The new 'northeastern region' comprises three provinces that refer to the PRC's traditional industrial belt: Liaoning, Jilin and Heilongjiang, which are the focus of economic recovery strategies. The eastern economic region refers to the economically developed municipalities of Beijing, Tianjin and Shanghai, and the provinces of Hebei, Shandong, Jiangsu, Zhejiang, Fujian, Guangdong and Hainan. The central region refers to the inland developing provinces of Shanxi, Henan, Anhui, Hubei, Hunan and Jiangxi. The western region comprises the municipality of Chongqing and 11 developing provinces and autonomous regions: Inner Mongolia, Shaanxi, Gansu, Ningxia, Qinghai, Xinjiang, Sichuan, Guangxi, Guizhou, Yunnan and Tibet.

Spatial analyses of China's internal migration flows indicate that people have predominantly migrated from poor and rural inland provinces to developing cities on the eastern seaboard. According to data from the 2010 Sixth National Population Census of the PRC, around 30 per cent of internal migrants come from the inland provinces of Anhui, Henan and Sichuan (National Bureau of Statistics of China 2012). The top three destinations for inter-provincial migration are Shanghai and the provinces of Guangdong and Zhejiang.

Such population flows may alter eventually, along with the expansion of the PRC's western development strategy. In October 2000, the State Council issued a circular which marked the formal launch of the campaign to 'Open-up the West' (*Xibudakaifa*) (Goodman 2004; Guowuyuan 2000). The policy, as affirmed by the Eleventh and Twelfth Five-Year Guidelines for National Economic and Social Development for 2006–2015, aims to offset the worsening regional inequity between eastern and western regions by promoting rapid development in China's western regions (National People's Congress 2006, 2011).

Economic data illustrate the recent shift in growth from the developed eastern regions towards more developing regions in the central, western and northern regions of China, which occurred in tandem with government stimulus policies in the aftermath of the Global Financial Crisis and the broader western development strategy. Between 2001 and 2007, the gross domestic product (GDP) growth in China's eastern cities and provinces averaged 13.1 per cent per annum compared with 11.8 for the northeastern region, 11.9 per cent for the central provinces, and 12.2 per cent for the western regions. Between 2008 and 2014, the GDP growth averaged 10.2 per cent per annum in the eastern cities and provinces compared with 10.9 for the northeastern region, 11.5 per cent in the central provinces and 12.4 per cent in the western regions.[1]

Such growth will eventually impact on migration flows. Internal migration flows are expected to continue to be directed towards the eastern economic region, and especially the mega urban clusters of Beijing-Tianjin, Shanghai and Guangzhou. However, future migration is also expected to be directed towards the inland city of Wuhan (Hubei Province) and the emerging inland megacities of Kunming (Yunnan Province), Xi'an (Shaanxi Province), Urumqi (Xinjiang Uyghur Autonomous Region) and Harbin (Heilongjiang Province) (Gransow 2012: 3, 5; see Figure 7.1).

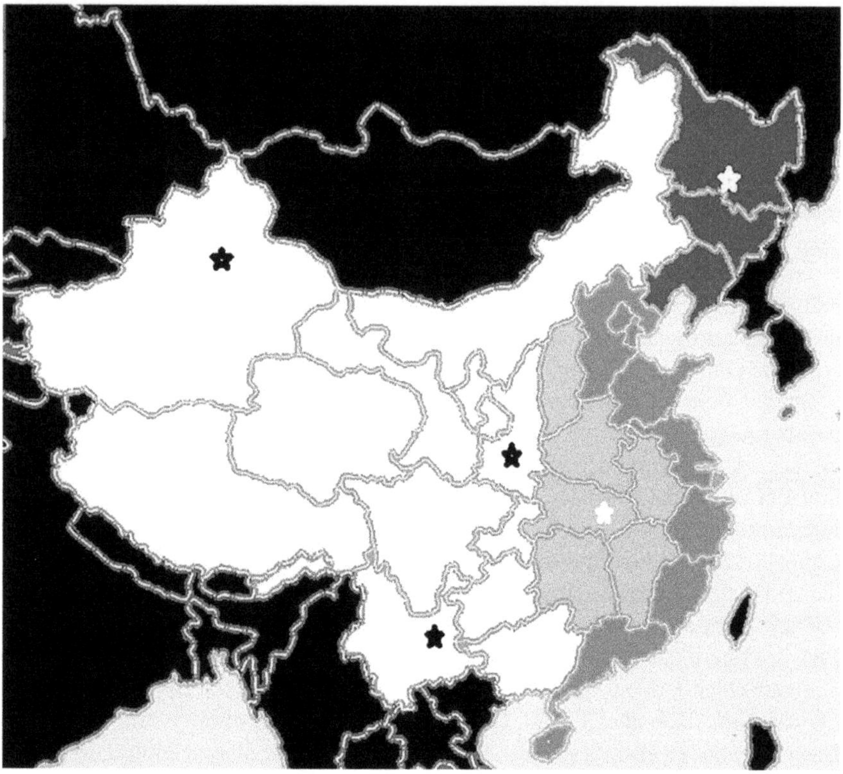

Figure 7.1 China's four main economic regions and developing megacities.

Key: white – western, underdeveloped region; light grey – central, developing region; grey – eastern, developed region; dark grey – northeastern region; stars – emerging megacities.

A major factor propelling internal population mobility is the continued income gap between urban and rural residents. The PRC has one of the largest urban-rural divides in the world in terms of living standards, according to a 2012 report by the China Academy of Social Sciences, a 'think tank'. The report claimed that the ratio of per capita disposable income between urban and rural residents in 2011 was 3.13:1 ('Income gap widens: report' 2012). In 2014, the per capita income of urban households was still 2.75 times higher than that of rural households (National Bureau of Statistics 2015). The per capita net income of rural residents was less than CNY 500 per month, but rural-to-urban migrants earned a monthly average of more than CNY 2,800 (Ibid.). Rural-born citizens thus often migrate to urban centres for work because they can earn substantially more money than they would earn by remaining in their hometown.

However, many rural-to-urban migrant workers are 'pushed' into relatively 'poor' employment choices by their limited educational background (Wong, Li and Song 2007: 33). Data from the 2010 Census reveal that more men than women migrate for work; around 114 men compared to 100 women, which is higher than the gendered breakdown of the population of 105 women to 100 men (National Bureau of Statistics of China 2012). The 2000 Census indicated that 88 per cent of rural-to-urban migrants had not completed high school – 64 per cent had a junior high school certificate and 24 per cent had only a primary school education (Ding Zhihong 2009). Data from the 2010 Census similarly suggest that more than 80 per cent of workers in the construction industry had not completed high school (National Bureau of Statistics of China 2012).

Rural-to-urban migration was associated for many years with a tolerance of any task work and poor working conditions, with migrants working in temporary or menial jobs described as 'dangerous, dirty and demeaning' (Kong 2016: 4). Rural-born migrants typically work in industries that are unattractive to urban residents, such as construction work and domestic housekeeping, or become self-employed as peddlers or owners of small businesses (Carrillo 2004; Gransow 2012; Solinger 1999a). In 2009, more than 90 per cent of rural-born migrants worked as production or service workers, compared to 35 per cent of urban residents (Xin Meng 2012). Only 3 per cent of rural-born migrants held a professional or managerial job compared to 31 per cent of urban residents. Generally speaking, therefore, rural-to-urban migrants are disadvantaged compared to urban residents.

New generations of rural-to-urban migrant workers are more 'preferential in the work they choose' and may move to urban centres for improved quality of life. Young migrant workers are more likely to switch jobs if they feel they are being underpaid, overworked, treated too harshly, and given limited opportunities for individual development (Hu Xiaochu 2012). They also increasingly relocate for 'fun', 'to be with friends', to have the 'freedom' to choose careers and sexual and life partners away from families, to experience the 'excitement' of city life as presented by media and returning migrants, and to obtain material goods and luxury items (Ibid.).

But one effect of such incitements is that many rural-born people are unwilling to complete or pay for schooling when urban job opportunities become available. This could entrench systemic inequality among certain migrant groups. Yet rural-to-urban migrant workers are considered to be at greater risk of contracting an STI, including HIV, than permanent residents of Chinese cities, largely as a result of structural inequality.

Rural-born migrants' HIV vulnerability

Rural-to-urban migrant labourers are viewed as more vulnerable to HIV infection than permanent rural and urban residents of China as a result of structural inequality, reflected in poor access to good education, employment and social services (Dai *et al.* 2015: 2; Sudhinaraset, Astone and Blum 2012: S72–3; Yang, Derlega and Luo 2007: 284). Relative poverty and limited education encourage many rural-born men to leave their native homes to engage in temporary work in factories and on construction sites in developing cities. Low wages and poor living conditions, often in the form of dormitories or campsites, mean that many such migrants leave their wives and partners behind in rural villages for extended periods of time, and only return home infrequently (Carrillo 2004: 17–19; Solinger 1999b: 15–23). Disrupted links to familial and stable sexual relationships, combined with anonymity, loneliness and financial difficulties, encourage some migrant workers to seek alternative sexual partners, potentially heightening their vulnerability to HIV infection (Dai *et al.* 2015: 2; Hayes 2010: 95; Li, Morrow and Kermode 2010: 383; Wu Junqing 2010: 415).

Numerous small-scale surveys of migrant workers' sexual behaviours conducted in the 2000s suggested that male migrants often engaged in unprotected sex with multiple partners, including sex workers. A 2002 survey of HIV risk behaviours among male migrant workers in Beijing, Nanjing and Shanghai, recruited over 1,300 men from community settings and over 450 men who had attended STI clinics (Wang *et al.* 2007: 58). It revealed that 10 per cent of men in the community group and nearly a third of the men in the clinic group had paid for sexual services, with 20 and 60 per cent having a history of STI, respectively. However, a third of the men from both groups reported that they did not like to use condoms. Between 14–19 per cent had used condoms in their last three sexual encounters and at least 25 per cent did not know how to use condoms correctly (Ibid.: 65–6). A 2005 survey of 163 male migrant workers aged between 18–35 years in Sichuan Province similarly found that 30 per cent had had two or more partners and 20 per cent had paid for sex, but only 36 per cent had used a condom during the most recent sexual encounter with a sex worker (Li, Morrow and Kermode 2007: 1288). Media reports further suggested that male rural-to-urban migrant workers regularly visited cheap hair and foot-massage salons, which are known venues for commercial sex (Wang Caili 2006). Such surveys and reports concluded that providing AIDS education to migrant workers should be a public health priority.

More recent and larger-scale studies indicate that rural-to-urban migrant workers have access to information about AIDS. In 2008, the CDC provided AIDS education to more than 43,000 migrant workers aged between 18 and 49 years, working in Beijing and 12 provincial capital cities across China (Lü Ke *et al.* 2010: 157). A post-intervention survey unsurprisingly found that between 50 and 85 per cent of the respondents had a basic knowledge of AIDS and modes of HIV transmission (Ibid.: 158). This is an expected result given that monitoring typically follows shortly after the delivery of education materials to priority populations (see also He and Wu 2013). The median level of knowledge for the survey was 74 per cent, which met the national target of 70 per cent as stipulated in China's second Action Plan (2006–2010) for the Containment and Prevention of HIV/AIDS (Guowuyuan 2006c).

But follow-up studies suggest that rural-born migrant workers may be aware of HIV transmission routes and still fail to use condoms consistently. A 2010 survey of more than 17,000 migrant workers in Zhejiang Province found that 76 per cent were aware that HIV could be prevented by using condoms (Pan *et al.* 2013: 3). However, of the 11,500 sexually active respondents, 51 per cent had never used condoms when engaging in sexual intercourse with spouses or regular sexual partners, and 74 per cent and 60 per cent reported inconsistent condoms use when engaging in sexual intercourse with non-regular partners and sex workers respectively (Ibid.). A 2010–2011 survey of 2,000 migrant workers aged around 20 years in Guangdong Province similarly revealed that 60 per cent of the respondents had engaged in sexual intercourse, and 11 per cent had had sexual experiences with multiple partners, but only 63 per cent of the respondents who had engaged in sexual intercourse had used condoms (He Xiaohong *et al.* 2013: 84). This apparent reluctance to internalize and act on AIDS communication may be correlated with age, as other surveys found that migrant workers aged between 40 and 59 years engaged in unprotected sexual intercourse more often than those aged between 20 and 29 years (Yang *et al.* 2009: 428; see also Dai *et al.* 2015: 4–6).

Low rates of condom use are also reported in surveys of the sexual behaviours of female migrant workers. A 2007 survey of married female migrants in Yancheng City, Jiangsu Province, showed that only 15 per cent of more than 500 respondents said that their spouses had used condoms and could afford condoms (Yin Qin *et al.* 2009: 149). Rural-born women typically use intrauterine devices for contraception, which are provided free of charge to married women of childbearing age through family planning services. But intrauterine devices offer women no protection against HIV infection from partners who have engaged in unprotected sex with other people (Chang Mingxiu 2009: 532–5; Peng and Chen 2013: 87).

Surveys of the sexual behaviours of unmarried female migrant workers similarly underscore low rates of condom use. According to a 2008 survey of 850 unmarried female migrants aged between 19 and 29 years in Qingdao City, Shandong Province, over 60 per cent of the respondents had engaged in sexual intercourse, some with multiple partners, but only 25 per cent of those respondents had experience with condoms, and less than 12 per cent said their partners always used condoms (Zhang Yuhan *et al.* 2010: 963). An investigation based on migrant population data from Hangzhou City, Zhejiang Province, in 2010, found that only 18 per cent of migrant women had experienced sex with condoms (Peng and Chen 2013: 88). A 2012 survey of nearly 6,000 migrant workers in Shanghai, with both genders roughly equally represented, revealed a low proportion of condom use among both genders; nearly 60 per cent had never used condoms during sexual encounters (Dai *et al.* 2015: 6).

Adding to the perceived potential of internal migration to contribute to the spread of HIV across China, rural-born migrant workers reportedly seldom seek STI and HIV testing and treatment services at government-run hospitals because of financial concerns and fear of what might happen should they test positive (Wang *et al.* 2010: 902). Despite policy changes designed to improve social services for internal migrants, many migrant workers are not entitled to subsidized medical welfare in areas other than their place of household registration (Pan *et al.* 2013: 2). A study of approximately 4,000 migrant workers in southern China revealed that only 7 per cent of respondents with symptoms of an STI had been to a government-run clinic to get treatment. The others had done nothing, bought non-prescription medicine, or had gone to private clinics offering cheap and often unlicensed medical services (Wang Wenjie *et al.* 2009: 86).

Rural-born migrant workers living with HIV are also often unable to access free antiretroviral drugs, even though access to such drugs is mandated by a policy known as the 'Four Frees and One Care' (*simianyiguanhuai*). The policy was introduced in 2003 as a trial in selected areas of China and adopted as a national policy in 2006 (Guowuyuan 2006a: Article 44; Thompson 2004). For example, in Beijing, a major destination for migrant workers, free antiretroviral drugs were only made available to migrant workers in 2010, and then only to migrant workers with a temporary residential certificate (Li Guiying *et al.* 2011: 687). These restrictions aim to spread the burden of cost for AIDS prevention and care across local governments. However, many migrants do not possess a temporary resident card, which means they may remain 'outside of' the system for HIV testing and treatment. Rural-born migrants working in major cities such as Beijing often do not apply for a temporary resident card. A card costs money, it requires original documentation that must be obtained in person from local governments in one's place of birth, and it is chiefly used to obtain a driver's licence or to purchase property (Li and Chui 2011: 13). The Thirteenth Five-Year Guidelines for National Economic and Social Development (2016–2020), and China's Action Plan for the Containment and Prevention of HIV and AIDS (2016–2020), therefore propose improving migrant access to subsidized testing and treatment services for HIV and AIDS (Guowuyuan bangongting 2017; National People's Congress 2016b).

The findings of surveys of migrant workers' sexual behaviours are routinely translated into calls for more, improved and broader public health interventions. Positive evaluations of AIDS education for rural-born migrant workers suggest that the provision of such education leads to increased knowledge of STI and modes of HIV transmission. After analyzing 20 reports on interventions involving migrant workers across different parts of China, He Lin and Wu Zunyou (2013) found that migrant worker knowledge of HIV transmission and prevention had improved. Post-intervention testing indicated that migrant workers knew that HIV can be transmitted sexually and that using condoms correctly can prevent HIV transmission. He and Wu also found that the reported use by migrant workers of condoms when last having sex with sex workers had increased.

Negative evaluations, such as studies that show that migrants are aware of modes of HIV transmission but still fail to use condoms consistently, generate calls for additional health interventions supported by improved policy frameworks and research methodologies. Proposed improvements include expanding policy frameworks to support large-scale health interventions into migrant workplaces and communities, focusing on migrant-sending rather than migrant-receiving locations to ensure that AIDS education also reaches spouses and other family members, developing better survey and condom-use questions, and conducting in-depth interviews with migrant workers about their sexual attitudes and practices (Dai *et al.* 2015; Pan *et al.* 2013; Zhuang *et al.* 2012: 5). They also include calls to popularize HIV prevention messages through broadcast and social media in easy-to-read or visually accessible formats that are regularly updated and provided more frequently, in order to reach broad sectors of the Chinese population, including new migrants (Li *et al.* 2009). Hence the following sections look first at the development of AIDS-related policy frameworks and then at public service advertising focused on migrant workers.

Evolving policy frameworks

China's Medium- and Long-Term Strategic Plan for HIV/AIDS Prevention and Control (1998–2010) mentioned internal migration, along with the underground sex industry and drug addiction, as a potential driver of AIDS (Guowuyuan 1998). Although the document urged government authorities to intensify the work of AIDS prevention, it did not specify what measures they should take with regard to internal migrants (Guowuyuan 1998: Section 1). China's first Action Plan (2001–2005) for the Containment and Prevention of HIV/AIDS outlined major plans for controlling the collection and sale of blood plasma products, and for funding and developing the PRC's AIDS response with international cooperation. It also recommended expanding AIDS communication, in part by displaying educational materials at transport hubs, and thus by implication in locations frequented by mobile populations (Guowuyuan bangongting 2001: Section 3, Item 2). However, the document only mentioned one specific migrant group – Chinese citizens returning from work or holidays overseas (Ibid.).

Internal migrants (*guonei liudong renkou*) were first listed as an active priority population for AIDS intervention programs in China's second Action Plan (2006–2010) for the Containment and Prevention of HIV/AIDS (Guowuyuan 2006c). Among other goals, the document urged local government authorities to promote education about AIDS prevention, testing and treatments for rural-to-urban migrants, with the aim of reaching 70 per cent of the migrant population by the end of 2007 and 80 per cent by the end of 2010 (Ibid.: Section 2). It advocated expanding AIDS communication in the broadcast media and in public spaces (residential communities, shopping centres, transport hubs, parks, hotels, tourism spots, etc.) (Ibid.: Section 3). It also recommended providing AIDS education in schools and workplaces and as part of occupational work trainings for rural-to-urban migrant workers. The latter recommendations follow UN suggestions that HIV infections mostly occur in productive people aged between 15 and 49 years, and 'lack of awareness and understanding of HIV, resulting in fear and negative attitudes among employees and managers, can cause workplace conflict as well as stigmatization, discrimination and mismanagement of HIV-positive employees' (Asian Business Coalition on AIDS 2002: 1). But they also point to the inclusion of private employers and members of residential community organizations in the work of AIDS prevention.

China's third Action Plan (2011–2015) for the Containment and Prevention of HIV/AIDS advocated scaling up the country's AIDS response and listed internal migrant workers, youth, women and key populations as the main focus of HIV prevention work (Guowuyuan bangongting 2012). The plan aimed to reduce the number of new HIV infections and control the number of people living with HIV at around 1.2 million people by 2015, in keeping with the UN vision of 'Zero new HIV infections. Zero discrimination. Zero AIDS-related deaths' (UNAIDS

2010). To do so, it noted that rates of new HIV infection had stabilized, access to testing and treatment had improved, and people with HIV were living longer due to the wider availability of better medical treatment and care services (Guowuyuan bangongting 2012). However, it added that AIDS prevention presented new challenges, with the prevalence of new infections from sexual transmission rising among certain sectors of the population. It therefore recommended that 80 per cent of rural residents, 85 per cent of internal migrants and women aged between 15 and 49 years, and 90 per cent of key populations and adolescents should have a working knowledge of AIDS transmission routes and prevention methods by 2016 (Ibid. Section 2, Item 1). Similar targets are outlined in the fourth Action Plan for 2016–2020 (Guowuyuan bangongting 2017).

Among other directives, the third and fourth Action Plans recommend using a wide range of government, private, community and technological resources to enhance the work of HIV prevention in migrant workplaces and communities, including: family planning departments; state-owned and private businesses; Party-affiliated mass organizations, which act as a medium for conveying policies to the public and ensuring their local implementation; community, fundraising and volunteer organizations; and the Internet. They urge government departments and businesses to provide AIDS-education materials and condoms in educational institutions and workplaces, and during health and safety and vocational skills training. They also recommend using public figures and people affected by AIDS in extensive public service advertising designed to popularize knowledge of HIV prevention, and reduce the stigma attached to people living with HIV.

The National Population and Family Planning Commission (NPFPC) issued a series of policy documents between 2009 and 2011 that supports some of these goals, by encouraging local authorities to adopt a more inclusive approach towards service provision for migrants. In 2009, the Regulations on Family Planning Work for Migrant Populations (*liudongrenkou jihuashengyu gongzuo tiaoli*) introduced a major change in the work of family planning authorities (Guowuyuan 2009). The regulations stipulated that the authorities where migrants *worked* rather than the authorities in their *place of birth* should be responsible for migrant-related family planning work (Ibid.: Item 4). In 2010, the NPFPC, the Central Public Security Comprehensive Management Commission, the Ministry of Finance, and the Ministry of Human Resources and Social Security, jointly promulgated a document on improving the provision of family planning services for migrant workers in urban centres. The document, titled Guidelines on Innovating the Management and Provision of Services to Migrant Populations: Piloting Equal Family Planning Service Provision, suggested that urban authorities should treat migrant workers as urban residents for the purposes of family planning work (*Guanyu chuangxin liudongrenkou fuwu guanli tizhi, tuijin liudongrenkou jihuashengyu jiben gonggongfuwu jundenghua shidian gongzuo de zhidao yijian*) (Li Xiaohong 2010: 2). In 2011, the NPFPC implemented a program called National Family Planning: Providing Nationwide Public Services and Free Contraceptives (*Quanguo jihuashengyu yaoju mianfei fafang gonggongfuwu quanfugai*) (Bai Yunting 2011: 1).

These policy changes have enabled rural migrants in urban areas to access family planning services such as government-subsidized condoms, irrespective of whether they have local residence permits or not. Condoms of different quality and cost are readily available online and in supermarkets, convenience stores and adult goods shops across China. Vending machines have been installed in urban public spaces, including shopping centres, that provide free condoms to people aged over 18 who swipe an identification card, irrespective of their residential status (Wu and Shi 2012: 2). Media reports suggest that such services are being used, with stocks of condoms being depleted daily in vending machines located in areas where migrants work, for example, wholesale markets in the city of Nanjing ('Shua "erdaizheng" ke mianfei ling anquantao' 2012).

Municipal authorities have used online and other methods to facilitate the distribution of government-subsidized condoms. Shanghai family planning authorities designed a smartphone application that provides users with the telephone numbers, service hours and addresses, of locations where free condoms are available (Wang Hongyi 2013). Beijing family planning authorities developed an iPhone application that enables users to order 30 free condoms online every two months. These are delivered by courier for the cost of CNY 1 (USD 0.15) to areas within the city's fifth ring road and CNY 2 to areas outside of that ring road ('Free condom' n.d.).

Although the main goal of providing condoms in such contexts is to curb China's high rate of unwanted pregnancies and subsequent abortions, it contributes to the normalization of condom use and HIV prevention. Hence altered policy frameworks and new technologies have improved public access to inexpensive condoms. They have also led to the expansion of AIDS communication focused on migrant workplaces and communities, in accordance with national AIDS action plans.

AIDS education for migrant workers

The PRC's first national AIDS education campaign focused on rural-to-urban migrant workers was launched in late 2005, and was preceded by broader media coverage of issues related to internal migrants and AIDS prevention. An editorial published in the state-run *Guangming Daily*, in January 2005, expressed concern about the limited nature of free condom distribution for migrant workers (Yan Yang 2005). The editor noted that migrant construction workers in Beijing had readily taken free condoms from health workers during World AIDS Day activities in 2004, whereas activities conducted on university campuses had met with a lukewarm reception from students. The editor concluded that migrant workers as a vulnerable population should be the first priority of public health interventions (Ibid.).

In March 2005, an article in the *Beifang Chenbao* (*North China Morning News*) stated that a medical doctor, Sun Yunhuan, had written a letter to Premier Wen Jiabao recommending that the government should provide cheap accommodations for migrant workers, so that families could remain together when people with rural household registration were working in the cities (Wang Shiming 2007, 2010). Sun said that she had become concerned about the prevalence of STI among migrant workers after working in a Liaoning community hospital, adding that long-term separation from family made migrants vulnerable to engaging in risky sexual behaviours. The letter attracted widespread discussion on the Internet, turning Sun Yunhuan into an 'overnight celebrity' who was voted as Sina.com's 'Person of the Month' for April 2005 (Ibid.).

The National Rural-to-Urban Migrant Workers' AIDS Prevention Education Project (hereinafter the 2005 Project) was launched around World AIDS Day, and preceded by an implementation plan issued on 21 November 2005. The plan was jointly released by the State Council AIDS Working Committee Office with the Publicity Department of the CCP Central Committee; the Ministries of Agriculture, Construction, Health, and Labour and Social Security; the NPFPC; the State Administration for Industry and Commerce; the All-China Federation of Trade Unions; the Central Committee of the Communist Youth League; the All-China Women's Federation; and the All-China Federation of Industry and Commerce (Quanguo nongmingong yufang aizibing xuanchuan jiaoyu gongcheng shishi fang'an 2005). This institutional cooperation reflects the complexity of administering AIDS prevention measures for China's massive migrant population.

The implementation plan outlined the various responsibilities of different ministries, government departments and Party-affiliated mass organizations with regard to promoting AIDS awareness among migrant workers (Ibid.). The Ministry of Health had to provide AIDS education materials and coordinate peer training sessions for members of relevant government departments and Party organizations. China's state-controlled media were to broadcast or publish at least 10 hours or 10 items of AIDS education during major holidays and agricultural planting/harvesting seasons. Departments associated with the Ministry of Agriculture were obliged to provide migrant workers with training about HIV prevention as part of vocational skills programs. Departments associated with the Ministry of Construction (now the Ministry of Housing and Urban-Rural Development) had to distribute AIDS awareness and HIV prevention booklets to migrant workers on construction sites, and conduct related on-site training and peer education. Departments associated with the Ministry of Labour and Social Security were required to offer migrant workers at least two hours of AIDS education as part of pre-job training programs. The NPFPC was charged with distributing a letter, AIDS booklet and two free condoms, to migrant workers returning home to undertake seasonal agricultural work and for the New Year holidays. Departments associated with the State Administration for Industry and Commerce were directed to provide AIDS awareness programs for migrant workers in private enterprises at least twice a year (Ibid.).

Party-affiliated mass organizations had to extend AIDS education for migrant workers at the local level. The All-China Federation of Industry and Commerce was instructed to organize real-estate developers and managers of beauty, hair and massage salons to provide AIDS education to people working in the construction industry and in service-industry sectors such as beauty, hair and massage salons.

These industries employ rural-to-urban migrant workers, and are also associated with the demand for and supply of commercial sexual services. The All-China Federation of Trade Unions had to provide workplace AIDS education for migrant workers and to support workers living with HIV. The Central Committee of the Communist Youth League was to coordinate AIDS education for migrant youths through existing training programs for young workers. The All-China Women's Federation was instructed to make migrant women a focus of its national 'Healthy Families, Preventing AIDS' project (*yufang aizibing jiankang quanjiaren*) (Ibid.).

In December 2005, the Ministry of Construction demonstrated its commitment to the implementation plan by issuing a Notice on Doing AIDS Prevention Work in the Construction Industry (*Guanyu zuohao jianshehangye aizibing fangzhi gongzuo de tongzhi*) (Jianshebu bangongting 2005). The Notice instructed construction enterprises to include AIDS education in work-related training courses. As many construction sites employed untrained staff, and offered basic skills-training for workers, the inclusion of AIDS education in vocational training programs aimed to reach large sectors of the male migrant workforce. China's migrant construction workers usually reside collectively in temporary and rudimentary accommodations provided by their employers, with behavioural surveys indicating that they often visit sex establishments after work hours. Hence, the Notice instructed construction enterprises to build onsite activity rooms with entertainment facilities for workers. Companies were specifically instructed to provide televisions, playing cards, books and magazines for migrant construction workers, so as to encourage 'healthy' leisure activities after work (Jianshebu bangongting 2005).

In January 2007, the Ministry of Labour and Social Security launched a project called AIDS Education in the Workplace (*Zhongguo aizibing gongzuochangsuo jiaoyu*) (Zheng Yong 2007). Funded by the US Department of Labor, the project was directed at migrant workers and implemented in three AIDS-affected provinces: Anhui, Guangdong and Yunnan. It aimed to help migrant workers and their family members learn about modes of HIV transmission, reduce risk-related behaviours, and reduce workplace discrimination against people living with HIV (Ibid.: 7).

On 29 November 2007, the Ministry of Agriculture launched a spin-off project at the Xinfadi agriculture goods wholesale market in Beijing, called the Red Ribbon in Village Homes Project (*Hongsidai jincunruhu gongcheng*). The red ribbon is an international symbol of awareness and support for those living with HIV, and has been associated with AIDS activities in China since the late 1990s when the Beijing Ditan Hospital established a Red Ribbon House. The Village Homes Project was launched at the market during a ceremony with representatives from the Ministry of Agriculture and the State Council AIDS Committee, and was attended by hundreds of market stall keepers (Wang Xiaojing 2007: 2). The Xinfadi market attracts around 4,000 stall keepers, chiefly rural-to-urban migrant workers, and an average of 50,000 customers per day.

The Ministry of Agriculture also distributed a series of low literacy cartoon-style booklets focused on AIDS education for migrant workers in 2009 with funding from the China Global Fund AIDS Program, the China HIV/AIDS Roadmap

Tactical Support Project and the National HIV/AIDS Prevention Mobilization Project. These booklets provide basic knowledge about AIDS and prevention methods through the use of simple stories with pictures.

One such booklet, 'Picturing AIDS Prevention' ('*Hua'shuo fang'ai*), explains the main modes of HIV transmission, how to prevent infection, how to use and dispose of condoms safely, and how to access testing and treatment services (Zhongguo nongxuehui 2009). It notes that HIV is a problem in rural areas, which is related to lack of knowledge and misconceptions about HIV transmission. For example, it suggests that rural residents incorrectly think that HIV is transmitted through 'outside influences' (mosquitoes, coughing and contact with foreigners), rather than through sexual contact between local people (male-female and male-male), sharing non-sterile injecting equipment and mother-to-child transmission (Ibid.: 4–5; see also Li, Morrow and Kermode 2007: 1290). The booklet thus aims to counter perceptions that AIDS is a disease that affects non-local people. It also contains information about how to reduce the risk of contracting HIV, for example, by using condoms, being faithful and using sterile injecting equipment.

The booklet also provides a positive, anti-discriminatory tale about 'Xiao Zhang', a handsome, young migrant construction site worker who has returned to the countryside after learning that he is HIV-positive. Although the booklet does not explicitly mention the source of Zhang's infection, it implies that he has contracted HIV through engagement in unprotected commercial sex. The first image at the top-left-hand corner of Figure 7.2 shows Zhang with two young women in a venue that provides massage services. The image at the top-right-hand corner of Figure 7.2 shows Zhang with a medical doctor. Zhang, who wishes to donate blood, is informed that he is not an eligible blood donor because preliminary testing has revealed that he is HIV-positive. The image at the bottom-left-hand corner of Figure 7.2 shows a dispirited looking Zhang asking himself: 'How did I get such a terrible disease?' (*Wo zenme huide zheme kepa de bing ne?*). An image in Zhang's head shows him in bed with a woman and thus suggests from sexual transmission. In the image at the bottom-right-hand corner of Figure 7.2, the doctor tells Zhang that HIV is not as terrible as he thinks and that antiretroviral drug treatment is very effective [in terms of reducing HIV-related illnesses and death].

After Xiao Zhang returns to his rural home, and contrary perhaps to reader expectations, his life improves; in other words, the story provides an example of someone living with HIV and having a successful career and family life. Zhang goes on to run a flourishing small business, gets married and has a child. His wife is aware of his HIV-positive status, and hence they use condoms when having sex. They also seek medical assistance to become pregnant and have a child. The overall message is clear: it is possible to live with HIV and to have a normal social and family life without harming others. The story concludes with Zhang becoming a peer educator for AIDS awareness and HIV prevention in rural areas.

The story of Xiao Zhang provides easy-to-understand information about modes of HIV transmission and prevention, and encourages more positive approaches to people living with HIV. Xiao Zhang is presented as a functioning, capable person with a business and a family who publicly admits that he is living with HIV. This is a marked departure from early negative constructions of AIDS in China

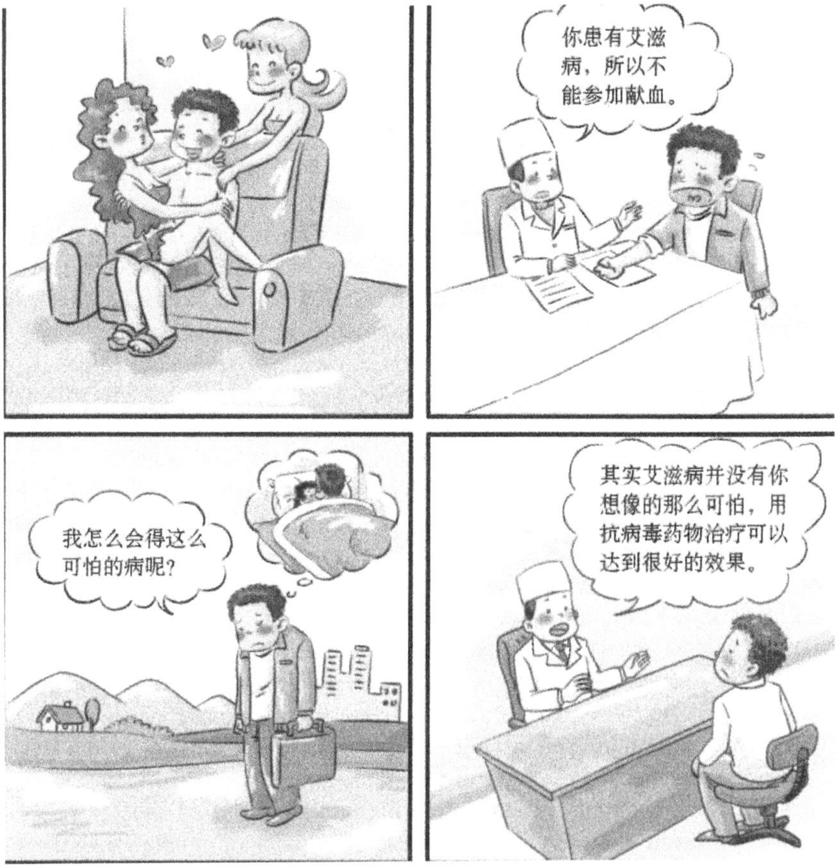
你患有艾滋病，所以不能参加献血。
我怎么会得这么可怕的病呢？
其实艾滋病并没有你想像的那么可怕，用抗病毒药物治疗可以达到很好的效果。

Figure 7.2 Zhang's story.

Source: Zhongguo nongxuehui [China Association of Agricultural Science Societies] (2009) '*Hua' shuo fang'ai* [Picturing AIDS Prevention], Beijing: Zhongguo Nongye Kexue Jishu Chubanshe, p. 54; reproduced with permission from the chief editors Niu Wenyi, Sun Zhe and Wang Chaoying.

as a 'terrifying disease existing mainly outside the country', which encouraged people to fear people living with HIV (Hood 2012: 127, 129). In other sections, the booklet presents 'incorrect', discriminatory ways of behaving towards people living with HIV and AIDS, for example, shunning them and refusing them service at hospitals and in restaurants (Zhongguo nongxuehui 2009: 44). It also advises readers that people living with HIV and AIDS should be treated with respect and have the right to legal protection from discriminatory treatment.

The Chinese Communist Youth League has facilitated the distribution of such materials through an initiative called the Youth Red Ribbon (*Qingchun hongsidai*). The original project, which started in 2002, aimed to increase AIDS awareness among youth to support the education of children in AIDS-affected areas, and promote AIDS awareness among rural youth populations, by training volunteer university students to disseminate AIDS education materials among youth in general. At the launch of an iteration of this project in April 2013 at the Beijing Forestry University, Wang Shuyan, Secretary of the Central Committee of the Communist Youth League, urged university students to volunteer to distribute AIDS education materials and conduct awareness activities in residential and migrant worker communities (Wang Shikun 2013: 6). This was part of a 2013 project theme known as the 'three enters' (*sanjin*); that is, 'entering campuses, construction sites and communities' (Ibid.). Additional initiatives were conducted in 2014, with volunteers from the All-China Women's Federation and more than 150 tertiary education institutions distributing 'Red Ribbon Health Packages' to migrants in workplaces and residential communities (National Health and Family Planning Commission of the PRC 2015: 12). These initiatives highlight the ongoing expansion of the work of AIDS education in China through Party-affiliated mass organizations, peer education and the developing medium of government-organized volunteering, in accordance with national AIDS action plans.

In summary, numerous initiatives involving cooperation between multiple government departments, Party-affiliated mass organizations and volunteers have been organized since 2005 to raise the AIDS awareness of rural-to-urban migrant workers. These initiatives involve the expansion of vocational trainings to include AIDS education. They also involve the provision of condoms and low literacy AIDS education materials in workplaces and residential areas where migrant workers are concentrated. These materials provide both basic information about HIV prevention, testing and treatments, and counter popular misconceptions about HIV transmission routes, and provide positive stories of people living with HIV.

AIDS communication focused on rural-to-urban migrant workers has also expanded. Such communication is intensified during holidays and agricultural planting/harvesting seasons, when hundreds of millions of people travel across the country. Apart from media publicity in specific locations, it includes celebrity-endorsed government advertising on broadcast, digital and social media.

Celebrity-endorsed AIDS communication

The use of celebrities in government health communication is a relatively recent phenomenon in the PRC. To the extent that mainland Chinese celebrities have been involved in AIDS awareness activities, they have typically acted as image ambassadors for PRC government and United Nations initiatives. The use of celebrity advocacy highlights a shift towards engaging citizens in sustained behavioural change to achieve AIDS-related policy goals through the indirect means of public service advertising, as opposed to interventions conducted through Party-affiliated mass organizations in workplaces and local communities.

Actor Pu Cunxin is widely credited as being the first A-list celebrity to be involved in a PSA about AIDS produced and distributed in mainland China (Hood 2010: 88–9). Pu, a Communist Party member, became an official advocate (*xuanchuanyuan*) for HIV prevention for the Ministry of Health in 2000, when he featured in Chinese-language poster and television PSAs for World AIDS Day (Ibid.; Li Ying 2000: 10–11). The poster promoted male responsibility for HIV prevention as part of UNAIDS' two-year campaign theme of Men Make a Difference, stating: 'Men have an unshirkable responsibility for helping to prevent AIDS' (*Yufang aizibing, nanshi zewupangdai*). A television PSA titled 'Care For, Don't Discriminate Against People Living with HIV and AIDS' (*guan'ai, bu qishi aizibingbingren*) showed Pu visiting an AIDS patient in hospital and rearranging the man's pillows to make him more comfortable (Ibid.). The PSA clearly aimed to counter public perceptions of people living with AIDS as a population who had to be shunned or quarantined to prevent further contamination.

Guidelines on AIDS prevention issued by the Publicity Department of the CCP Central Committee and the Ministry of Health in 2004 recommended enlisting public figures, and people affected by HIV and AIDS, in public service advertising (Zhonggong zhongyang xuanchuanbu, weishengbu 2004). The expressed aim was threefold. First, it would help to prevent the spread of HIV through broad publicity about modes of transmission. Second, it would reduce AIDS-related discrimination, create support for affected people and encourage public uptake of testing and treatment services. Third, it would generate public support for organizations working with people affected by HIV and AIDS.

In May 2006, the State Council AIDS Working Committee Office held a meeting to discuss the role of celebrities in HIV and AIDS prevention, which was attended by actor Pu Cunxin and soprano Peng Liyuan – the wife of PRC President Xi Jinping. Peng Liyuan became an official advocate for AIDS prevention for the Ministry of Health in 2006, and was named as a Goodwill Ambassador for Tuberculosis and HIV/AIDS for the World Health Organization in 2011 (Liu Na 2011; see also Hood 2015a). The May 2006 meeting of the State Council AIDS Working Committee Office discussed how best to use the public visibility of celebrities to extend the work of HIV prevention. That meeting was later cited as an example of progress in a joint report by the State Council AIDS Working Committee Office and UN Theme Group on AIDS in China (2007: 15). Peng Liyuan featured in a PSA produced by China Central Television in December 2014, which showed the first lady touching and hugging rural children living with AIDS, and asking people to care for children affected by AIDS instead of shunning them ('Meiyou qishi yongyuan zai yiqi guan'ai aizibing ertong gongyi guanggao' 2014). Her involvement signifies central government support for AIDS prevention and anti-discrimination measures in China and globally, albeit by focusing on children as 'innocent victims'.

Actor Wang Baoqiang, a migrant construction worker and rags-to-riches film star, has featured in PSAs explicitly designed to promote HIV prevention and anti-discrimination messages among male rural-to-urban workers. Born in a village in Hebei Province, Wang left home as a young boy to study martial arts at the Shaolin Temple in Henan Province in 1992, inspired by the film *Shaolin Temple* which stars the internationally renowned Chinese actor Jet Li (Li, J. 2013; on Jet Li, see Farquhar 2010). At that time, the Shaolin Temple was not as commercialized as it is today, and Wang would have studied there cheaply. Wang subsequently went to work on a construction site in Beijing, where he also regularly queued outside the front gate of the Beijing Film Studio, hoping to find work as a film extra. He was later chosen to star in a low-budget but award-winning 2002 movie about the mining industry called *Blind Shaft* (Li Jianmin 2003: 64–5). Wang Baoqiang went on to become a household name in 2006–2007 as a village boy-turned-soldier called Xu Sanduo, the lead character in a cult DVD series called *Soldiers Sortie* (*Shibing tuji*) (Kang Honglei 2006).

Wang Baoqiang became a celebrity advocate for issues affecting migrant workers in 2008. He sang songs written for migrant workers on CCTV's Spring Festival Gala – a Chinese New Year special and the PRC's most-watched television show (Zhai Shanliang 2008). In March 2008, he was appointed as a spokesperson for the Migrant Worker Assistance Fund (*Nongmingong yuanzhu jijin*) in Shanghai, which is linked to the Chinese Red Cross Foundation. He subsequently made appeals in Beijing for donations for cataract patients ('Wang Baoqiang chuxi gongyi huodong mengyan tiyan mangren shenghuo' 2008).

In 2008, Wang Baoqiang also became a spokesperson for an AIDS education project called Hometown Fellows Help Hometown Fellows (*laoxiang bang laoxiang*), involving domestic and international and public and private collaborations (International Labour Organization Country Office for China and Mongolia 2008). The project was coordinated by the International Labour Organization, in partnership with the PRC's Ministry of Human Resources and Social Security, the State Council AIDS Working Committee Organization, and 19 large-scale enterprises in the construction, mining and transport sectors in Chinese provinces most affected by HIV. It aimed to tap into migrant social networks to deliver AIDS education in the workplace, work-related accommodations and nearby entertainment and leisure venues, in accordance with UNAIDS' directives and China's action plans.

Wang starred in a 7-minute video PSA directed by the award-winning director Gu Changwei, called *Never Abandon, Never Give Up*, which aims to counter discrimination against migrant workers living with HIV by providing visual messages communicating that HIV is not transmitted through general physical contact (Gu Changwei 2008). That message was delivered using the concept of hometown fellowship and 'migrant voices'. This approach turned on the understanding that rural-to-urban migrants typically have strong social bonds based on common provincial origin, which is potentially influential in terms of changing attitudes and behaviours (UNAIDS 2009b). In contrast, migrants often hold negative perceptions of government health officials, company managers and migrant-receiving communities, and hence may be less inclined to accept anti-discriminatory messages from them.

Released in November 2008, the PSA was broadcast on Chinese television channels and shown on video-sharing websites such as Youku.com and Ku6.com, at factories, labour markets and vocational training centres, and on railway television networks (Gu Changwei 2008; Youku 2008). For example, starting in May 2009, the ILO and Mega-info Media, which runs the PRC's national railway station television network, screened the PSA for a period of three months to an estimated 40 million viewers in 500 stations in 450 cities across China (UNAIDS 2009b). Other reports suggest that the PSA was viewed by 50 million migrant workers (Leng Qifeng 2009). This example highlights the expansion of AIDS communication at transport hubs and other public spaces to include digital advertising.

Wang Baoqiang stars in the PSA as a rural-born migrant who has come to Beijing to visit a HIV-positive male migrant worker from his hometown, played by migrant-worker actor, Wang Zhenting, whose real-life HIV-positive status adds to the PSA's realism and anti-discriminatory messages. Wang Zhenting plays a construction worker stigmatized because he is living with HIV, which mirrors his real-life situation as China's first migrant worker to speak out publicly about his HIV-positive status and experience of discrimination from colleagues. In Wang Zhenting's words: 'No one wanted to work with me, eat with me or share a dormitory' (UNAIDS 2009b). The PSA's protagonist is similarly shunned by his work colleagues who are afraid of his HIV-positive status. However, the PSA shows Wang Baoqiang and Wang Zhenting hand-wrestling and dancing together, sharing food and towels, and dipping their heads in the same basin of water to see who can hold their breath the longest. Wang Baoqiang also delivers a speech in which he calls on construction-site workers, and hence male migrant workers in general, to care for rather than abandon their colleagues (brothers) living with HIV (Gu Changwei 2008).

These anti-discrimination messages were repeated on Wang Baoqiang's blog, which has more than 3.8 million visitors (Wang Baoqiang 2008). Shortly after the release of the PSA, Wang posted a blog titled 'Don't be scared of AIDS' (*Aizibing, ni bingbu kepa*), with photographs of Wang Baoqiang and Wang Zhenting dancing with their arms around each other. He encouraged 'fellow' migrant workers not to be afraid of AIDS, stating that 'the worse thing about AIDS is the human suffering caused by lack of understanding' [of its modes of transmission and how to prevent its spread].

The PRC's turn to celebrity advocacy highlights the use of new, broader-based communication in AIDS education. It demonstrates a shift towards communication that emphasizes both the domestically transmitted and manageable nature of HIV, as opposed to early representations of AIDS in China as an external and untreatable disease that could only be dealt with by quarantine (see Hood 2011). It also aims to reach large audiences, being delivered by entertainment celebrities, and distributed through television and social media.

The State Council has since issued notices and action plans promoting celebrity advocacy as a means to enhance public awareness of AIDS and create a more accepting social environment for people living with HIV and AIDS. The 2010 Notice on Strengthening the Work of Containing and Preventing AIDS (*Guowuyuan guanyu jinyibu jiaqiang aizibingfangzhi gongzuo de tongzhi guofa (2010) 48 hao*) states that promoting the work of AIDS prevention, and generating public support for people living with HIV, means reaching more audiences. It therefore recommends leveraging celebrity (Guowuyuan 2010: Section 2, Item 3). The use of famous people in 'easy-to-understand' PSAs about preventing AIDS is also promoted in China's two action plans for the containment and prevention of HIV and AIDS for 2011–2020 (Guowuyuan bangongting 2012, 2017). As this suggests, the use of diverse media and celebrity-endorsed messaging to raise public awareness of modes of HIV transmission and combat AIDS-related stigma will continue. In 2011, the PRC's official news agency, Xinhua, also partnered with UNAIDS to promote communication about HIV prevention globally ('UNAIDS and Xinhua' 2016).

Concluding remarks

Although official statistics indicate that the HIV prevalence among China's large internal population of rural-to-urban migrant workers is low, research aimed at 'knowing' the sexual behaviours of male migrant workers suggests that many such men engage in multiple and risky sexual intercourse, irrespective of whether they are single, married, divorced or widowed (He Xiaohong *et al.* 2013; Li, Morrow and Kermode 2007; Pan *et al.* 2013). Many of these men have limited education, precarious employment and reduced access to government-subsidized services in urban centres. These factors, when combined with social and institutional discrimination against people living with HIV, mean that many rural-to-urban migrant labourers do not use testing and treatment services, and therefore the prevalence of infection among certain sectors of this population may be higher than is documented.

Migrant workers are listed as a priority focus of HIV prevention work in China's actions plans for preventing AIDS and male migrants became a focus of HIV sentinel surveillance in 2009 (Wen *et al.* 2012: 79). The two action plans between 2006 and 2015 directed relevant government departments and employers to display AIDS education materials and provide condoms in workplaces, and also to make AIDS education a feature of vocational skills and health and safety trainings (Guowuyuan 2006c; Guowuyuan bangongting 2012). The ongoing nature of such activities is demonstrated by media reports of 'Red Ribbon' activities being held on-site for subway line construction workers in Wuhan City around World AIDS Day in 2016 ('"Hong sidai" qingxi nongmingong fang'ai zhishi zou jin gongdi' 2016). The expansion of such activities is further recommended in China's action plan for the containment and prevention of HIV/AIDS between 2016 and 2020, which proposes that 90 per cent of migrant workers should be equipped with basic knowledge of HIV prevention and access to testing and treatments (Guowuyuan bangongting 2017).

The action plans recommend using a wide range of government, private, community and technological resources to enhance the work of HIV prevention in migrant workplaces and communities, including family planning departments; state and private businesses; Party-affiliated mass organizations; community, fundraising and volunteer organizations; and the Internet. Policy documents issued by the National Health and Family Planning Commission (formerly the NPFPC) require local authorities to adopt a more inclusive approach to service provision for migrant workers. Among other services, this involves providing government-subsidized condoms through vending machines and online outlets in major urban centres.

AIDS communication focused on rural-to-urban migrant labourers also involves celebrity-fronted public service advertising. Celebrity-fronted PSAs offer informal and entertaining educational tools that large sectors of the population can access informally through broadcast, digital and social media, rather than referring to top-down medicalized health interventions focused on sex workers and men who have sex with men in discreet venues. They are also a novel attempt to combat prejudice and discrimination against migrant workers living with HIV in the Chinese context.

But the focus on rural-born migrant workers, a large population group that is already stereotyped as marginalized, second-class citizens, may reinforce the perception among urban residents of major cities that HIV attacks 'other and lesser people' (Jeffreys and Huang 2009: 167). This focus may encourage new forms of discrimination against rural-to-urban migrant labourers by presenting them as a sexually promiscuous and immoral group, when only a small proportion of such workers engage in risky and extramarital sexual behaviours. It may also reinforce the perception that HIV is not a problem for people migrating between Chinese cities to take up higher-paid work in government and corporate sectors, thereby perpetuating the association of AIDS with poverty, prostitution and homosexuality.

Note

1 Authors' calculations based on provincial national accounts data collected from the website of the National Bureau of Statistics of China, http://data.stats.gov.cn/english (accessed 25 September 2015).

8 Afterword

Ending AIDS?

This book examines the development since the early 2000s of public health campaigns to stop the spread of HIV, and hence AIDS, in the People's Republic of China. It explores the evolution of behavioural health interventions that provide information about how to use condoms to help prevent the sexual transmission of HIV, showing how particular populations have been identified as in need of such education, and the methods and media used to communicate that information. It focuses on the representation of the sexual behaviours of female sex workers, men who have sex with men and male migrant labourers, as a problem for public health, and thus of government, flowing from the PRC's engagement with global AIDS governance.

The United Nations' current mission of ending the AIDS epidemic as a global health threat by 2030, as affirmed in the 2016 Political Declaration on HIV and AIDS, involves 'fast-tracking' the national health policies of participating countries such as China to reach three milestones by 2020 (United Nations General Assembly 2016). The three milestones are eliminating HIV-related discrimination, and reducing both the number of people newly infected with HIV and those dying from AIDS-related causes to fewer than 500,000 respectively (UNAIDS 2016b). Achieving this mission entails reducing the prevalence of HIV among key and vulnerable populations, who are defined as key to the epidemic's dynamics and hence national and international responses (WHO 2014, 2015; UNAIDS 2015b). Key populations are currently sex workers, men who have sex with men, people who inject drugs using non-sterile injecting equipment, transgender people, and people in prisons and other closed settings (WHO 2014; UNAIDS 2016b: 7). Key populations are viewed as facing increased risk, vulnerability and burden with respect to HIV and AIDS because of a combination of biological, socio-economic and structural factors. Vulnerable populations such as women, migrants and mobile workers do not necessarily face the same epidemiological risk as members of key populations, but they are often vulnerable to infection because of societal pressures or social circumstances.

UNAIDS' plan to end AIDS as a public health threat exemplifies the organizing theme of this book – the links between new governmentalities, classificatory practices and the 'making up' of people. Michel Foucault (1991: 93, 95) coined the term 'governmentality' to describe the overarching concern of modern

DOI: 10.4324/9781315175546-8

government with 'the conduct of conduct', that is, efforts to guide the possibility of human conduct in order to achieve optimal outcomes for the 'things' that are to be governed. The plan to end AIDS aims to transform national governmental frameworks and social environments to enable those people classified as members of key populations to modify their individual decision-making and behaviours, for example, by using condoms in every sexual encounter. In doing so, it seeks to rid the world of and save future generations from the human and economic cost of AIDS.

Our history of such health interventions in China demonstrates that their effects extend beyond the reduction of HIV prevalence and AIDS-related deaths. They change the nature and form of government, for example, by requiring new types of government agencies, interdepartmental cooperation, legal frameworks, funding arrangements, and professional and community expertise and training. They alter broader social behaviours and attitudes in relation to issues of sex and sexuality, by making non-marital sexual behaviours more publicly visible and in some instances normalizing them. They also create both 'moving targets' in terms of the objects of government and kinds of people that in certain senses and contexts did not exist before (Hacking 2006). Sometimes what starts off as a norm to be instilled into members of key populations (to protect their health and that of the nation by using condoms) can be reconfigured as politicized demands that citizens can make of authorities. Members of key populations, or those claiming to speak on their behalf, may demand the right, instead of government authorities, to inculcate such norms in others as 'experts of themselves' or relevant community members. They may even demand an end to government and social practices that are viewed as preventing 'the end of AIDS', such as bans on the sex industry and discrimination against same-sex attracted people. Ian Hacking (2002: 99) refers to this 'reversibility' of relations of authority as 'the looping effect'.

We revisit these conclusions in the following sections by looking at the issues raised for China's HIV governance by UNAIDS' plan to end the AIDS epidemic as a global health threat by 2030. The first section looks at guidelines released by the World Health Organization to support this goal. The guidelines offer a 'global blueprint for ending AIDS' by consolidating information about how to conduct health interventions focused on key populations, and by providing detailed instructions about how to monitor, evaluate and 'score' the responses of participating countries. The second section shows how the linking of HIV to key populations via related health campaigns not only creates 'moving targets' in terms of the objects and subjects of government, but also promotes a logic of inclusion and exclusion that may discourage attention to potential local variants. The third section focuses on the WHO's recent determination that transgender people are key to the global AIDS response, in order to illustrate how health interventions may create kinds of people that in certain senses did not exist before. We conclude that the plan to end the AIDS epidemic as a global health threat will depend on the development of habits of conduct and consumption technologies that encourage sexually active people in general, and youth in particular, to practice correct and consistent condom use, and undertake regular HIV testing.

The global blueprint

In 2016, the National Health and Family Planning Commission of the People's Republic of China (NHFPC) and the World Health Organization Western Pacific Region (WHO/WPR) released the China–WHO Country Cooperation Strategy 2016–2020 (NHFPC and WHO/WPR 2016). The document provides a basis for the WHO to strengthen China's national health-care system and for the PRC to make greater contributions to global health. It states that China became the world's second-largest economy in terms of gross domestic product and joined the upper-middle-income country group in 2010 (Ibid.: 2). It adds that the PRC is entering into a new era of health literacy and health consumerism, along with the increased purchasing power, Internet connectivity and awareness of health risks of Chinese citizens. At the same time, the PRC has shifted from being primarily a beneficiary of development aid to serving as a development partner to other developing countries using its own finances and technical expertise (NHFPC and WHO/WPR 2016: viii).

Confirming its newfound role as a participant in global health governance, the PRC government has committed to UNAIDS' mission of ending the AIDS epidemic as a global health threat by 2030. This requires the nationwide scale-up of essential HIV prevention, testing and treatment approaches by 2020, which is mandated in the PRC's Thirteenth Five-Year Guidelines for National Economic and Social Development for 2016–2020, and in the PRC's 2016–2020 Action Plan for the Containment and Prevention of HIV and AIDS (Guowuyuan bangongting 2017; National People's Congress 2016b). The goal established by UNAIDS (2015b) is to ensure that 90 per cent of all people living with HIV know their HIV status, 90 per cent of all people diagnosed with HIV have access to antiretroviral therapy, and 90 per cent of all people on HIV treatment have a suppressed viral load so that their immune system remains strong and they are no longer infectious. AIDS prevention programs promoting condom use are also expected to achieve a compliance rate of at least 90 per cent.

Meeting UNAIDS' 90 per cent targets demands universal access to rapid HIV testing and treatments, and high levels of media coverage for programs that promote consistent condom use, with close to saturation coverage of outreach programs focused on key populations (Ibid.). Five populations are classified as key to the global AIDS epidemic and response. Key populations include the established categories of sex workers, men who have sex with men and people who inject drugs using non-sterile injecting equipment. They also include the new categories of transgender people, and people in prisons and other closed settings (UNAIDS 2016b; WHO 2014).

The World Health Organization (2014, 2015) has issued two documents that provide a 'blueprint' for scaling up and evaluating national responses to HIV prevention among key populations. These documents are the Consolidated Guidelines on HIV Prevention, Diagnosis, Treatment and Care for Key Populations, issued in July 2014; and the Tool to Set and Monitor Targets for HIV Prevention,

Diagnosis, Treatment and Care for Key Populations, issued in July 2015 (hereinafter the WHO Guidelines). The two documents bring together all existing WHO guidance relevant to health interventions focused on the five groups of people classified as key populations, and provide instructions about how to monitor, evaluate and 'score' the responses of participating countries.

The WHO Guidelines are based on the biopolitical logic that 'ending AIDS' requires major changes in the ways that national governments attempt to guide the conduct of citizens, and hence in modes of governance and self-government. Participating countries are expected to increase access to information about HIV prevention, and access to testing and treatments, at the micro-level through community-engaged service delivery. This means involving members of key populations, and their families and friends, in the design, implementation and monitoring of HIV prevention and condom use promotion programs. The rationale is that fostering a sense of community ownership in service delivery will aid successful outcomes, which implies the expansion of non-governmental organizations and associated cause-marketing through social media.

The WHO Guidelines further expect that participating countries will facilitate community-engaged service delivery by creating enabling environments for key populations at the macro-level. This involves not only financial commitment to increase access to AIDS-related information, testing and treatments, but also a political commitment to effecting legal and social change. The guidelines recommend decriminalizing behaviours associated with injecting drug use, sex work, same-sex activity and nonconforming gender identities. They also recommend monitoring and evaluating the stigma and discrimination experienced by key populations, and transforming the conduct of service providers, law enforcement officers and the general community towards members of key populations. Indicators and checklists are provided to develop 'country scorecards', based on the involvement of key populations in relevant national policy and strategy formulation, the extent of legal and other support services for key populations, and the extent of sensitization training on key populations for law enforcement officers. In other words, they provide checklists for evaluating changes in the conduct of 'the governed' and 'government'.

The global blueprint is a governmental program for corrective social transformation that also highlights the links between classificatory practices and the 'making up' of people. As we illustrate, key populations are often presented as defined groups of people with fixed properties whose conduct can be transformed, for example, by being exposed to the information provided in the global blueprint, and in the manner prescribed by that blueprint. But these populations are also 'moving targets' in that techniques for representing and intervening on key populations may alter those populations in anticipated and unintended ways, and deflect attention away from potential local variations. Health interventions promoting AIDS awareness and consistent condom use may even change the space of possibilities for personhood, creating what are in certain senses and contexts 'new kinds' of people.

Moving targets

The international AIDS governance system has presented a universalizing blueprint for *final* action to end the AIDS epidemic as a global health threat. It is recognized that national responses have to be localized to prevent bottlenecks in service delivery. But the blueprint mandates particular forms of governmental action on particular types of people, who are usually presented as defined groups with fixed properties.

Yet AIDS epidemics have varied considerably within and between countries and regions, and may even evolve in ways that require different forms of attention. Improved health interventions and medical technologies have ensured that sexual transmission is the most common route for HIV transmission. However, the majority of new cases of HIV infection in the PRC prior to 2009 were related to contaminated blood transfusions, mother-to-child transmission and the sharing of drug injecting equipment. The number of infections from these transmission routes has been radically reduced by closing down commercial blood centres, improving antenatal services, and providing needle exchange and methadone treatment programs for people who inject drugs.

Sexual transmission now accounts for more than 94 per cent of all new cases of HIV infection in the PRC. The national HIV prevalence remains low at less than 0.06 per cent, but meeting UNAIDS' 90 per cent targets still presents evident challenges (Guowuyuan bangongting 2017). The rate of new infection from sexual transmission is rising, a third of the estimated people living with HIV are not aware of their HIV status and access to HIV treatment is not universal (Ibid.; NHFPC and WHO/WPR 2016: 4). As of 2015, approximately only 50 per cent of people living with HIV in China had received antiretroviral therapy (UNAIDS 2016b: 35–7). Although 94 per cent of surveyed sex workers reported consistent condom use, the figure was slightly lower for men who have sex with men (88 per cent) (UNAIDS 2016a). The reported rate of condom use also varies significantly between different types of sex workers and men who have sex with men (Zhongguo jibing yufang kongzhi zhongxin, xingbing aizibing yufang kongzhi zhongxin 2016a, 2016b).

The growing rate of HIV infection through sexual transmission has encouraged what Haiqing Yu (2016: 185–6) describes as the hierarchical 'sexualization' of China's AIDS response, with HIV becoming attached to those classified as members of key and vulnerable populations, rather than 'the rest of us'. Since the 2000s, health authorities in the PRC have worked with the UN and other international agencies, and with local governments, the private sector and the media, to design, implement and publicize AIDS awareness and condom use programs. These public-private collaborations initially focused on female sex workers. They subsequently shifted to include men who have sex with men and male rural-to-urban migrant labourers. In keeping with the WHO Guidelines, new iterations will include people in prisons and transgender people, the latter as a disaggregation of interventions focused on sex workers and men who have sex with men. The Guidelines for Interventions to Prevent AIDS Among Men Who Have Sex With Men, issued by the CDC in 2016, propose extending such interventions to include transgender people (Zhongguo jibing yufang kongzhi zhongxin, xingbing aizibing yufang kongzhi zhongxin 2016a).

Although the global blueprint recommends eliminating AIDS-related stigma, the attaching of HIV in China to people classified as members of key and vulnerable populations has typically exacerbated and only occasionally challenged their socio-political marginalization. Public health campaigns focused on female sex workers reinforce the stigma attached to prostitution as an illicit means of earning a livelihood and a perceived conduit of disease. Health campaigns for men who have sex with men reinforce negative constructions of homosexuality in terms of 'improper', 'unclean' or 'promiscuous' behaviours. The association of HIV with rural-to-urban migrant labourers entrenches the stereotyping of them as uneducated, second-class citizens. These populations are presented as the most economical and efficient focus of HIV prevention and testing programs based on the assumption that they are 'almost always already infected' (Fan 2014: 86; see also Hildebrandt 2011: 983–4).

At the same time, the work of AIDS prevention has encouraged a rise in domestic advocacy for more inclusive social policies for migrant workers and homosexuals, and occasionally for sex workers. Some studies draw on interviews with Chinese men who have sex with men to suggest that HIV prevention would be enhanced by the governmental act of promoting gay venues with legal protections, legalizing same-sex marriage, and presenting both homosexuals and people living with HIV as positive role models in mass media (Chen *et al.* 2012: 6; Shang *et al.* 2012: 577). Behavioural health interventions focused on sex workers have contributed to the diversification of debates about the sex industry, by introducing new terminology to describe people who sell sexual services, and new ideas about how the sex industry might be better managed. Lawyers, retired Communist Party officials, NGOs and sex workers alike, have argued in different political forums that legalizing the sex industry in China will promote public health and sex workers' rights (Jeffreys 2012b). The 2016 Guidelines for AIDS Prevention Interventions Among Groups at High-risk Through Heterosexual Sexual Transmission state that the contracting of social organizations/NGOs to access female sex workers, and the training of sex workers as peer educators, has become an 'irreplaceable' part of such interventions since the State Council permitted government departments to contract private social services in 2013 (Zhongguo jibing yufang kongzhi zhongxin, xingbing aizibing yufang kongzhi zhongxin 2016b: 8). The PRC's evolving AIDS response has thus promoted new ways of 'knowing' particular sectors of the population, and new ideas about how those sectors of the population should be governed or might govern themselves.

The linking of HIV to key and vulnerable populations also promotes a logic of inclusion and exclusion that may deflect attention away from potential local variants. In China, it perpetuates the view that AIDS is something that happens to marginalized or 'other' people. This has ensured that male government and corporate elites are not prioritized by AIDS prevention programs by default.

Anthropologists Elanah Uretsky (2008, 2016) and Zheng Tiantian (2006) maintain that a significant proportion of elite men in China are vulnerable to HIV infection because they are highly mobile for work purposes, and regularly engage in commercial sex as part of masculinist practices associated with the 'entertaining' of business partners. But there is no quantitative data on the HIV prevalence among such men, nor are there multiple surveys of their sexual behaviours and condom use patterns, for the simple reason that they are not a focus of sentinel surveillance and public health interventions. In other words, elite men may be a 'missing target' of public health campaigns because their sexual behaviours have not been constructed as a necessary object of knowledge and government intervention.

The vulnerability of elite men to HIV infection may have been reduced in recent years by the introduction of government anti-corruption measures (Uretsky 2016: 207–12). In December 2013, the central government introduced regulations curbing extravagant spending on the part of government officials on wining and dining, and frequenting entertainment and leisure venues (Zhonggong zhongyang bangongting, guowuyuan bangongting yinfa 'dang zheng jiguan guonei gongwu jiedai guanli guiding' 2013). This has limited the extent of public funds that can be spent in entertainment and leisure venues, and subsequently on commercial sex, because people who provide sexual services in such venues are often paid through 'tips' and 'commission' associated with the costs of rooms, services, food and beverages.

Alternatively, anti-corruption measures may enhance the vulnerability of elite men to HIV infection. Although many high-grade entertainment and leisure venues have closed down because of reduced custom, local government officials may be frequenting lower-grade venues, many of which function as indirect sex establishments. Such venues typically operate on a short-term basis, with a high turnover of staff, to avoid police detection. Thus health officials are unlikely to have the kinds of established relationships with venue owners and managers that facilitate the implementation of location-based AIDS awareness programs.

Whichever the case may be, elite men are unlikely to voluntarily present for HIV testing because a positive result is likely to have a negative impact on their careers. Article 18 of the PRC's civil service recruitment criteria precludes people with AIDS or a serious STI from entering the civil service ('Gongwuyuan luyong tijian tongyong biaozhun (shixing)' 2005). This remains the case despite some efforts by lawyers and advocacy groups to have Article 18 repealed as outdated and discriminatory (Qiao Long 2016). Government employees have annual health checks, but these do not include STI and HIV testing. However, engagement in 'improper' (*bu zhengdang*) sexual relations can result in demotion or loss of employment according to the Chinese Communist Party disciplinary regulations, and most civil servants are Party members ('Zhonggong fabu zui yan dangji lie chu 6 lei fumian qingdan (quanwen) 2015). This means that elite men are unlikely to voluntarily present for HIV testing because a positive result may bring to light their involvement in extramarital and commercial sex, and thereby demonstrate their 'unsuitability' for Party membership and government employment. Hence, the emphasis of the global blueprint on key populations may overlook the influence of masculinist business cultures on the sexual transmission of HIV in China (Uretsky 2016).

The global blueprint is clearly also embedded in the neoliberal governmentality of Western liberal-democratic societies. It promotes privatized service delivery mediated through communities and associated social media marketing to create self-governing individuals who will actively govern their own health and occupational and lifestyle risks. Yet the communities, and community networks and organizations that are expected to facilitate such outcomes are incipient or even non-existent in many local contexts.

We demonstrate this argument with reference to the WHO's recent determination that transgender people are key to the global AIDS response.

'Making up' people

The classification of transgender people as key to the global AIDS response illustrates how health interventions both depend on a knowledge of that which is to be governed, and may create kinds of people that in certain senses and contexts did not exist before (Hacking 2006). 'Transgender' is defined as 'an umbrella term for people whose gender identity and expression does not conform to the norms and expectations traditionally associated with the sex assigned to them at birth; it includes people who are transsexual, transgender or otherwise gender non-conforming' (World Health Organization 2014: xiii).

Transgender people have been classified as key to the global AIDS response based on information from epidemiological surveys. International surveys conducted with support from the Global Fund suggest that the HIV prevalence among transgender women (male to female), and among transgender men (female to male) who have receptive anal intercourse with men, is equivalent to, or even higher than, the prevalence of HIV among men who have sex with men. The WHO therefore recommends that countries implement individual- and community-level behavioural health interventions to increase consistent condom and lubricant use, and regular HIV testing, among transgender people who have sex with men, and especially among those who are sex workers. It further recommends that countries should provide legal recognition for transgender people, if they have not already done so.

The recommendations assume that participating countries have a distinct population of people who self-identify and/or are identified by others as transgender. The corollary demands for legal recognition of transgender people, and the roll-out of health interventions promoting AIDS awareness and condom use, similarly presuppose the existence of organizations advocating for, or on behalf of, transgender people, typically in the context of activism by lesbian, gay, bisexual and transgender (LGBT) individuals and communities. Such organizations are expected to conduct or support sex venue-based outreach, and to offer targeted Internet-based information using social marketing strategies that provide sexual health training for diverse transgender communities, and generate public awareness of issues affecting transgender people. Transgender people and their family members are also expected to be involved in the design, implementation and monitoring of such programs, to foster a sense of community ownership in their outcomes.

These directives may prove to be unrealistic or difficult to act on immediately in the PRC, given the absence of affirmative LGBT legislation and lack of public recognition of transgender people. Unlike in Thailand, transgender people have limited public visibility in the PRC, with the exception of celebrity Jin Xing. Jin was the PRC's best male dancer while performing with the People's Liberation Army troupe in the 1970s. Jin is now an internationally acclaimed female dancer, married mother of three adopted children, and hosts her own television talk-show host, following a popular stint as a 'hard' judge on China's *So You Think You Can Dance* (Davies and Davies 2010; Jin Xing tuokou xiu 2015). Public interest in Jin's life story has augmented her celebrity and opened the space for discussions of transgender people. However, her life is typically presented in the media in terms of gender conformity – the struggle of a woman trapped in a man's body to become her true self and realize her dreams – rather than challenging the male/female gender binary and heteronormativity (Davies and Davies 2010). Her parent's acceptance of her decision to have sex reassignment surgery, and her rich, glamorous lifestyle, also stand in marked contrast to the lives of most transgender people in China who cannot afford costly hormone replacement therapy and surgery, which are difficult to access through the official health care system. As with other transgender people in the PRC, Jin Xing is generally referred to as a person who underwent a sex change (*bianxingren*), rather than as a person who transgresses gender boundaries (*kuaxingbiezhe*), although the latter terminology is used in 2016 public health intervention guidelines focused on men who have sex with men (Zhongguo jibing yufang kongzhi zhongxin, xingbing aizibing yufang kongzhi zhongxin 2016a).

There are also no formally registered transgender organizations in the PRC, nor are any government departments specifically tasked with managing issues relating to sexual and gender minorities (Asia Catalyst 2015: 6, 49–50; UNDP, USAID 2014: 13, 25). A few informal transgender communities exist in the form of online chat groups and through occupational socialization in urban gay-themed entertainment and leisure venues (UNDP, USAID 2014: 64). Some organizations also work with transgender sex workers as an extension of AIDS prevention programs for men who have sex with men (Ibid.: 18). However, the absence of tailored health services and anti-discrimination laws means that transgender people without considerable financial resources are left without effective health (and legal) protections. This is especially the case for female-presenting transgender sex workers. Yet transgender people who have sex with men are viewed as likely to constitute the majority of all new HIV infections in the Asia-Pacific region by 2020 (Asia Catalyst 2015: 1 & 9; see also Best *et al.* 2015).

The global blueprint thus requires PRC authorities to develop strategies for the government of public health and techniques for self-government that are situated within new relations of mutual obligation: a community (of LGBT people). Yet community-based mobilization and intervention is complicated by the 'hidden' and heterogeneous nature of transgender sex workers, comprising men who have sex with men, transgender individuals and transsexuals who self-identify as homosexual, heterosexual and bisexual. It is further complicated by hostile attitudes towards them on the part of some members of local gay and sex worker communities, who view them as 'not gay' and as 'competitors for clients' (Asia Catalyst 2015: 34–5). Many transgender sex workers reportedly first provide commercial sex to men who have sex with men and then shift towards a heterosexual clientele (presented as rural-to-urban migrant labourers), either because they find the sex work easier to manage or because they identify as female and heterosexual. The high turnover and mobility of transgender sex workers raises additional problems for prospective intervention efforts, which cannot anticipate consistent support from 'community' volunteers or peer educators (Ibid.: 50).

The global blueprint also requires the PRC government to develop national legislation that will empower LGBT people, which means creating responsible government agencies with the capacity to create relevant laws, and the authority to monitor and enforce them. This may happen in the near future. In December 2013, the PRC government accepted recommendations made to the Human Rights Council of the UN that it establish anti-discrimination legislation to ensure that lesbian, gay, bisexual and transgender persons enjoy equal treatment, including at schools and in the workplace, and also prohibit workplace discrimination based on sexual orientation and gender identity, among other considerations (United Nations General Assembly 2013). Research collaborations between international and domestic NGOs on issues affecting LGBT people and organizational development have increased in this context (Asia Catalyst 2015; UNDP, USAID 2014). The acceptance also prompted a series of small-scale activist efforts designed to obtain media publicity for and raise public awareness of issues affecting Chinese LGBT people. Between 2014 and 2016, a series of landmark legal cases were filed with the Chinese courts against different government agencies to demand the legalization of same-sex marriage, and prevent homophobic textbooks, workplace discrimination and censorship of homosexual media content (Phillips 2016).

The roll-out of the global blueprint may therefore help to increase the space of possibilities for personhood for Chinese people who self-identify or are identified as LGBT. But this is not going to happen overnight, given the absence in mainland China of both self-identified transgender communities, and government agencies and community organizations that support such communities. Coordinated LGBT organization and activism is also underdeveloped to date.

Concluding remarks

Ending AIDS as a public health threat in China and elsewhere ultimately depends on the development of habits of conduct and consumption technologies that encourage sexually active people in general, and youth in particular, to practice correct and consistent condom use, and undertake regular HIV testing. While sex education is notoriously inadequate in Chinese schools, educated youth can and do access information about sex and HIV prevention from the Internet (Muessig *et al.* 2015). Domestically produced and imported condoms of different quality and cost are now readily available online and in supermarkets and convenience stores across China, providing interested consumers with easy and anonymous access to such goods.

However, the recent growth of HIV infection among high school and college students, and among young men in particular, demonstrates that, as in other parts of the world, the availability of condoms and AIDS information is not necessarily resulting in safer-sex practices (Guowuyuan 2017). Condoms may be a simple protective barrier against HIV infection, but most individuals are unable to sustain consistent condom use over the course of a relationship, never mind a lifetime. This suggests the need for continued AIDS communication and easy access to rapid HIV testing and early treatment, as is mandated in the PRC's 2016–2020 action plan for the containment and prevention of HIV and AIDS (Guowuyuan bangongting 2017).

More young condom consumers will have to be created by forming connections between sexual passions, sexual ethics and public and personal health, and specific features of condoms and lubricants, and particular consumption practices and lifestyles. This demands more than better sex education in schools and colleges. It requires reliable age- and sex-disaggregated data on young people's sexual behaviours and reproductive health. It also requires the creation and public delivery of youth-friendly information about sex, condoms and HIV prevention, and HIV testing and treatment services.

Ending AIDS as a public health threat means creating and mobilizing particular types of self-governing, self-consciously sexualized and ethical consumers through appeals to diverse desires and lifestyle communities, as well as funding, implementing and publicizing improved public health campaigns. It requires the creation of a global population of sexualized citizens-consumers who can individually demonstrate educated sexual restraint and the educated and ethical pursuit of sexual pleasures.

References

'2011nian shijie ribao faxingliang qian100ming paihangbang 2011' [2011 top 100 world daily papers by circulation] (2011) *Xinwen Jizhe*, 10: 8–10.

'654,000 living with HIV/AIDS in China' (2016) *Xinhua*, 1 December. Online. Available: www.china.org.cn/china/2016-12/01/content_39824758.htm (accessed 16 December 2016).

'99575 Beijing tongzhi rexian' [Beijing Tongzhi Hotline] (2005) 'Yinggai yindizhiyi xietiaofazhan [Coordinate development to suit local conditions], in Beijing jiande jiankang jiaoyu yanjiusuo [Beijing Gender Health Education Institute] (ed.) *Tongzhi shequ huodong de zuzhi yu xietiao jingyan huibian* [Compilation on Organizing and Coordinating Activities in Gay Communities], Beijing.

Abrams, H.K. (2001) 'The resurgence of sexually transmitted disease in China', *Journal of Public Health Policy*, 22, 4: 429–40.

Ainsworth, M., Beyrer, C., and Soucat, A. (2003) 'AIDS and public policy: The lessons and challenges of "success" in Thailand', *Health Policy*, 64, 1: 13–37.

All-China Youth Federation (2009) 'Basic data'. Online. Available: www.acyf.org.cn/2009-12/29/content_3319246.htm (accessed 22 February 2017).

Amin, A. (2005) *Violence Against Sex Workers and HIV Prevention*, Geneva: World Health Organization.

Anagnost, A. (2006) 'Strange circulations: The blood economy in rural China', *Economy and Society*, 35, 4: 509–29.

Anderson, A.F., and Gil, V.E. (1998) 'China's modernization and the decline of communitarianism: The control of sex crimes and implications for the fate of informal social control', *Journal of Contemporary Criminal Justice*, 14, 3: 248–61.

'Anquantao fang aizi, "xing" fu you jiankang' [Condoms prevent AIDS: 'Sex' be happy and healthy] (2015) Chinese Center for Disease Control and Prevention. Online. Available: http://v.ku6.com/show/fsdZw6mOrUk41VwhMB0KdQ . . . html (accessed 16 December 2016).

Asia Catalyst (2015) 'My life is too dark to see the light': A survey of the living conditions of transgender female sex workers in Beijing and Shanghai. Online. Available: http://asiacatalyst.org/wp-content/uploads/2014/09/Asia-Catalyst-TG-SW-Report.pdf (accessed 22 February 2017).

Asian Business Coalition on AIDS (2002) 'Business taking action to manage HIV/AIDS', 1–22. Online. Available: www.hivpolicy.org/Library/HPP000308.pdf (accessed 16 December 2016).

AVERT (2013) 'Introduction to HIV and AIDS education', AVERT.org. Online. Available: www.avert.org/introduction-hiv-and-aids-education.htm (accessed 22 February 2017).

AVERT (2016) 'Global HIV and AIDS statistics', AVERT.org. Online. Available: www.avert.org/global-hiv-and-aids-statistics (accessed 22 February 2017).

Bai, J. (2000) 'Zhongguo gaodu zhongshi aizibing fangzhi' [China places high value on preventing AIDS], *Jiankangbao*, 26 July, p. 1.

Bai, J. (2009) 'Weishengbu gongbu aizibing yiqing pinggu' [Ministry of Health releases information on AIDS epidemic], *Renmin Ribao*, 1 December, p. 7.

Bai, T. (2016) '190 Chinese LGBT groups condemn Orlando club shooting', *Global Times*, 14 June. Online. Available: www.globaltimes.cn/content/988160.shtml (accessed 23 February 2017).

Bai, Y. (2011) 'Tisheng guanli shuiping, tigao fuwu zhiliang' [Improving management and quality of service], *Zhongguo Renkoubao*, 28 November, p. 1.

Bao, H. (2012) 'Querying/ queering cosmopolitanism: Queer spaces in Shanghai', *Culture Unbound: Journal of Current Cultural Research*, 4: 97–120.

Beijing aizhixing jiankang jiaoyu yanjiusuo [Beijing Aizhixing Institute for Health Education] (2009) *Zhongguo xinggongzuo yu xinggongzuozhe jiankang yu falü renquan baogao* (2008–2009) [Report on the health, legality and human rights of sex workers and the sex industry in China], Beijing: Beijing Aizhixing Jiankang Jiaoyu Yanjiusuo.

Beijing aizhixing jiankang jiaoyu yanjiusuo he Wuhan xinyuan [Beijing Aizhixing Institute for Health Education and Wuhan Xinyuan] (2009) 'Nantongxinglian yuchi kaizhan yufang aizi xingwei ganyu gongzuo jingyan jiaoliu yu yanjiu' [Behaviour interventions focused on HIV prevention in male gay bathhouses], Beijing: Beijing Aizhixing Jiankang Jiaoyu Yanjiusuo.

Beijingshi jibing yufang kongzhi zhongxin [Beijing Center for Disease Control and Prevention] (n.d.-a)' MSM renqun HIV ganran anli' [Cases of HIV infection among MSM], Beijing Center for Disease Control and Prevention.

Beijingshi jibing yufang kongzhi zhongxin [Beijing Center for Disease Control and Prevention] (n.d.-b) 'Ziyuan zixun jiance' [Voluntary participation in consulting and testing services], Beijing Center for Disease Control and Prevention.

Beijingshi jibing yufang kongzhi zhongxin [Beijing Center for Disease Control and Prevention] (n.d.-c) 'Xingbing aizibing yufang zhishi' [Knowledge about STI and AIDS prevention], Beijing Center for Disease Control and Prevention.

Benney, J. (2012) 'How to avoid the centre: The strategies of a small feminist workshop in rural China', *International Journal of China Studies*, 3, 3: 383–410.

Best, J., Tang, W. M., Zhang, Y., Han, L., Fengying M. S., Huang, S. J., Yang, B., Wei, C. Y., and Tucker, J. D. (2015) 'Sexual behaviors and HIV/Syphilis testing among transgender individuals in China: Implications for expanding HIV testing services, *Sexually Transmitted Diseases*, 42, 5: 281–5.

Biddulph, S. (1993) 'Review of police powers of administrative detention in the People's Republic of China', *Crime and Delinquency*, 39, 3: 337–54.

Biddulph, S. (2007) *Legal Reform and Administrative Detention Powers in China*, Cambridge: Cambridge University Press.

Binson, D., Woods, W. J., Pollack, L., Paul, J., Stall, R., and Catania, J. A. (2001) 'Differential HIV risk in bathhouses and public cruising areas', *American Journal of Public Health*, 91, 9: 1482–6.

Boittin, M. (2013) 'New perspectives from the oldest profession: Abuse and the legal consciousness of sex workers in China', *Law and Society Review*, 47, 2: 245–78.

Brady, A-M. (2012) 'Market-friendly, scientific, high tech, and politics-lite: China's new approach to propaganda', in A-M. Brady (ed.) *China's Thought Management*, Abingdon: Routledge, pp. 1–10.

Branigan, T. (2010) 'Chinese sex workers protest against crackdown', *The Guardian*, 4 August, p. 15.

Bray, D. (2005) *Social Space and Governance in Urban China: The Danwei System from Origins to Reform*, Stanford: Stanford University Press.

Bray, D., and Jeffreys, E. (2016) 'New mentalities of government in China: An introduction', in D. Bray and E. Jeffreys (eds) *New Mentalities of Government in China*, Abingdon: Routledge, pp. 1–15.

Bray, D. and Jeffreys, E. (eds) (2016) *New Mentalities of Government in China*, Abingdon: Routledge.

Cao, L., and Stack, S. (2010) 'Exploring terra incognita: Family values and prostitution acceptance in China', *Journal of Criminal Justice*, 38, 4: 531–7.

Carrillo, B.G. (2004) 'Rural-urban migration in China: Temporary migrants in search of permanent settlement', *Portal*, 1, 1: 1–26. Online. Available: http://opus.lib.uts.edu.au/bitstream/10453/3324/1/2004001471.pdf (accessed 16 December 2016).

CDC Centers for Disease Control and Prevention (2015) 'STDs and HIV – CDC Fact Sheet'. Online. Available: www.cdc.gov/std/hiv/stdfact-std-hiv.htm (accessed 22 February 2017).

Chamratrithirong, A., Thongthai, V., Boonchalaski, W., Guest, P., Kanchanachitra, C., and Varangrat, A. (1999) *The Success of the 100% Condom Use Promotion Programme in Thailand: Survey Results of the Evaluation of the 100% Condom Promotion Programme*, Salaya, Mahidol University.

Chan, K.W., and Zhang, L. (1999) 'The *hukou* system and rural-urban migration in China: Processes and changes', *China Quarterly*, 160: 818–55.

Chang, Mingxiu (2009) 'Henansheng nongcun funü biyun jieyü ji jieshou xiangguan fuwu de xiankuang diaocha' [Survey on the reception of contraception and related services among rural women in Henan Province], *Zhongguo Jihuashengyuxue Zazhi*, 9: 532–5.

Chapman, J., Cai, Y., Hillier, S., and Estcourt, C. (2009) 'Sex and sexuality in the Shenzhen '*tongzhi*' circle: HIV risk context and migrant men who have sex with men in China', *Culture, Health and Sexuality*, 11, 7: 689–702.

Chen, G., Li, Y., Beichuan, Z., Zengzhao, Y., Xiufang, L., Lixin, W., and Ziming, Y. (2012) 'Psychological characteristics in high-risk MSM in China', *BMC Public Health*, 12: 58 (7 pp.).

Chen, Guangman (2000) 'Dapo chenmo gongtong yingzhan aizibing' [Ending the silence: Meeting AIDS head-on], *Guangming Ribao*, 4 December. Online. Available: www.gmw.cn/01gmrb/2000-12/04/GB/12%5E18624%5E0%5EGMB2-006.htm (accessed 23 February 2017).

Chen, Jieren (2002) 'Ping Lixian 'yulechangsuo 100% shiyong anquantao xiangmu bangongshi' [Comment on 'Li County 100 Per Cent Condom Use Office'], *Zhongguo Qingnianbao*, 20 September 2002. Online. Available: www.people.com.cn/GB/guandian/28/20020920/826950.html (accessed 16 December 2016).

Chen, N. (2010) 'Gonganbu jiang "changtaihua" anfang yulechangsuo' [Ministry of Public Security will make regular 'secret' checks at entertainment and leisure venues], *Xinjingbao*, 12 December, p. A14.

Chen, W. (2011) 'Tongxinglian quanli burongqinfan' [The rights of homosexual should not be violated], *Xinwen Chenbao*, 6 July, p. B2.

Chen, Z. (2005) 'Tongxinglian de falü diwei yinqi guanzhu' [The legal status of homosexuals raises concern], *Minzhu yu Fazhi Shibao*, 13 September, p. 2.

Chen, Z., Schilling, R., Wei, S., Cai, C., Zhou, W., and Shan, J. (2008) The 100% condom use programme: A demonstration in Wuhan China, *Evaluation and Programme Planning*, 31, 1: 10–21.

Chen, Z.Q., Zhang, G.C., Gong, X.D., Lin, C., Gao, X., Liang, G.J., Yue, X.L., Chen, X.S., and Cohen, M.S. (2007) 'Syphilis in China: Results of a national surveillance programme', *Lancet*, 369, 9556: 132–8.Cheng, T.J., and Selden, M. (1994) 'The origins and social-consequences of China *hukou* system', *China Quarterly*, 139: 644–68.

Cheng, X., and Xiaoshu, C. (2008) 'Dongguan: yige xinggongzuozhe lianshang de daoba' [Dongguan: Scar on the face of a female sex worker], *Zhongguo Xinwen Zhoukan*, 13: 46–8.

'China: Beijing starts promoting condom use to fight HIV/AIDS' (2004) *Agence France Presse*, 23 November. Online. Available: www.thebody.com/content/art26194.html (accessed 14 December 2016).

China Central Television (2004) 'Shehui jilu: jingcha yisheng xiezhu yulechangsuo tuiguang anquantao' [Social records: Police and doctors assist condom promotion in entertainment venues]. Online. Available: http://news.sina.com.cn/s/2004-04-21/15313152204.shtml (accessed 14 December 2016).

'China's entertainment venues checked for drugs, prostitutes and gangsters' (2006) People's Daily Online, 16 March. Online. Available http://en.people.cn/200603/16/print20060316_250905.html (accessed 3 July 2017).

'China launches AIDS prevention among migrant workers' (2007) *Xinhua*, 26 January. Online. Available: www.chinadaily.com.cn/china/2007-01/26/content_794231.htm (accessed 16 December 2016).

'China's anti-AIDS, HIV practices successful: Experts' (2016) *China Daily*, 2 December. Online. Available: www.chinadaily.com.cn/china/2016-12/02/content_27548656.htm (accessed 27 January 2017).

Chinese Society of Psychiatry (2001) *Zhongguo jingshen zhang'ai fenlei yu zhenduan biaozhun disanban* [Chinese Classification for Mental Disorders Version 3 (CCMD-3)], Jinan: Shandong Kexuejishu Chubanshe.

Choi, S.Y.P. (2011) 'State control, female prostitution and HIV prevention in China', *China Quarterly*, 205: 96–114.

Choi, S.Y.P., and Holroyd, E. (2007) 'The influence of power, poverty and agency in the negotiation of condom use for female sex workers in mainland China', *Culture, Health and Sexuality*, 9, 5: 489–503.

Chou, W.-S. (2000) *Tongzhi: Politics of Same-Sex Eroticism in Chinese Societies*, Binghamton: The Haworth Press.

Chou, W.-S. (2001) 'Homosexuality and the cultural politics of *tongzhi* in Chinese societies', *Journal of Homosexuality*, 40, 3–4: 27–46.

Chow, E., Iu, K., Fu, X., Wilson, D., and Zhang, L. (2012) 'HIV and sexually transmissible infections among money boys in China: A data synthesis and meta-analysis, *PLoS ONE*, 7, 11: e48025.

Chow, E., Lau, J., Zhuang, X., Zhang, X., Wang, Y., and Zhang, L. (2014) 'HIV prevalence trends, risky behaviours, and governmental and community responses to the epidemic among men who have sex with men in China', *BioMed Research International*, 19 pp. Online. Available: www.hindawi.com/journals/bmri/2014/607261/ (accessed 16 December 2016).

Cliff, A.D., and Smallman-Raynor, M.R. (2003) 'The AIDS pandemic: Global geographical patterns and local spatial processes', *The Geographical Journal*, 158, 2: 182–98.

Cohen, M.S., Henderson, G.E., Aiello, P., and Zheng, H.Y. (1996) 'Successful eradication of sexually transmitted diseases in the People's Republic of China: Implications for the 21st century', *Journal of Infectious Diseases*, 174: S223–9.

'Condoms no longer evidence of prostitution in China' (2007) Gov.cn. Online. Available: www.gov.cn/english/2007-12/01/content_822404.htm (accessed 16 December 2016).

Criminal Law of the People's Republic of China (1997) Adopted by the Second Session of the Fifth National People's Congress on 1 July 1979 and amended by the Fifth Session of the Eighth National People's Congress on 14 March 1997. Online. Available: www.fmprc.gov.cn/ce/cgvienna/eng/dbtyw/jdwt/crimelaw/t209043.htm (accessed 1 February 2017).

Da, Dan (1990) 'Maiyinpiaochang wenti de diaocha fenxi yu zhili duice' [The problem of prostitution: An investigative survey and proposed countermeasures], *Shenzhen daxue xuebao*, 2: 90–8.

Dai, W., Gao, J., Gong, J., Xia, X-P., Yang, H., Shen, Y., Gu, J., Wang, T-H., Liu, Y., Zhou, J., Shen, Z-P. Zhu, Z-S., and Pan, Z-G. (2015) 'Sexual behavior of migrant workers in Shanghai, China', *BMC Public Health*, 15, 1067: 1–9.

Davies, G., and Davies, M.E. (2010) 'Jin Xing: China's transexual star of dance', in L. Edwards and E. Jeffreys (eds) *Celebrity in China*, Hong Kong: Hong Kong University Press, pp. 169–91.

Deng, L. (2003) 'Ganshou chongji: anquantao jinru yulecheng' [Feel the impact: Condoms enter entertainment and leisure venues in mountainous areas], *Jiangkang Bidu*, 10: 48–51.

Deng, X. (1979) 'Speech greeting the Fourth Congress of Chinese writers and artists (30 October)', *The Selected Works of Deng Xiaoping*. Online. Available: https://dengxiaopingworks.wordpress.com/2013/02/25/speech-greeting-the-fourth-congress-of-chinese-writers-and-artists/ (accessed 16 December 2016).

Deng, X. (2014) 'Dongguan fushizhang gongan juzhang bei mianzhi' [The Deputy Mayor and Police Chief of Dongguan have been sacked], *Fazhi Ribao*, 15 February, p. 2.

Detels, R., Wu, Z.Y., Rotheram, M.J., Li, L., Guan, J.H., Yin, Y.P., Liang, G.J., Lee, M., Hu, L.H., and the National Institute of Mental Health Collaborative HIV/STD Prevention Trial Group. (2003) 'Sexually transmitted disease prevalence and characteristics of market vendors in eastern China', *Sexually Transmitted Diseases*, 30, 11: 803–8.

Ding, Z. (2009) 'Woguo xinshengdai nongmingong de tezheng fenxi' [Analysis of the characteristics of a new generation of migrant workers in China], *Lanzhou Xuekan*, 7: 71–3.

Doland, A. (2015) 'Masters of sex and satire: How Durex wins in China with digital tactics range from humor on social to personalized condoms via e-commerce', *Advertising Age*, 12 October. Online. Available: http://adage.com/article/additional-industry-events/masters-sex-satire-durex-wins-china-digital/300844/ (accessed 16 December 2016).

Dong, D., Chang, T.K., and Chen, D. (2008) 'Reporting AIDS and the invisible victims in China: Official knowledge as news in the People's Daily, 1986–2002', *Journal of Health Communication*, 13, 4: 357–74.

Dong, H., Xing, H., Shao, Y., and Ruan, Y. (2014) 'HIV, syphilis, and behavioral risk factors among female sex workers before and after implementation of harm reduction programs in a high drug-using area of China', *PLoS ONE*, 9, 1: 1–6.

Downing, M.J.J. (2010) 'Perception of risk, sexual behaviors, and HIV prevention in commercial and public sex venues: A study of MSM venue attendees', PhD thesis, The City University of New York, New York.

Duan, B., and Mingyi, Z. (eds) (2004) *Beijing nianjian* [Beijing Almanac], Beijing: Beijing nianjianshe.

Duan, Y. (2002) 'Zhengfu ganyu buzu: yingdui aizibing de zhimingshang' [Lack of government intervention: A fatal response to AIDS], *21Shiji Huanqiu Baodao*, 3 December. Online. Available: http://news.sina.com.cn/c/2002-12-03/1316827828.html (accessed 16 December 2016).

Dutton, M. (2009) 'Passionately governmental: Maoism and the structured intensities of revolutionary government', in E. Jeffreys (ed.) *China's Governmentalities: Governing Change, Changing Government*, Abingdon: Routledge, pp. 24–37.

Edwards, M., Thomsen, S., and Toroitich-Ruto, C. (2005) 'Thinking aloud to create better condom use questions', *Field Methods*, 17: 183–99.

Evans, H. (1995) 'Defining difference: The "scientific" construction of sexuality and gender in the People's Republic of China', *Signs*, 20, 2: 357–94.

Fan, C.C. (1995) 'Of belts and ladders: State policy and uneven regional development in post-Mao China', *Annals of the Association of American Geographers*, 85, 3: 421–49.

Fan, C.C. (2003) 'Rural-urban migration and gender division of labor in transitional China', *International Journal of Urban and Regional Research*, 27, 1: 24–47.

Fan, E.L. (2014) 'HIV testing as prevention among MSM in China: The business of scaling-up', *Global Public Health*, 9, 1–2: 85–97.

Fan, X., Fanzhu, H., Jiejun, L., and Xiaoling, M. (2004) 'Xiaojie chenghuyu de yuyong tezheng dili fenbu jiqi zouxiang' [The uses, features and geographic distribution of the appellation "xiaojie" (Miss)], *Yuyan Wenzi Yingyong*, 4: 41–7.

Fang, Meng (2002) '"100% shiyong anquantao xiangmu" Jingjiang geqian' [100 Per Cent Condom Use Program comes to a standstill in Jingjiang], *The Bund*, 27 January. Online. Available: www.hangzhou.com.cn/20020127/ca178113.htm (accessed 16 December 2016).

Farquhar, M. (2010) 'Jet Li: wushu master' in sports and film', in L. Edwards and E. Jeffreys (eds) *Celebrity in China*, Hong Kong: Hong Kong University Press.

Feng, W., Yuqiu, W., Lin, W., Qihou, W., and Guisu, S. (2006) 'Guangxi Liuzhoushi aizibing liuxing tezheng yu liuxing qushi fenxi' [Characteristics and trend analysis of the AIDS epidemic in Liuzhou, Guangxi], *Gonggongweisheng yu Yufangyixue*, 17, 5: 6–7.

'Few people well informed about AIDS: Survey' (2004) *Xinhua*. Online. Available: www.chinadaily.com.cn/english/doc/2004-08/09/content_363490.htm (accessed 16 December 2016).

Foucault, M. (1991 [1978]) 'Governmentality' (Lecture at the Collège de France, 1 February 1978), in G. Burchell, C. Gordon and P. Miller (eds), *The Foucault Effect: Studies in Governmentality*, Chicago: University of Chicago Press, pp. 87–104.

Foucault, M. (1998) *The Will to Knowledge: The History of Sexuality: 1*, London: Penguin Books.

Foucault, M. (2007) *Security, Territory, Population: Lectures at the Collège de France 1977–1978*, Houndsmills: Palgrave MacMillan.

'Free condom' (n.d.) National Health and Family Planning Commission. Online. Available: https://itunes.apple.com/app/id468314123?mt=8 (accessed 16 December 2016).

Fu, D. (2005) 'Tongxinglian zhide guanzhu de quanli suqiu' [Homosexuals concerned with rights], *Jiancha Ribao*, 2 November, p. 6.

Gåsemyr, H.J. (2015) 'Twenty years of mobilising around AIDS in China: The main actors and influences behind organisational growth', *Asian Studies Review*, 39, 4: 609–27.

Ge, Zongyu (2002) 'Guanzhu aizibing fangzhi zhengce' [Focus on AIDS prevention policy], *Guangming Ribao*, 29 November. Online. Available: www.nwccw.gov.cn/html/52/n-137152.html (accessed 16 December 2016).

Gil, V.E., Wang, M.S., Anderson, A.F., Lin, G.M., and Wu, Z.J.O. (1996) 'Prostitutes, prostitution and STD/HIV transmission in mainland China', *Social Science and Medicine*, 42, 1: 141–52.

Gittings, J. (2001) 'The AIDS scandal China could not hush up: Health officials' blood-for-cash scheme breeds HIV tragedy', *The Guardian*, 11 June. Online. Available: www.

guardian.co.uk/world/2001/jun/11/china.internationaleducationnews (accessed 16 December 2016).

The Global Fund (2006) Amended and Restated Program Grant Agreement. Online. Available: www.theglobalfund.org/en/portfolio/country/grant/?grant=CHN-506-G06-H (accessed 16 December 2016).

Gong, W. (1984) 'Dui funü maiyin dingzui wenti de tantao' [Discussion of the problems associated with convicting women who provide sexual services], *Faxue Zazhi*, 1: 28–9.

Gonganbu [Ministry of Public Security] (1981) 'Gonganbu guanyu jianjue zhizhi maiyin huodong de tongzhi' (jielu) [Ministry of Public Security: Notice on resolutely curbing prostitution (excerpt)], 10 June. Online. Available: http://210.73.66.144:4601/law?fn=chl057s080.txt&truetag=1&titles=&contents=&dbt=chl (accessed 16 December 2016).

Gonganbu [Ministry of Public Security] (1988) 'Gonganbu yinfa: jinyibu daji qudi maiyinpiaochang huodong he zuohao shourong jiaoyu gongzuo zuotanhui jiyao' [Ministry of Public Security issues the 'Minutes of the symposium on advancing campaigns against prostitution activities and improving re-education work']. Online. Available: http://law.lawtime.cn/d541430546524.html (accessed 16 December 2016).

Gonganbu [Ministry of Public Security] (1993) 'Guanyu qudi tongxinglian wenhua shalong 'nanren de shijie' de qingkuang tongbao' [Notice on the closure of the "Men's World" homosexual culture salon], Gong tong zi [1993] 62hao. Online. Available: www.chinaacc.com/new/63%2F71%2F2006%2F3%2Fxu6735315913360023029-0.htm (accessed 16 December 2016).

Gonganbu [Ministry of Public Security] (2010) 'Guanyu bu de caiqu youjieshizhongdeng yousun gongmin rengezunyan de zhifa fangshi de tongzhi' [Notice on prohibiting the use of law enforcement practices that violate citizen's rights, such as parading suspects in public], Gonganbu zhian guanli ju gong zhi mingfa 2010, 198 hao.

Goodman, D.S.G. (2004) 'The campaign to "open up the West": National, provincial-level and local perspectives', *The China Quarterly*, 178: 317–34.

Goodman, D.S.G. (2014) *Class in Contemporary China*, Cambridge: Polity.

Gransow, B. (2012) 'Internal migration in China – opportunity or trap?', Policy Brief, *Focus Migration*, 19: 1–10.

Green, M. (2014) ;China to abolish re-education through labor', *The Diplomat*, 5 January. Online. Available: http://thediplomat.com/2014/01/china-to-abolish-re-education-through-labor/ (accessed 16 December 2016).

Greenberg, D.F. (1988) *The Construction of Homosexuality*, Chicago: University of Chicago Press.

Greenhalgh, S., and Winckler, E.A. (2005) *Governing China's Population: From Leninist to Neoliberal Biopolitics*, Stanford: Stanford University Press.

Gu, C. (director) (2008) *Laoxiang bang laoxiang* [Hometown Fellow Help Hometown Fellow], China. Distributed by the International Labour Organization and All-China Federation of Trade Unions. Online. Available: http://v.youku.com/v_show/id_XMTEMjcxNzQ4.html?spm=a2h0j.8191423.module_basic_relation.5~5!2~5~5!3~5~5~A&from=y1.2-1-84.3.1-1.1-1-1-0-0 (accessed 17 December 2016).

Gu, J., and Renwick, N. (2008) 'China's fight against HIV/AIDS', *Journal of Contemporary China*, 17, 54: 85–106.

Guangdong Province Health Department (2010) '2010nian Guangdongsheng aizibing fangzhi gongzuo qingkuang tongbao' [Notice on 2010 AIDS prevention work in Guangdong Province], 29 November. Online. Available: www.gdwst.gov.cn/a/zwxw/201011298373.html (accessed 17 December 2016).

'Guangzhou fang'ai renyuan jiaban piaoke jiao maiyinnü yong anquantao' [Guangzhou AIDS prevention workers disguise themselves as clients in order to teach sex worker how to use condoms] (2006) *Xinxi Shibao*, 26 November. Online. Available: http://news.sina.com.cn/s/2006-11-28/090710616191s.shtml (accessed 16 December 2016).

'Guanyu yinfa: "Gongwuyuan luyong tijian tongyong biaozhun (shixing)" de tongzhi' [Civil service recruitment examination standard (Trial)] (2005) Renshibu, Weishengbu, 17 January. Online. Available: www.mohrss.gov.cn/gkml/xxgk/201407/t20140717_136044.html (accessed 16 December 2016).

Guo, X. (2007) *Zhongguo fa shiyexia de tongxinglian* [Homosexuality From the Perspective of Chinese Law], Beijing: Zhishichanquan Chubanshe.

Guo, Y., Li, X.M., and Stanton, B. (2011) 'HIV-Related behavioral studies of men who have sex with men in China: A systematic review and recommendations for future research', *AIDS and Behavior*, 15, 3: 521–34.

Guowuyuan [State Council] (1986) 'Guowuyuan guanyu jianjue qudi maiyin huodong he zhizhi xingbing manyan de tongzhi' [Notice of the State Council on resolutely banning prostitution and curbing the spread of sexually transmitted disease], 1 September. Online. Available: www.medste.gd.cn/Html/Article/165849.html (accessed 16 December 2016).

Guowuyuan [State Council] (1993) 'Maiyinpiaochang renyuan shourong jiaoyu banfa' [Notice on detention and education of people who engage in prostitution activites]. Online. Available: http://baike.baidu.com/view/4960938.htm (accessed 16 December 2016).

Guowuyuan [State Council] (1998) 'Zhongguo yufang yu kongzhi aizibing zhongchangqi guihua (1998–2010)' [China's medium- and long-term strategic plan for HIV/AIDS prevention and control (1998–2010)], 26 October. Online. Available: http://news.xinhuanet.com/zhengfu/2002-09/29/content_579877.htm (accessed 16 December 2016).

Guowuyuan [State Council] (2000) 'Guowuyuan guanyu shishi xibu dakaifa ruogan zhengce de tongzhi' [Circular of the State Council on policies and measures pertaining to the development of the western region], 28 November. Online. Available: www.gov.cn/gongbao/content/2001/content_60854.htm (accessed 16 December 2016).

Guowuyuan [State Council] (2006a) Aizibing fangzhi tiaoli [Regulations on AIDS Prevention and Treatment], issued 18 January, effective 1 March. Online. Available: www.gov.cn/flfg/2006-02/12/content_186324.htm (accessed 1 February 2017).

Guowuyuan [State Council] (2006b) 'Yulechangsuo guanli tiaoli' [Regulations on the Management of Entertainment and Leisure Venues], 1 March. Online. Available: www.gov.cn/zwgk/2006-02/13/content_187029.htm (accessed 16 December 2016).

Guowuyuan [State Council] (2006c) 'Zhongguo ezhi yu fangzhi aizibing xingdong jihua (2006–2010)' [China's Action Plan (2006–2010) for the Containment and Prevention of HIV/AIDS], 27 February. Online. Available: www.gov.cn/gongbao/content/2006/content_284340.htm (accessed 12 December 2016).

Guowuyuan [State Council] (2009) 'Liudongrenkou jihuashengyu gongzuo tiaoli' [Regulations on family planning work for migrant populations], 29 April. Online. Available: www.gov.cn/zwgk/2009-05/20/content_1320203.htm (accessed 16 December 2016).

Guowuyuan [State Council] (2010) 'Guowuyuan guanyu jinyibu jiaqiang aizibing fangzhi gongzuo de tongzhi' [2010 Notice of the State Council on strengthening the work of containing and preventing AIDS], 31 December. Online. Available: www.gov.cn/zwgk/2011-02/16/content_1804536.htm (accessed 16 December 2016).

Guowuyuan bangongting [General Office of the State Council] (2001) 'Zhongguo ezhi yu fangzhi aizibing xingdong jihua (2001–2005)' [China's Action Plan (2001–2005) for the Containment and Prevention of HIV/AIDS], 25 May. Online. Available: www.gov.cn/gongbao/content/2001/content_60908.htm (accessed 16 December 2016).

Guowuyuan bangongting [General Office of the State Council] (2012) 'Guowuyuan bangongting guanyu yinfa Zhongguo ezhi yu fangzhi aizibing "shierwu" xingdong jihua de tongzhi' [General Office of the State Council: Notice on China's action plan for the containment and prevention of HIV/AIDS 'during the period of the twelfth five-year economic plan' [2011–2015], 13 January. Online. Available: www.gov.cn/zwgk/2012-02/29/content_2079097.htm (accessed 6 January 2017).

Guowuyuan bangongting [General Office of the State Council] (2013) 'Guowuyuan bangongting guanyu zhengfu xiang shehui liliang goumai fuwu de zhidao yijian' [Guiding Opinions of the State Council on the Government Purchase of Services from Social Forces], 26 September. Online. Available: www.gov.cn/zwgk/2013-09/30/content_2498186.htm (accessed 1 February 2017).

Guowuyuan bangongting [General Office of the State Council] (2017) 'Zhongguo ezhi yu fangzhi aizibing "shisanwu" xingdong jihua' [China's Action Plan for the Containment and Prevention of HIV/AIDS for the Period of the 'Thirteenth Five-Year Guidelines for National Economic and Social Development' [2016–2020], 19 January. Online. Available: www.gov.cn/zhengce/content/2017-02/05/content_5165514.htm (accessed 22 February 2017).

Hacking, I. (2002) *Historical Ontology*, Cambridge, MA: Harvard University Press.

Hacking, I. (2006) 'Making up people', *London Review of Books*, 28, 16: 23–6.

'Haerbin zhiyuanzhe huizhi anchang fenbutu fangfan aizibing' [Harbin volunteers to map distribution of illicit sex workers to prevent AIDS] (2006) *Shenghuobao*, 19 September. Online. Available: http://news.sina.com.cn/c/h/2006-09-10/135510971147.shtml (accessed 16 December 2016).

Han, Fudong (2002) '"Anquantao xiangmu" de pinghengdian hezai?' [Where does the balance of 'the condom project' lie?], *Nanfang Dushibao*, 23 September. Online. Available: www.southcn.com/news/china/gdspcn/200209230675.htm (accessed 16 December 2016).

Hanenberg, R. S., Rojanapithayakorn, W., Kunasol, P., and Sokal, D. C. (1994) 'Impact of Thailand HIV-control program as indicated by the decline of sexually-transmitted diseases', *Lancet*, 344, 8917: 243–5.

'Harbin zhiyuanzhe dui tongxinglian xuanchuan fang'ai huizhi anchang fenbutu' [Volunteers in Harbin draw maps of illicit sex work venues and promote HIV prevention education among men who have sex with men] (2006) *Shenghuo Bao*, 19 September. Online. Available: http://news.sohu.com/20060910/n245259791.shtml (accessed 30 June 2016).

Hayes, A. (2005) 'AIDS, bloodheads and cover-ups: The "abc" of Henan's AIDS epidemic', *Australian Quarterly*, 77, 3: 12–6.

Hayes, A. (2010) 'Gender, migration and human security: HIV vulnerability among rural to urban migrants in the People's Republic of China', paper presented to the Migrant Security 2010: Citizenship and Social Inclusion in a Transnational Era, Toowoomba, Australia, 15–16 July 2010. Online. Available: http://eprints.usq.edu.au/9303/1/Hayes_Migrant_Security_2010_PV.pdf (accessed 16 December 2016).

He, G. (2002a) 'Lixian yulechangsuo "anquan" diyi' [Li County entertainment and leisure venues put 'safety' first], *Xiaoxiang Chenbao*. Online. Available: www.xxcb.cn/show.asp?id=125253 (accessed 5 September 2011).

He, G. (2002b) 'Yulechangsuo 100% shiyong anquantao de taiqianmuhou' [What's behind the promotion of 100% condom use in entertainment and leisure venues?], *Beijing Qingnianbao*. Online. Available: www.people.com.cn/GB/guandian/20020925/831117.html (accessed 16 December 2016).

He, L. and Zunyou, W. (2013) 'Zhongguo nongmingong aizibing jiankang jiaoyu ganyu xiaoguo de Meta fenxi' [Meta-analysis of HIV/AIDS interventions for migrant workers in China], *Zhongguo Aizibing Xingbing*, 19, 8: 585–9.

He, N., Detels, R., Chen, Z., Jiang, Q.W., Zhu, J.D., Dai, Y.Q., Wu, M., Zhong, X., Fu, C.W., and Gui, D.X. (2006) 'Sexual behavior among employed male rural migrants in Shanghai, China', *AIDS Education and Prevention*, 18, 2: 176–86.

He, N., Wong, F.Y., Huang, Z.J., Ding, Y.Y., Fu, C.W., Smith, B.D., Young, D., and Jiang, Q.W. (2007) 'HIV risks among two types of male migrants in Shanghai, China: money boys vs. general male migrants', *AIDS*, 21: S73 – S9.

He, X., Yuanyuan, W., Jin, C., Jiangtao, H., and Qingjian, Z. (2013) 'Guangdongsheng weihun qingshaonian liudongrenkou xingjiangkang xingweiganyu yanjiu' [A study of sexual health and behavioural interventions for unmarried migrant youth in Guangdong Province], *Zhongguo Xingkexue*, 22, 1: 82–90.

He, Z. (1989) 'Tongxinglian zai Zhongguo de bukejieshouxing' [The unacceptable aspects of homosexuality in China], *Daode yu Wenming*, 4: 31–3.

Hershatter, G. (1997) *Dangerous Pleasures: Prostitution and Modernity in Twentieth-century Shanghai*, Berkeley; Los Angeles: University of California Press.

Hesketh, T., Ye, X., and Zhu, W. (2008) 'Syphilis in China: The great come back', *Emerging Health Threats Journal*, 1: 1–6.

Hildebrandt, T. (2011) 'The political economy of social organization registration in China', *The China Quarterly*, 208: 970–89.

Hildebrandt, T. (2012) 'Development and division: The effect of transnational linkages and local politics on LGBT activism in China', *Journal of Contemporary China*, 21, 77: 845–62.

'HIV in Thailand: the 100% Condom Use Program' (2011) Case in Global Health Delivery, Harvard Medical School and Brigham and Women's Hospital. Online. Available: https://ghca.jp/files/fm/5153d4421p7jjb1vnfhy_0_8.pdf (accessed 16 December 2016).

'HIV in the United States: At a glance' (2015) CDC, National Center for HIV/AIDS, Viral Hepatitis, STD, and TB Prevention, Division of HIV/AIDS Prevention, July. Online. Available: www.cdc.gov/hiv/pdf/statistics_basics_ataglance_factsheet.pdf (accessed 21 December 2016).

Hong, Y., Stanton, B., Li, X.M., Yang, H.M., Lin, D.H., Fang, X.Y., Wang, J., and Mao, R. (2006) 'Rural-to-urban migrants and the HIV epidemic in China', *AIDS and Behavior*, 10, 4: 421–30.

Hong, Y., Zhang, C., Li, X-M., Zhou, Y-J., and Guo, W-G, (2014) 'Female sex workers and their gatekeepers in China: Implications for HIV/STI prevention', *Qualitative Health Research*, 24, 10: 1431–9.

'"Hong sidai" qingxi nongmingong fang'ai zhishi zou jin gongdi' ['Red Ribbon' message of love brought knowledge about AIDS prevention to migrant workers onsite] (2016) *Xinhuawang*, 29 November. Online. Available: www.hb.xinhuanet.com/2016-11/29/c_1120014400.htm (accessed 13 January 2017).

Hood, J. (2010) 'Celebrity philanthropy: The cultivation of China's HIV/AIDS heroes', in L. Edwards and E. Jeffreys (eds) *Celebrity in China*, Hong Kong: Hong Kong University Press.

Hood, J. (2011) *HIV/AIDS, Health, and Media in China: Imagined Immunity Through Racialized Disease,* Abingdon: Routledge.

Hood, J. (2012) 'HIV/AIDS and shifting urban China's sociomoral landscape: Engendering bio-activism and resistance through stories of suffering', *IJAPS*, 8, 1: 125–44.

Hood, J. (2015a) 'Peng Liyuan's humanitarianism: Morality, politics and eyeing the present and past', *Celebrity Studies*, 6, 4: 414–29.

Hood, J. (2015b) 'Untangling HIV in China: Social, political, economic, and global-local factors', in M. McLelland and V. Mackie (eds) *The Routledge Handbook of Sexuality Studies in East Asia*, Abingdon: Routledge, pp. 356–71.

Hu, M. (2004) 'Huangpi shidian tongguo pinggu Wuhan 100% anquantao shiyong xiangmu zouxiang qiantai' [Huangpi pilot passes evaluation, Wuhan's 100% Condom Use Program goes public], *Hubei Ribao*, 28 April.

Hu, W. (2004) 'Anquantao guanggao kaishi songbang' [Relaxing controls on condom advertising], *Zhongguo Yiyaobao*, 19 October, p. B1.

Hu, X. (2012) 'China's young rural-to-urban migrants: In search of fortune, happiness, and independence', Migration Policy Institute, 4 January. Online. Available: www.migrationpolicy.org/article/chinas-young-rural-urban-migrants-search-fortune-happiness-and-independence (accessed 16 December 2016).

Hu, X., Shilong, T., Xin, X., Xiajuan, X., Xin, D., Bei, W., and Tian, G. (2011) 'Hubeisheng nüxing xinggongzuozhe shehuiwangluo zhichi zhuangkuang yanjiu' [Study of social network support for female sex workers in Hubei Province], *Yixue yu Shehui*, 24, 2: 44–5.

Huang, K. (2006) 'Lectures held for sex workers and gays', *South China Morning Post*, 12 September, p. 8.

Huang, Y. (2013) *Governing Health in Contemporary China*, Abingdon: Routledge.

Huang, Z. J., He, N., Nehl, E. J., Zheng, T., Smith, B. D., Zhang, J., McNabb, S., and Wong, F. Y. (2012) 'Social network and other correlates of HIV testing: Findings from male sex workers and other MSM in Shanghai, China', *AIDS Behaviour*, 16, 4:858–71.

'Huibi buru zhengshi' [Acknowledgement is better than avoidance] (2004) China Central Television, 2 December. Online. Available: http://v.youku.com/v_show/id_XNDA1NDA4MTI=.html (accessed 16 December 2016).

Human Rights Watch (2013) ' "Swept Away": Abuses against sex workers in China', May, USA. Online. Available: www.hrw.org/report/2013/05/14/swept-away/abuses-against-sex-workers-china (accessed 16 December 2016).

Hutcheon, S. (2008) 'Olympic condoms ads', Beijing08Blogs, Fairfax Digital. Online. Available: http://blogs.smh.com.au/olympics/stephenhutcheon/2008/07/28/olympiccondom.html (accessed 16 December 2016).

Hyde, S. T. (2007) *Eating Spring Rice: The Cultural Politics of AIDS in Southwest China*, Berkeley, Los Angeles: University of California Press.

'Income gap widens: Report' (2012) Xinhua, 15 August. Online. Available: www.china.org.cn/chinese/2012-08/15/content_26244816.htm (accessed 16 December 2015).

International Labour Organization Country Office for China and Mongolia (2008) 'The first targeted HIV/AIDS prevention campaign in China featuring migrant workers for their hometown fellows'. Online. Available: www.ilo.org/beijing/information-resources/public-information/press-releases/WCMS_142075/lang – en/index.htm (accessed 16 December 2016).

International Organization for Migration, Global Migration Data Analysis Centre (2016) '2015 global migration trends factsheet', April. Online. Available: http://iomgmdac.org/wp-content/uploads/2016/06/Global-Migration-Trends-2015-Factsheet.pdf (accessed 22 December 2016).

Jacobs, A. (2009) 'H.I.V. tests turn blood into cash in China', *The New York Times*, 3 December, p. A6. Online. Available: www.nytimes.com/2009/12/03/health/policy/03china.html?_r=1&sq=hiv%20china&st=cse&scp=1&pagewanted=print (accessed 16 December 2016).

Jeffreys, E. (2004) *China, Sex and Prostitution*, London; New York: Routledge.

Jeffreys, E. (2006) 'Governing buyers of sex in the People's Republic of China', *Economy and Society*, 35, 4: 571–93.

Jeffreys, E. (2008) 'Advanced producers or moral polluters? China's bureaucrat-entrepreneurs and sexual corruption', in D.S.G. Goodman (ed.) *The New Rich in China: Future Rulers, Present Lives*, Abingdon: Routledge, pp. 229–44.

Jeffreys, E. (2009) 'Serial prostitute homicide in the Chinese media', in L.M. Cuklanz and S. Moorti (eds) *Local Violence, Global Media: Feminist Analyses of Gendered Representations*, New York: Peter Lang, pp. 27–46.

Jeffreys, E. (2010) 'Exposing police corruption and malfeasance: China's virgin prostitution cases', *China Journal*, 63: 127–49.

Jeffreys, E. (2012a) 'Prostitution and propaganda in the People's Republic of China', in A-M. Brady (ed.) *China's Thought Management*, Abingdon: Routledge, pp. 146–63.

Jeffreys, E. (2012b) *Prostitution Scandals in China: Policing, Media and Society*, Abingdon: Routledge.

Jeffreys, E., and Huang, Y. (2009) 'Governing sexual health in the People's Republic of China', in E. Jeffreys (ed.) *China's Governmentalities: Governing Change, Changing Government*, Abingdon: Routledge.

Jeffreys, E., and Sigley, G. (2009) 'Governmentality, governance and China', in E. Jeffreys (ed.) *China's Governmentalities: Governing Change, Changing Government*, Abingdon: Routledge, pp. 1–23.

Jeffreys, E., and Su, G. (2011) 'China's 100 per cent condom use program: Customising the Thai experience', *Asian Studies Review*, 35, 3: 315–33.

Jeffreys, E., and Yu, H. (2015) *Sex in China*, Cambridge: Polity.

Jia, M., Yunhua, K., Xiangsheng, K., Yuebo, L., Jing, A., Qiongying, L., Jumei, X., Jin, S., Hongfeng, X., and Zunyou, W. (1999) 'Yunnansheng mouxian yulechangsuo zhong aizibing yufang xingwei ganyu yanjiu' [Research on AIDS prevention behavioural interventions in entertainment and leisure venues in a county in Yunnan Province], *Zhongguo Aizibing Xingbing Fangzhi*, 5, 2: 62–4.

Jia, Y. (1995) 'ICD9,10,CCMD-2, CCMD-2-R, DSM III, IV he SMD zhenduan, fenlei, bianma de xianghu duizhao' [ICD9,10,CCMD-2, CCMD-2-R, DSM III, IV and SMD: Comparision of diagnosis, classification and coding], *Shanghai Jingshen Yixue*, 2: 128–57.

Jiang, H., Lu, C.D., Wei, W., Jianxin, Z., Yi, G., Dickson, S.R., and Hui, J. (2009) 'Zhongguo nananxingxingwei qunti HIV ganyu mianlin de tiaozhan: jiyu shequ he yi fabiao zhengju de xunzheng yanjiu' [The challenges of China's HIV/AIDS interventions for men who have sex with men: An appraisal based on evidence from community, behavioural and sociological research], *Yufang Yixue Qingbao Zazhi*, 25, 7: 499–503.

Jianshebu bangongting [General Office of the Ministry of Construction] (2005) Guanyu zuohao jianshe hangye aizibing fangzhi gongzuo de tongzhi [Notice on the work of HIV/AIDS prevention in the construction Industry], 14 December. Online. Available: www.mohurd.gov.cn/zcfg/jsbwj_0/jsbwjrsjy/200611/t20061101_153033.html (accessed 16 December 2016).

Jin, S. (2002) 'Wuhan jinxing anquantao shiyong shidian xiangmu, xingbing fashenglü mingxian xiajiang' [The incidence of sexually transmitted infection has declined sharply following the implementation of a pilot condom use program in Wuhan], *Chutian Jinbao*, 29 June. Online. Available: http://news.sina.com.cn/s/2002-06-29/1119620186.html (accessed 16 December 2016).

Jin Xing tuokou xiu [The Jin Xing Show] (2015) 'Sohu', Online. Available: http://tv.sohu.com/s2014/jxtkx/ (accessed 16 December 2016).

Joint UNFPA Joint United Nations Programme on HIV/AIDS and World Health Organization (2009) *AIDS Epidemic Update: November 2009*, Geneva: UNAIDS.

Kang, H. (2006) *Shibing Tuji* [Soldiers Sortie], China. Distributed by Bayi Film Studio and Huayi Bros. Media Group.

Kaufman, J. (2011) 'HIV, sex work, and civil society in China', *Journal of Infectious Diseases*, 204: S1218–22.

Kaufman, J. (2012) 'China's evolving AIDS policy: The influence of global norms and transnational non-governmental organizations', *Contemporary Politics*, 18, 2: 225–38.

Kilvington, J., Day, S., and Ward, H. (2001) 'Prostitution policy in Europe: A time of change?', *Feminist Review*, 67: 78–93.

Kong, T.S.K. (2009) 'More than a sex machine: Accomplishing masculinity among Chinese male sex workers in the Hong Kong sex industry', *Deviant Behavior*, 30, 8: 715–45.

Kong, T.S.K. (2012) 'Reinventing the self under socialism migrant – male sex workers ("money boys") in China', *Critical Asian Studies*, 44, 2: 283–308.

Kong, T.S.K. (2016) 'Sex and work on the move: Money boys in post-socialist China', *Urban Studies*, 1–17. DOI: 10.1177/0042098016658411

Lan, Y. (2002) 'Zhuanjia: tuiguang anquantao shi zhengfu de zeren, juefei moxu maiyinpiaochang' [Expert: It is the government's responsibility to promote condom use; it is not about permitting prostitution], *Zhongguo Qingnianbao*, 25 September. Online. Available: www.chinanews.com.cn/2002-09-25/26/226381.html (accessed 16 December 2016).

Lee, M. (2011) 'Love for Life: Film review', *Hollywood Reporter*, 7 August. Online. Available: www.hollywoodreporter.com/review/love-life-film-review-209353 (accessed 16 December 2016).

Leng, Q. (2009) 'Laoxiang bang laoxiang, yufang aizibing' jiankang xingdong chujian chengxiao' [Hometown fellows help hometown fellows to prevent HIV/AIDS: Health action achieves preliminary success], *CRI Online*, 3 August. Online. Available: http://gb.cri.cn/27824/2009/08/03/3245s2581437.htm (accessed 16 December 2016).

Li, G., Yanming, S., Hongyan, L., Min, X., Gang, Z., and Fan, L. (2011) 'Fei Jing huji HIV ganranzhe/AIDS bingren mianfei kangbingduzhiliao de xianzhuang wenti ji duice' [Problems and solutions relating to the provision of free antiretroviral therapy for people living with HIV/AIDS in Beijing who are not registered permanent residents], *Zhongguo Aizibing Xingbing*, 17, 6: 686–88.

Li, H. (2010) 'Zai ba xianfan youjie shizhong zhuijiu jingfang lingdao zeren' [Police chiefs will be held responsible if suspects are paraded in public again], *Dahe Bao*, 26 July, p. A07.

Li, H., Kuo, N.T., Liu, H., Korhonen, C., Pond, E., Guo, H.Y., Smith, L., Xue, H., and Sun, J.P. (2010) 'From spectators to implementers: Civil society organizations involved in AIDS programmes in China', *International Journal of Epidemiology*, 39: II65–II71.

Li, H.C., Lau, J.T.F., Holroyd, E., and Yi, H.S. (2010) 'Sociocultural facilitators and barriers to condom use during anal sex among men who have sex with men in Guangzhou, China: An ethnographic study', *Aids Care*, 22, 12: 1481–6.

Li, J. (2003) 'Heiren' Li Yang' ['Underground man', Li Yang], *Xinwen Zhoukan*, 9: 64–5.

Li, J. (2013) 'Wang Baoqiang: From screen to political stage', China.org.cn, 25 January. Online. Available: www.china.org.cn/arts/2013-01/25/content_27793252.htm (accessed 16 December 2016).

Li, L., Morrow, M., and Kermode, M. (2007) 'Vulnerable but feeling safe: HIV risk among male rural-to-urban migrant workers in Chengdu, China', *AIDS Care*, 19, 10: 1288–95.

Li, L., Morrow, M., and Kermode, M. (2010) 'Rural-to-urban male migrant workers' vulnerability to HIV infection in Chengdu, China: Qualitative findings from a mixed-method study', *Work-A Journal of Prevention Assessment and Rehabilitation*, 37, 4: 375–86.

Li, L., Wu, Z., Lin, C., Guan, J., Rotheram-Borus, M., Lu, Y., and NIMH Collaborative HIV/STD Prevention Trial Group (2009) 'Mass media and HIV/AIDS in China', *Journal of Health Communication*, 14, 5: 424–38.

Li, Q. (2009) 'Wosheng nongcun aizibing duowei "shuruxing"' [AIDS in the rural areas of our province is is mostly "imported"], *Changjiang Ribao*, 1 November. Online.

Available: http://e.cjn.cn/whcb/html/2009-11/02/content_2164021.htm (accessed 16 December 2016).

Li, S. (1986) 'Jinmou de maiyin xingwei yi ding liumangzui' [Jin's act of prostitution can be classified as hooliganism], *Faxue*, 7: 45–6.

Li, X. (2006) 'Haerbin peixun "xiaojie" de fengbo' [The storm created by the 'working girl' training class in Harbin], *Xiaokang*, 12: 40–2.

Li, X. (2010) 'Tuidong liudongrenkou shiminhua' [Promoting citizenship for the migrant population group], *Renmin Ribao*, 18 October, p. 2.

Li, Y. (2000) 'Guan'ai, bu qishi aizibing bingren' [Care for people living with HIV and AIDS, don't discriminate against them], *Zhongguo Keji Yuebao*, 12: 10–11.

Li, Y. (2006) 'Regulating male same-sex relationships in the People's Republic of China', in E. Jeffreys (ed.) *Sex and Sexuality in China*, Abingdon: Routledge, pp. 82–101.

Li, Y. (2006) 'Wo tiyi zhendui anchang lifa' [My proposal is directed at prostitution laws], *Falü yu Shenghuo*, 4: 7–9.

Li, Y. (2009) 'Dali tongxinglian jiuba bei fou you zhengfu chuzi, wei ruqikaiye' [Dali gay bar opening is delayed, municipal government says it did not provide funding], *China Daily*, 2 December. Online. Available: www.chinadaily.com.cn/zgrbjx/2009-12/02/content_9096790.htm (accessed 16 December 2016).

Li, Y. (2015) 'Zhongguo heshi pizhun tongxinghunyin?' [When will China approve same-sex marriage?], 27 June. Online. Available: http://blog.sina.com.cn/s/blog_473d53360102vub7.html (accessed 20 January 2017).

Li, Y., and Chui, E. (2011) 'China's policy on rural-urban migrants and urban social harmony', *Asian Social Science*, 7, 7: 12–22.

Li, Y., and Xiaobo, W. (1992) *Tamen de shijie* [Their World], Taiyuan: Shanxi Renmin Chubanshe.

Li, Y., and Xiaobo, W. (1998) *Tongxinglian yawenhua* [The Sub-culture of Homosexuality], Beijing: Jinri Zhongguo Chubanshe.

Liang, J. (2008) 'Bie rang "xiaojie xuanshi" jiaole aizibing fangzhi daju' [Don't let the sex workers' pledge compromise the work of HIV/AIDS prevention], *Zhongguo Qingnianbao*, 3 December. Online. Available: http://news.163.com/08/1203/05/4S7E6K2F000120GU.html (accessed 16 December 2016).

Liao, S.S., He, Q.Y., Choi, K.H., Hudes, E.S., Liao, J.F., Wang, X.C., Liu, M., Pan, W.L. and Mandel, J.S. (2006) 'Working to prevent HIV/STIs among women in the sex industry in a rural town of Hainan, China', *AIDS and Behavior*, 10: S35–S45.

Liebman, B.L. (2005) 'Watchdog or demagogue? the media in the Chinese legal system', *Columbia Law Review*, 105, 1: 1–157.

'Life is too good' (2007) United Nations Development Program: China. Online. Available: www.youtube.com/watch?v=BZe264972jM (accessed 16 December 2016).

Liu, G., Yunyan, L., Yong, C., Dan, L., and Na, J. (2004) 'Jingcai wuhan 2004 bianhua' [Wonderful Wuhan, changes in 2004], *Wuhan Chenbao*. Online. Available: www.cnhan.com/gb/content/2004-12/27/content_414164.htm (accessed 16 December 2016).

Liu, H.J., Liu, H., Cai, Y.M., Rhodes, A.G., and Hong, F.C. (2009) 'Money boys, HIV risks, and the associations between norms and safer sex: *A respondent-driven sampling study in Shenzhen, China', AIDS and Behavior*, 13, 4: 652–62.

Liu, J. (2009) 'Yunnan Dali nantongxinglian jiuba yanqi kaiye diaocha' [Investigation: Why the opening of a gay bar in Yunnan Dali was delayed], *Xinhua*, 8 December, Online. Available: http://news.xinhuanet.com/focus/2009-12/08/content_12572890.htm (accessed 16 December 2016).

Liu, M. (2011) *Migration, Prostitution, and Human Trafficking*: The Voice of Chinese Women, New Brunswick; London: Transaction Publishers.

Liu, N. (2011) 'Peng Liyuan de xin shiming' [Peng Liyuan's new mission], *Huanqiu Renwu*, 17. Online. Available: http://news.china.com.cn/rollnews/2011-07/05/content_8727170.htm (accessed 16 December 2016).

Liu, Y. (1989) 'Woguo meidu liuxing ji fangzhi jianshi' [A short history of China's syphilis epidemic and prevention], *Yixue yu Zhexue*, 10: 50–3.

Liu, Y. (2003) 'Shehui yulun rijian kuansong tongxinglianzhe xianshen Yangzhou xinlimenzhen' [Public opinion is softening: Homosexuals come to Yangzhou psychology clinic], *Xinhua Ribao*, 10 December, p. 5.

Liu, Z. (2005) 'Institution and inequality: The *hukou* system in China', *Journal of Comparative Economics*, 33, 1: 133–57.

Liu, Z. (2015) 'Gonganbu zhian guanli ju xia fa tongzhi, yaoqiu yange yule fuwu changsuo zhian guanli, yanda shehuang shedu weifa fanzui huodong' [Ministry of Public Security notice on the strict management of venues providing leisure and entertainment services, and cracking down on the criminal activities of prostitution and gambling], *Renmin Gonganbao*, 25 November. Online. Available: http://jz.sxgov.cn/content/2015-11/25/content_6485981.htm (accessed 16 December 2016).

Liu, Z., Xiaoke, Z., Peng, X., Maohe, Y., and Shaohui, C. (2009) 'Tianjinshi xingfuwu nanhai de HIV he meidu ganran zhuangkuang fenxi' [Analyzing the prevalence of HIV and syphilis among money boys in Tianjin], *Zhongguo Aizibing Xingbing*, 15, 3: 279–81.

Lixian xiangmuban [Li County Project Office] (2004) Zhongguo Lixian/WHO 100% CUP shishi qingkuang de baogao [China Li County/WHO 100% CUP implementation report], Li County.

Lü, F. (2004) 'Zhongguo shouci gongbu nantongxinglian renshu ji ganran HIV bingdu qingkuang' [China's first announcement regarding the number of men who have sex with men and HIV infection rates], *Xinhua*, 12 January. Online. Available: http://news.xinhuanet.com/newscenter/2004-12/01/content_2280169.htm (accessed 16 December 2016).

Lü, K., Yifei, H., Ran, X., Yingpeng, M., Jing, L., and Hong, H. (2010) 'Woguo 13 gesheng nongmingong aizibing jiben zhishi zhixiaolü de diaocha yu fenxi' [Survey and analysis of HIV/AIDS awareness among migrant workers in 13 Chinese provinces], *Zhongguo Aizibing Xingbing*, 16, 2: 157–9.

Lu, L., Aisheng, P., Jianguo, C., Xiaokang, L., Wangui, L., and Huayu, W. (1992) 'Tongxinglian 1000li linchuang fenxi' [Clinical analysis of 1,000 homosexual cases], *Zhongguo Xinli Weishen Zazhi*, 6, 3: 132–4.

Ma, S. (2005) 'Zhongguo biyun yaoju de gongying yu shiyong' [Development of contraceptive supply in China], *Zhongguo Jihuashengyuxue Zazhi*, 10: 602–3.

Ma, S., Dukers, N., van den Hoek, A., Fu, Y.-L., Chen, Z.-H., Feng, J.-T., Zhang, L., and Zhang, X.-X. (2002) 'Decreasing STD incidence and increasing condom use among Chinese sex workers following a short term intervention: A prospective cohort study', *Sexually Transmitted Infections*, 78, 2: 110–14.

Ma, W. (1994) 'Jianguo chuqi jinchang shulüe' [A brief introduction: Prohibiting prostitution following the founding of the People's Republic of China], *Gongan Yanjiu*, 2: 56–8.

Mao, J. (2008) 'Xiaojie xuanshi' de heise youmo' [The black humour of the 'working-girl pledge'], *CRI Online*. Online. Available: http://gb.cri.cn/26004/2008/12/01/2165s2344879.htm (accessed 16 December 2016).

McDaid, L., and Hart, G. (2010) 'Sexual risk behaviour for transmission of HIV in men who have sex with men: Recent findings and potential interventions', *Current Opinion in HIV and AIDS*, 5:311–15.

'Meiyou qishi yongyuan zai yiqi guan'ai aizibing ertong gongyi guanggao' [No discrimination: Forever care for children with AIDS public service advertisement] (2014) *CCTV.com*, 3 December. Online. Available: http://igongyi.cntv.cn/2014/12/03/VIDE1417600085978809.shtml (accessed 16 December 2016).

Meng, J. (2012) 'HIV governance through law: Achievements and challenges of China's legal environment', *International Journal of Asia Pacific Studies*, 8, 1: 57–75.

Meng, J. (2013) *On the Decriminalization of Sex Work in China: HIV and Patients' Rights*, New York: Palgrave Macmillan.

Meng, N., and Yan, L. (2003) 'Rang aizibing cong xingshenghuo zhong zoukai' [AIDS is separated from sexual life, Liuzhou launches a '100 Per Cent Condom Use Program'], *Nanguo Jinbao*, 1 August. Online. Available: http://news.sina.com.cn/c/2003-08-01/13431458543.html (accessed 25 January 2017).

Meng, Q., Qiulan, Y., Lingqiao, Z., and Jianwei, L. (2004) 'Jinjuli kan ganyu' [A close look at the intervention], *Jiankangbao*, 24 November.

Micollier, E. (2012) 'Sexualised illness and gendered narratives: The problematic of social sciences and humanities in China's HIV and AIDS governance', *International Journal of Asia Pacific Studies*, 8, 1: 103–24.

Miller, P., and Rose, N. (2008) *Governing the Present*, Cambridge: Polity.

Mills, S., Benjarattanaporn, P., Bennett, A., Pattalung, R. N., Sundhagul, D., Trongsawad, P., Gregorich, S. E., Hearst, N., and Mandel, J. S. (1997) 'HIV risk behavioral surveillance in Bangkok, Thailand: Sexual behavior trends among eight population groups', *AIDS*, 11: S43–51.

Ministry of Health of the People's Republic of China (2004) 'Guanyu zai geji jibing yufang kongzhi zhongxin (weisheng fangyizhan) jianli gaoweirenqun ganyu gongzuodui de tongzhi' [Notice on forming intervention teams at different levels of the CDC to target high-risk groups], 20 August, Beijing. Online. Available: www.moh.gov.cn/mohbgt/pw10409/200804/27106.shtml (accessed 1 February 2017).

Ministry of Health of the People's Republic of China (2005) 'Gaoweixingwei ganyu gongzuo zhidao fang'an (shixing) [Guidelines for interventions among those at high risk (trial)]', *Weiban jikongfa* [2005] 102 hao, 9 June, Beijing. Online. Available: www.china.com.cn/chinese/PI-c/885526.htm (accessed 1 February 2017).

Ministry of Health of the People's Republic of China (2012) *2012 China AIDS Response Report*, 31 March. Online. Available: www.unaids.org/sites/default/files/country/documents/ce_CN_Narrative_Report%5B1%5D.pdf (accessed 16 December 2016).

Ministry of Health, People's Republic of China, Joint United Nations Programme on HIV/AIDS and World Health Organization (2006) 2005 Update on the HIV/AIDS Epidemic and Response in China, Beijing: National Center for AIDS/STD Control and Prevention.

Ministry of Health, People's Republic of China, Joint United Nations Programme on HIV/AIDS and World Health Organization (2010) '2009 Estimates for the HIV/AIDS epidemic in China', Beijing: National Center for AIDS/STD Control and Prevention.

Ministry of Health, People's Republic of China, Joint United Nations Programme on HIV/AIDS and World Health Organization (2012) '2011nian Zhongguo aizibing yiqing guji 2011' [Estimation of HIV/AIDS epidemic in China in 2011], *Zhongguo aizibing xingbing*, 18, 1: 1–5.

Mu, H., and Ming, X. (2006) 'Haerbin jizhong gongkai peixun nüxing xinggongzuozhe yufang xingbing aizibing [Harbin's CDC staff focus on STI and HIV prevention trainings for female sex workers], *Harbin Ribao*, 15 October. Online. Available: http://news.sohu.com/20061015/n245797216.shtml (accessed 16 December 2016).

Mu, Y. (2003) '1949: Beijing quanmian jinchang' [1949: Beijing prohibited prostitution thoroughly], *Renmin Gongan*, 3: 46–50.

Muessig, K.E., Bien, C.H., Wei, C., Lo, E.J., Yang, M., Tucker, J.D., Yang, L., Meng, G., and Hightow-Weidman, L.B. (2015) 'A mixed-methods study on the acceptability of using eHealth for HIV prevention and sexual health care among men who have sex with men in China', *Journal of Medical Internet Research*, 17(4): e100. doi: 10.2196/jmir.3370.

Nan, J. (2008) 'Bukan xingbing zhemo ta qiannu maiyinnü' [Man tormented by STI takes out his anger on female sex sellers], *Jinri Zaobao*, 24 August, p. B2.

Nanjing shi gonganju pukou fenju [Nanjing City, Pukou Public Security Bureau] (2006) Guanyu banli maiyinpiaochang anjian de zhidao yijian [Guideline on handling cases related to the selling and buying of sex], 1 June. Online. Available: www.nanjing.gov.cn/njszf/qzf/pkq/njsgajpkfj/201012/t20101222_2018487.html (accessed 11 July 2016).

'"Nantong" ganran aizibing zengjia tongzhi shejiao pingtai huyu baohu ziji' [The prevalence of HIV is increasing among homosexual men: Gay social media platforms appeal to users to protect themselves] (2015) *Renminwang*, 27 November. Online. Available: http://health.people.com.cn/n/2015/1127/c398004-27863289.html (accessed 16 December 2016).

National Bureau of Statistics of China (2012) 'Woguo liudong renkou guoqu 10nian zengjia jin yi ren' [China's migrant population has increased by more than one hundred million people over the past ten years], *Zhongguo Xinxibao*, p. 1.

National Bureau of Statistics of China (2015) 'China's economy realized a new normal of stable growth in 2014', 20 January. Online. Available: www.stats.gov.cn/english/PressRelease/201501/t20150120_671038.html (accessed 16 December 2016).

National Center for AIDS/STD Control and Prevention, China CDC (2010) 'Xing'ai zhongxin guanyu yinfa "nannanxingxingweirenqun aizibing xingbing fangzhi xuanchuan cailiao" de han' [NCAIDS: on the issuing of AIDS prevention promotional materials for men who have sex with men], 21 December. Online. Available: http://ncaids.chinacdc.cn/fzdt/zxdt/201012/t20101221_1519120.htm (accessed 23 January 2017); reproduced with permission.

National Center for AIDS/STD Control and Prevention, China CDC (2010) 'Xing'ai zhongxin guanyu yinfa "nannanxingxingweirenqun aizibing xingbing fangzhi xuanchuan cailiao" de han' [NCAIDS: on the issuing of 'AIDS prevention promotional materials for men who have sex with men'], 21 December. Online. Available: http://ncaids.chinacdc.cn/fzdt/zxdt/201012/t20101221_1519120.htm (accessed 7 February 2017); reproduced with permission.

National Center for AIDS/STD Control and Prevention, China CDC (n.d.) 'General information'. Online Available: http://ncaids.chinacdc.cn/english/aboutncaids/angi/ (accessed 23 January 2017).

National Health and Family Planning Commission of the People's Republic of China (2014) '2014 China aids response progress report'. Online. Available: www.unaids.org/sites/default/files/documents/CHN_narrative_report_2014.pdf (accessed 16 December 2016).

National Health and Family Planning Commission of the People's Republic of China (2015) '2015 China aids response progress report'. Online. Available: www.unaids.org/sites/default/files/country/documents/CHN_narrative_report_2015.pdf (accessed 16 December 2016).

National Health and Family Planning Commission of the People's Republic of China and the World Health Organization Western Pacific Region (2016) 'CHINA-WHO country cooperation strategy 2016–2020', World Health Organization, July.

National People's Congress (2006) 'Zhonghua renmin gongheguo guomin jingji he shehui fazhan di shiyi ge wunian guihua gangyao' [PRC's Eleventh Five-Year Guidelines for National Economic and Social Development], 16 March. Online. Available: http://news.xinhuanet.com/misc/2006-03/16/content_4309517.htm (accessed 16 December 2016).

National People's Congress (2011) 'Zhonghua renmin gongheguo guomin jingji he shehui fazhan di shier ge wunian guihua gangyao' [PRC's Twelfth Five-Year Plan for National Economic and Social Development], 16 March. Online. Available: www.gov.cn/2011lh/content_1825838.htm (accessed 16 December 2016).

National People's Congress (2016a) 'Jingwai feizhengfuzuzhi guanlifa' (Law of the People's Republic of China on the management of overseas non-governmental organizations' activities within Mainland China), 28 April, effective 1 January 2017. Online. Available: http://chinalawtranslate.com/bilingual-fngo-law/?lang=en (accessed 1 February 2017).

National People's Congress (2016b) 'Zhonghua renmin gongheguo guomin jingji he shehui fazhan di shisan ge wunian guihua gangyao' [PRC's thirteenth five-year plan for national economic and social development], 17 March. Online. Available: www.gov.cn/xinwen/2016-03/17/content_5054992.htm (accessed 1 February 2017).

National People's Congress (2016c) 'Zhonghuarenmingongheguo cishanfa' (Charity law of the People's Republic of China), 16 March, effective 1 September 2016. Online. Available: www.npc.gov.cn/npc/dbdhhy/12_4/2016-03/21/content_1985714.htm (accessed 1 February 2017).

National Population and Family Planning Commission of China (2007) 'Cong chengnuo dao xingdong: aizibing yugfang yu shengzhi jiankang/jihua shengyu fuwu xiangjiehe' [From promise to action: Combine AIDS prevention and reproductive health/family planning]. Online. Available: www.docin.com/p-317863451.html&dpage=1&key=%E8%89%BE%E6%BB%8B%E7%97%85%E6%80%8E%E4%B9%88%E6%B2%BB (accessed 16 December 2016).

NCAIDS (n.d.) 'Aizibing jiankang jiaoyu zikeku' [AIDS health education resource database]. Online. Available: http://ncaids.chinacdc.cn/zsk/mbrq/index.html (accessed 12 January 2017).

NCAIDS, NCSTD, China CDC (2015) 'Update on the AIDS/STD epidemic in China and main response in control and prevention in July, 2015', *China Journal of AIDS STD*, 21, 9: 749.

Ni, Z., Jian, L., Dan'ge, X., Yan, Z., and Ting, C. (2011) 'Yuchi MSM requn aizibing ji meidu ganranlü diaocha' [Investigating the infection rates of syphilis and HIV among men who have sex with men in public bathhouses], *Zhejiang Yufang Yixue*, 23, 5: 14–6.

Osmond, D. (2003) 'Epidemiology of HIV/AIDS in the United States', *HIV Insite*. Online. Available: http://hivinsite.ucsf.edu/InSite?page=kb-01-03 (accessed 23 February 2017).

Pan, J., Bing, L., Jianhong, Z., and Ying, W. (2010) 'Nüxing xinggongzuozhe liyong aizibing ziyuan zixun jiance menzhen de yiyuan ji yingxiang yinsu dingxingfenxi' [Qualitative study on the factors influencing female sex workers' willingness to use clinics that provide counselling and voluntary HIV testing], *Jibing Jiance*, 25, 4: 308–11.

Pan, S. (1994) 'Zhongguo you "xingchanye" ma? Guanyu Zhongguo dixia "xingchanye" de diaocha yu sikao' [Does China have a 'sex industry'? Investigation and thoughts on China's underground 'sex industry'], *Falü yu Shenghuo*, 10: 23–5.

Pan, S. (2002) 'Xingchuanbo aizibing de keneng jiujing youduoda' [It is highly likely that sexual transmission will become the main mode of HIV transmission in China], *Baike Zhishi*, 4: 17–19.

Pan, S. (2007) 'Zhongguoren dui xingchanye riyi kuanrong' [Chinese people are becoming more tolerant of the sex industry], *Baike Zhishi*, 7: 53–4.

Pan, X.H., Zhu, Y.Y., Wang, Q., Zheng, H., Chen, X., Su, J., Peng, Z.H., Yu, R.B., and Wang, N. (2013) 'Prevalence of HIV, Syphilis, HCV and their high risk behaviors among migrant workers in eastern China', *Plos One*, 8, 2: 1–9.

Peng, W., and Xiaohui, C. (2013) 'Nüxing liudongrenkou shengzhijiankang fuwu xuqiuyanjiu-jiyu Hangzhoushi 2010nian liudongrenkou dongtai jiance diaocha' [Snowball reserarch on the need for reproductive health services for female migrants: 2010 dynamic monitoring survey of migrants in Hangzhou], *Zhongguo Xingkexue*, 22, 3: 84–90.

Perkins, D. (1994) 'Completing China's move to the market', *Journal of Economic Perspectives*, 8, 2: 23–46.

Peterson, J., and DiClemente, R.J. (eds) (2000) *Handbook of HIV Prevention*, New York: Kluwer Academic Publishers.

Phillips, T. (2016) 'Court hears China's first transgender discrimination case', *The Guardian*, 12 April. Online. Available: www.theguardian.com/world/2016/apr/12/court-hears-chinas-first-transgender-discrimination-case (accessed 16 December 2016).

Phoolcharoen, W. (2006) 'The Thai response to the HIV/AIDS epidemic', in D. Francis, J. Esparza and P. Thongcharoen (eds) *HIV Vaccine Research and Development in Thailand*, Bangkok: Amarin Printing and Publishing Public Co., pp. 53–82.

Punpanich, W., Ungchusak, K., and Detels, R. (2004) 'Thailand's response to the HIV epidemic: Yesterday, today, and tomorrow', *AIDS Education and Prevention*, 16, 3: 119–36.

Qiao, L. (2016) '50 ming lüshi lian shu guanzhu aizibing qishi cu xiugai gongwuyuan luyong tijian biaozhun' [50 lawyers draw attention to AIDS discrimination to promote reform of the health examination standards for civil servant recruitment], *Radio Free Asia*, 11 July. Online. Available: www.rfa.org/mandarin/yataibaodao/renquanfazhi/ql1-07112016101039.html (accessed 21 December 2016).

Qiu, Y. (2000) 'Shanghai qidong fangzhi aizibing zhongchangqi guihua' [Shanghai begins implementation of mid- to long-term AIDS prevention plans], *Xinhua Meiri Dianxun*, 30 November, p. 5.

Qiu, Y., and Yequan, W. (2006) 'Jiangsu jikong zhongxin jiaodao "xiaojie" youpian keren dai anquantao' [Jiangsu Center for Disease Control and Prevention instructs 'working girls' on how to coax clients into using condoms], *Zhongguo Jiangsuwang*, 18 October. Online. Available: http://news.sina.com.cn/s/2006-10-18/150210266866s.shtml (accessed 16 December 2016).

'Quanguo nongmingong yufang aizibing xuanchuan jiaoyu gongcheng shishi fang'an' [National rural-to-urban migrant workers AIDS Prevention education project] (2005) Guoaiban fa 2005, 53 hao, 21 November. Online. Available: www.china.com.cn/chinese/PI-c/1045184.htm (accessed 16 December 2016).

Quanguo renda changwu weiyuanhui [Standing Committee of the National People's Congress] (1986) 'Zhonghua renmin gongheguo zhian guanli chufa tiaoli' [Regulations of the People's Republic of China on Penalties for Administration of Public Security], 5 September. Online. Available: www.law-lib.com/law/law_view.asp?id=95355 (accessed 16 December 2016).

Quanguo renda changwu weiyuanhui [Standing Committee of the National People's Congress] (1991) 'Quanguo renmin daibiao dahui changwu weiyuanhui guanyu yanjin maiyinpiaochang de jueding' [Standing Committee of the National People's Congress: Decision on Strictly Forbidding the Selling and Buying of Sex]. Online. Available: www.npc.gov.cn/wxzl/gongbao/2000-12/05/content_5004558.htm (accessed 16 December 2016).

Quanguo renda changwu weiyuanhui [Standing Committee of the National People's Congress] (2005) 'Zhonghua renmin gongheguo zhian guanli chufa fa' [Law of the People's Republic of China on Penalties for Administration of Public Security], adopted at the 17th Meeting of the Standing Committee of the Tenth National People's Congress of the People's Republic of China on 28 August 2005, effective 1 March 2006. Online. Available: www.law-lib.com/law/law_view.asp?id=97597; www.npc.gov.cn/englishnpc/Law/2007-12/13/content_1384114.htm (accessed 16 December 2016).

Reingold, A., and Phares, C. (2006) 'Infectious diseases', in M. H. Merson, R. E. Black and A. Mills (eds) *International Public Health: Diseases, Programs, Systems and Policies*, Boston: Jones and Bartlett, pp. 127–86.

Ren, X. (1999) 'Prostitution and economic modernization in China', *Violence Against Women*, 5, 12: 1411–36.

Ren, X., Xiaoyan, L., and Duowen, R. (2005) 'Tongxinglian xingwei shiyufei xuyao falü shuofa' [Legal position required on whether homosexual behaviour is right or wrong], *Fazhi Ribao*, 27 October, p. 5.

'Renmin shiping: shuoshuo "100% anquantao" xiangmu' [Editorial comments: talking about the 100 Per Cent Condom Use Program] (2006) *People.cn*. Online. Available: http://news.sohu.com/20061202/n246756830.shtml (accessed 16 December 2016).

Revenga, A., Over, M., Masaki, E., Peerapatanapokin, W., Gold, J., Tangcharoensathien, V., and Thanprasertsuk, S. (2006) *The Economics of Effective AIDS Treatment: Evaluating Policy for Thailand*, Washington, DC: The World Bank.

Rofel, L. (2010) 'The traffic in money boys', *Positions: East Asia Cultures Critique*, 18, 2: 425–58.

Rogers, S. J., Ying, L., Xin, Y. T., Fung, K., and Kaufman, J. (2002) 'Reaching and identifying the STD/HIV risk of sex workers in Beijing', *AIDS Education and Prevention*, 14, 3: 217–27.

Rojanapithayakorn, W., and Hanenberg, R. (1996) 'The 100% condom program in Thailand', *AIDS*, 10, 1: 1–7.

Rojanapithayakorn W. (2006) 'The 100% condom use programme in Asia', *Reproductive Health Matters*, 14(28): 41–52.

Rou, K. M., Sullivan, S. G., Liu, P., and Wu, Z. Y. (2010) 'Scaling up prevention programmes to reduce the sexual transmission of HIV in China', *International Journal of Epidemiology*, 39: II38–II46.

Ru, X., Daxun, Q., Jiangfeng, G., Hongyan, L., Hongcai, H., Yan, L., and Xiaoming, S. (2007) 'Dui yulechangsuo congye nüxing shishi yufang xingbing/aizibing de zonghe ganyu xiangmu shishi baogao' [Project performance report on STI and AIDS interventions for female workers in entertainment and leisure venues], *Zhongguo Jihuashengyuxue Zazhi*, 2: 77–80.

Ruan, Qinghua (2009) 'Jianguo chuqi Shanghai feichang yundong zai renshi' [Reevaluating the prohibition of prostituion in Shanghai during the early stage of the founding of the People's Republic of China], *Huadong Shifan Daxue Xuebao*, 4: 30–7.

Rush, A. (2011) 'China's labour market', *Reserve Bank of Australia Bulletin*, September: 29–38.

Schreurs, M. (2015) 'Li Yinhe: Chinese sexologist opens up about the future for China's LGBT community', *The Beijinger*, 27 May. Online. Available: www.thebeijinger.com/blog/2015/05/27/li-yinhe-chinese-sexologist-opens-about-future-chinas-lgbt-community (accessed 20 January 2017).

'Serosorting and strategic positioning' (n.d.) MSMGF Technical Bulletin Series. Online. Available: www.msmgf.org/files/msmgf/documents/TechBulletins/EN/Sec5MSMGF_TechBulletins2012.pdf (accessed 16 December 2016).

Sexton, J. (2009) 'State-funded gay bar closes amid media storm', China.org.cn, 2 December. Online. Available: www.china.org.cn/china/2009-12/02/content_18994332.htm (accessed 16 December 2016).

Shang, H., Xu, J., Han, X., Spero, L., Arledge, K., and Zhang, L. (2012) 'HIV prevention: Bring safe sex to China', *Nature*, 485: 576–7.

'Shanghai qidong <yufang yu kongzhi aizibing zhongchangqi guihua>' [Shanghai starts AIDS Prevention and Control Long-term Plan] (2000) *Xinmin Wanbao*, 28 November. Online. Available: http://news.eastday.com/epublish/gb/paper103/19/class010300003/hwz253797.htm (accessed 16 December 2016).

'Shua "erdaizheng" ke mianfei ling anquantao meizhang meiyue xianling yihe' [Swipe a 'second-generation' ID card to get a free box of condoms every month] (2012) *Yangzi Wanbao*, 23 May. Online. Available: www.yangtse.com/system/2012/05/23/013392349.shtml (accessed 29 March 2016).

Sigley, G. 2009 [2006], 'Sex, politics and the policing of virtue in the People's Republic of China', in E. Jeffreys (ed.) *Sex and Sexuality in China*, Abingdon: Routledge, pp. 43–61.

Smith, C. J. (2005) 'Social geography of sexually transmitted diseases in China: Exploring the role of migration and urbanisation', *Asia Pacific Viewpoint*, 46, 1: 65–80.

Solinger, D. J. (1999a) 'Citizenship issues in China's internal migration: Comparisons with Germany and Japan', *Political Science Quarterly*, 114, 3: 455–78.

Solinger, D. J. (1999b) *Contesting Citizenship in Urban China: Peasant Migrants, the State and the Logic of the Market, Berkeley*, Los Angeles: University of California Press.

Song, W., Meili, T., Ping, Y., Xianming, G., and Mingzhu, X. (1995) 'Dui minyinfunü jingxing xingbing aizibing jiankang jiaoyu de xiaoguo pingjia' [Evaluating STI and AIDS education for female sex sellers], *Zhongguo Xingbing Aizibing Fangzhi*, 1, 1: 23–6.

Song, X., and Fangming, C. (1987) 'Woguo yufang aizibing de cuoshi' [China's AIDS prevention measures], *Liaowang*, 37: 46.

Starr, J.B. (2001) *Understanding China: A Guide to China's Economy, History and Political Structure,* London: Profile Books.

State Administration for Industry and Commerce (1989) 'Guanyu yanjin kanbo youguan xingshenghuo chanpin guanggao de guiding' [Regulations on prohibiting the advertisement of sexual life products]. Online. Available: http://china.findlaw.cn/fagui/p_1/195925.html (accessed 16 December 2016).

State Council (1987) Certain Regulations on the Monitoring and Control of AIDS. Approved 26 December 1987 by the State Council and jointly promulgated on 14 January 1988 by the Ministry of Public Health, the Ministry of Foreign Affairs, the Ministry of Public Security, the State Education Commission, the National Tourism Administration, the Civil Aviation Administration of China and the National Foreign Experts Bureau. Online. Available: http://en.pkulaw.cn/display.aspx?cgid=3664&lib=law (accessed 16 December 2016).

State Council AIDS Working Committee Office and UN Theme Group on HIV/AIDS in China (2004) A Joint Assessment of HIV/AIDS Prevention, Treatment and Care in China, Beijing. Online. Available: www.chinaaids.cn/ddpg/lhpgbg1/zgazbyq/201312/P020131210547942626797.pdf (accessed 16 December 2016).

State Council AIDS Working Committee Office and UN Theme Group on HIV/AIDS in China (2007) A Joint Assessment of HIV/AIDS Prevention, Treatment and Care in China, Beijing. Online. Available: www.unaids.org.cn/uploadfiles/20080725151739.pdf (accessed 16 December 2016).

Sudhinaraset, M., Astone, N., and Blum, R.W. (2012) 'Migration and unprotected sex in Shanghai, China: Correlates of condom use and contraceptive consistency across migrant and nonmigrant youth', *Journal of Adolescent Health*, 50, 3: S68–S74.

Sun, Z., Farrer, J., and Choi, K.-H. (2006) 'Sexual identity among men who have sex with men in Shanghai', *China Perspectives*, 64: 2–14.

Sun, J. P., Liu, H., Li, H., Wang, L. Q., Guo, H. Y., Shan, D., Bulterys, M., Korhonen, C., Hao, Y. and Ren, M. H. 2010, 'Contributions of international cooperation projects to the HIV/AIDS response in China', *International Journal of Epidemiology*, 39: II14–II20.

Tan, Z. (2010) 'Guangdong Dongguan jingfang sheng qian maiyinnü youjie re zhengyi' [Police in the Dongguan District of Guangdong leading a sex seller down the street by a rope causes controversy], *Nanfang Ribao*, 18 July.

Tang, H. (1989) 'Ezhi xingbing zai Zhongguo chongxin manyan' [Curbing the resurgence of sexually transmitted infection in China], *Liaowang*, 9: 20–1.

Tao, J., Ruan, Y., Yin, L., Vermund, S.H., Shepherd, B.E., Shao, Y., and Qian, H.-Z. (2013) 'Sex with women among men who have sex with men in China: Prevalence and sexual practices', *AIDS Patient Care and STDs*, 27, 9: 524–8.

Tao, X. R., Gai, R. Y., Zhang, N., Zheng, W., Zhang, X. F., Xu, A. Q., and Li, S. X. (2010) 'HIV infection and mental health of "money boys": A pilot study in Shandong Province, China', *Southeast Asian Journal of Tropical Medicine and Public Health*, 41, 2: 358–68.

'Thailand's new condom crusade' (n.d.) *Bulletin of the World Health Organization*. Online. Available: www.who.int/bulletin/volumes/88/6/10-010610/en/ (accessed 16 December 2016).

Thompson, D. (2004) Anti-AIDS Effort in Central China Focuses on Former Plasma Donors, Population Reference Bureau. Online. Available: www.prb.org/Publications/Articles/2004/AntiAIDSEffortinCentralChinaFocusesonFormerPlasmaDonors.aspx (accessed 16 December 2016).

Tian, Y., and Donggang, W. (2010) 'Weishengbuzhang Chen Zhu shicha Guangxi Lücheng caihong tongzhi huodong zhongxin' [Chen Zhu, Minister of Health, inspects HIV/AIDS prevention work at the Guangxi Lücheng Rainbow Homosexual Activity Centre], *Nanning Ribao*, 23 January. Online. Available: www.danlan.org/disparticle_26959_4_2.htm (accessed 16 December 2016).

Tong, D. (2002) 'Anquantao xiangmu' jiaogei mingjianzuzhi ban ruhe?' [How about letting NGOs implement 'the condom project'?], *Nanfang Dushibao*, 24 September. Online. Available: www.southcn.com/news/china/gdspcn/200209240663.htm (accessed 16 December 2016).

Tong, G. (2009) *Zhongguo nannan xingjiaoyi zhuangtai diaocha* [Investigating commercial sexual transactions among men who have sex with men in China], Beijing: Beijing Gender Health Education Institute.

Tong, G., Mei, L., Yaqi, G., and Pengfei, Z. (2005) *Zhongguo MSM shequn aizibing yufang gongzuo huigu* [Reviews of HIV/AIDS prevention among China's MSM community], unpublished article.

Trevaskes, S. (2003) ' "Strike Hard 2001": form and strategy in a Chinese anti-crime campaign', *Australian and New Zealand Journal of Criminology*, 36(3): 272–92.

Tse, C. W. (2016) 'Urban residents' prejudice and integration of rural migrants into urban China', *Journal of Contemporary China*, 25, 100: 579–95.

Tucker, J., Ren, X., and Sapio, F. (2010) 'Incarcerated sex workers and HIV prevention in China: Social suffering and social justice countermeasures', *Social Science and Medicine*, 70, 1: 121–9.

UNAIDS (2000) Evaluation of 100% Condom Programme in Thailand, UNAIDS, Geneva. Online. Available: http://data.unaids.org/publications/IRC-pub01/jc275-100pcondom_en.pdf (accessed 16 December 2016).

UNAIDS (2001) *Population Mobility and AIDS*, UNAIDS, Geneva. Online. Available: http://data.unaids.org/Publications/IRC-pub02/jc513-popmob-tu_en.pdf (accessed 16 December 2016).

UNAIDS (2004) 'The media and HIV/AIDS: Making a difference'. Online. Available: http://data.unaids.org/Publications/IRC-pub06/jc1000-media_en.pdf (accessed 16 December 2015).

UNAIDS (2009a) 'China to tackle HIV incidence amongst MSM', 16 January. Online. Available: www.unaids.org/en/resources/presscentre/featurestories/2009/january/20090116msmasia (accessed 16 December 2016).

UNAIDS (2009b) '"Never abandon, never give up": ILO film helps China's migrant workers challenge AIDS stigma', 30 April. Online. Available: www.unaids.org/en/resources/presscentre/featurestories/2009/april/20090430ilofilmschina (accessed 16 December 2015).

UNAIDS (2010) Global Report: UNAIDS Report on Global AIDS Epidemic 2010, Geneva: UNAIDS.

UNAIDS (2015a) 'Chinese Premier commits to ending the AIDS epidemic in China', 4 May. Online. Available: www.unaids.org/en/resources/presscentre/featurestories/2015/may/20150504_china (accessed 16 December 2016).

UNAIDS (2015b) 'UNAIDS 2016–2021 strategy: On the fast-track to end AIDS'. Online. Available: www.unaids.org/sites/default/files/media_asset/20151027_UNAIDS_PCB37_15_18_EN_rev1.pdf (accessed 16 December 2016).

UNAIDS (2015c) 'UNAIDS terminology guidelines'. Online. Available: www.unaids.org/sites/default/files/media_asset/2015_terminology_guidelines_en.pdf (accessed 16 December 2016).

UNAIDS (2016a) *China: Snapshot 2016*, Geneva: UNAIDS.

UNAIDS (2016b) *Prevention Gap Report*, Geneva: UNAIDS.

'UNAIDS and Xinhua renew their partnership towards ending AIDS by 2030' (2016) UNAIDS, 18 March. Online. Available: www.unaids.org/en/resources/presscentre/featurestories/2016/march/20160318_xinhua (accessed 16 December 2016).

UNAIDS, UNICEF, UNDP, UNFPA, UNESCO, WHO, and the World Bank (1998) 'Relationships of HIV and STD declines in Thailand to behavioural change: A synthesis of existing studies'. Online. Available: http://data.unaids.org/publications/irc-pub04/una98-2_en.pdf (accessed 16 December 2016).

UNDP, USAID (2014) Being LGBT in Asia: China Country Report, Bangkok.

United Nations Department of Economic and Social Affairs (2013) 'Number of international migrants rises above 232 million', 11 September. Online. Available: www.un.org/en/development/desa/news/population/number-of-international-migrants-rises.html (accessed 16 December 2016).

United Nations Development Programme (2004) *Thailand's Response to HIV: Progress and Challenges*, Bangkok: UNDP.

United Nations General Assembly (2013) Human Rights Council Twenty-fifth Session Agenda Item 6: Universal Periodic Review, Report of the Working Group on the Universal Periodic Review, China (including Hong Kong, China and Macao, China), 4 December.

United Nations General Assembly (2016) Seventieth Session, Agenda Item 11: Political Declaration on HIV and AIDS: On the Fast-Track to Accelerate the Fight against HIV and to End the AIDS Epidemic by 2030, 7 June.

The UN Theme Group on HIV/AIDS in China (2002) HIV/AIDS: China's Titanic Peril – 2001 Update of the AIDS Situation and Needs Assessment Report, Beijing: UNAIDS.

'Unused condoms no longer evidence of prostitution in NYC' (2014) *Associated Press*, 12 May. Online. Available: www.usatoday.com/story/news/nation/2014/05/12/nyc-cops-wont-seize-condoms/9002435/ (accessed 16 December 2016).

Uretsky, E. (2008) 'Mobile men with money: The socio-cultural and politico-economic context of "high-risk" behaviour among wealthy businessmen and government officials in urban China', *Culture Health and Sexuality*, 10, 8: 801–14.

Uretsky, E. (2016) *Occupational Hazards: Sex, Business, and HIV in Post-Mao China*, Stanford: Stanford University Press.

U.S. Department of Health and Human Services (n.d.) 'A timeline of HIV/AIDS'. Online. Available: www.aids.gov/hiv-aids-basics/hiv-aids-101/aids-timeline/ (accessed 16 December 2016).

U.S. Department of State (2009) '2009 Human Rights Report: China'. Online. Available: www.state.gov/g/drl/rls/hrrpt/2009/eap/135989.htm (accessed 16 December 2016).

Wan, Y. (2014) 'Aizhixing zouguo ershi chunqiu' [20 years of the Beijing Aizhixing Institute for Health Education], *Sina.com*, 14 June. Online. Available: http://blog.sina.com.cn/s/blog_4b87e3950101j2ph.html (accessed 16 December 2016).

Wan, Y.-H. (2001) 'Becoming a gay activist in contemporary China', *Journal of Homosexuality*, 40, 3: 47–64.

Wang, Shiming (2007) 'Wo wei chu zhege "fengtou" er gandao jiaoao' [I am proud of being in this 'limelight'], *Zhongguo Xinwenbao*, 30 November, p. C01.

Wang, B. (2008) 'Aizibing, ni bingbu kepa' [Don't be scared of AIDS], *Wang Baoqing de BLOG*, weblog, 28 November. Online. Available: http://blog.sina.com.cn/s/blog_4ac0673a0100bjec.html (accessed 16 February 2017).

Wang, B., Li, X. M., Stanton, B., Fang, X. Y., Liang, G. J., Liu, H., Lin, D. H., and Yang, H. M. (2007) 'Gender differences in HIV-related perceptions, sexual risk behaviors, and history of sexually transmitted diseases among Chinese migrants visiting public sexually transmitted disease clinics', *AIDS Patient Care and STDs*, 21, 1: 57–68.

Wang, B., Li, X. M., Stanton, B., and McGuire, J. (2010) 'Correlates of HIV/STD testing and willingness to test among rural-to-urban migrants in China', *AIDS and Behavior*, 14, 4: 891–903.

'Wang Baoqiang chuxi gongyi huodong mengyan tiyan mangren shenghuo' [Wang Baoqiang attends charity event blindfolded to experience life as a blind person] (2008) *Tengxun Yule*, 12 April. Online. Available: http://ent.qq.com/a/20080413/000064.htm (accessed 16 December 2016).

Wang, C. (2006) 'Nongminggong-ji cuiruo de aizibing yiganrenqun' [Rural-to-urban migrant workers: A very vulnerable group for HIV/AIDS infection], *Weisheng yu Shenghuo*, p. 1.

Wang, H. (2013) 'Shanghai: City develops app for contraceptives', *China Daily*, 11 July, p. 2.

Wang, J. (2004) 'Shangyexing xingfuwu/xiaofeizhe: yizhong xinde mingming' [Commercial sexual service provider/consumer: A new name], *Zhejiang Xuekan*, 4: 202–11.

Wang, N. (1998) 'Dangqian guonei dui tongxinglian wenti de butong guandian' [Current different perspectives on homosexuality in mainland China], *Yixue yu Zhexue*, 19, 6: 335–7.

Wang, N. (2000) 'Bie jiao wo xiaojie' [Do not call me *xiaojie* [Miss]], *Beijing Wanbao*, 17 October. Online. Available: www.people.com.cn/wsjk/update/10/18/A107.html (accessed 16 December 2016).

Wang, S. (2007) 'Wo wei chu zhege "fengtou" er gandao jiaoao' [I am proud of being in this 'limelight'], *Zhongguo Xinwenbao*, 30 November, p. C01.

Wang, S. (2008) 'Jingfang bude yi you anquantao zuowei maiyinpiaochang zhengju' [Police will not use condom possession as evidence of engaging in prostitution], *Xinhua Meiri Dianxun*, 30 March, p. 2.

Wang, S. (2013) '"Qingchun hongsidai" fang'ai xuanchuan huodong qidong' [Launch of 'Youth Red Ribbon' AIDS prevention campaign], *Zhongguo Qingnianbao*, 2 April, p. 6.

Wang, S., Song, D., Huang, W., He., H., Wang, M., Manning, D., Zaller, N., Zhang, H., and Operario, D. (2015) 'Heterosexual partnerships and the need for HIV prevention and testing for men who have sex with men and women in China: A qualitative study', *AIDS Education and Prevention*, 27, 2: 126–38.

Wang, T. (2011) 'Lü Liping fantong fengbo fajiao zhuanjiaxuezhe pinglun yingxiang' [Lü Liping's anti-gay actions cause a storm: Experts assess the impact], *Minzhu yu Fazhi Shibao*, 11 July, p. D03.

Wang, W. (2005) 'Zhongguo tongxinglian gaobie yinmi shidai 2005nian meiti tan gay shuo ai' [China's homosexuals say goodbye to the days of secrecy: Media discusses gay love in 2005], *Xinmin Zhoukan*, 14 September. Online. Available: http://news.sohu.com/20050914/n226957803.shtml (accessed 16 December 2016).

Wang, W., Fan, L., and Mo, H. (2009) 'Liudong renkou aizibing fangzhi gongzuo guanjian wenti de yanjiu' [Identification of the key problems in AIDS prevention and control among the internal migrant population], *Jibing Jiance*, 24, 2: 84–7.

Wang, X. (2007) 'Nongyebu "hongsidai jincun ruhu gongcheng" qidong xuanchuan yufang aizibing' [Ministry of Agriculture launches AIDS education, 'Red Ribbon in Village Homes Project'], *Nongmin Ribao*, 30 October, p. 2.

Wang, Y. (2002) 'Chutian jinbao faxing celüe qianxi' [Analysis of the circulation strategy of the *Golden Post*], in J. Song (ed.) *Zhongguo Baoye Nianjian*, Beijing: Zhongguo Gongshang Lianhe Chubanshe.

Wei, C. (2010) 'Beijing aizibing huanzhe 7chen waishengshi huji' [70 per cent of AIDS patients in Beijing hold household registration in areas other than Beijing], *Beijing Sheqübao*, 23 June, p. 2.

Wei, C.-Y., Yan, H.-J., Yang, C.-K., Raymond, H.F., Li, J.-J., Yang, H.-T., Zhao, J.-K., Huan, X.-P., and Stall, R. (2014) 'Accessing HIV testing and treatment among men who have sex with men in China: A qualitative study', *AIDS Care: Psychological and Socio-medical Aspects of AIDS/HIV*, 26, 3: 372–8.

Wei, M. (2008) 'Mai anquantao ke shua yikatong' [Condoms can be bought by swiping a city transport card], *Xinjingbao*, 17 December, p. A12.

Wei, M. (2011) 'Nantong fang'ai xuanchuanhua tiejin juminqu' [AIDS prevention posters for gays posted in residential areas], *Xinjingbao*, 6 December, p. A12.

Weishengbu [Ministry of Health] (2008) Nannanxingxingweirenqun aizibing zonghe fangzhi shidian gongzuo fang'an [MSM AIDS prevention pilot program]. Online. Available: www.law-lib.com/law/law_view.asp?id=253715 (accessed 16 December 2016).

Weishengbu, xuanchuanbu, guojia jiaoyuwei [Ministry of Health, Publicity Department and National Board of Education] (1998) Guanyu yinfa yufang aizibing xingbing xuanchuan jiaoyu yuanze de tongzhi [Principles for STD/AIDS Education and Prevention], Weijikong, 8 January. Online. Available: http://law.lawtime.cn/d474637479731.html (accessed 10 January 2017).

Wen, L. (2002) 'Maiyin qi neng jiao gongzuo' [How can we call prostitution work?], *Xinwen Sanmei*, p. 20.

Wen, L., Chen, S., Seguy, N., Chen, Z-D., Sabin, K., Calleja, J., and Bulterys, M. (2012) 'Is the HIV sentinel surveillance system adequate in China? Findings from an evaluation of the national HIV sentinel surveillance system', *Western Pacific Surveillance and Response Journal*, 3, 4: 78–85.

'What do condoms mean to the Chinese' (2002) *People's Daily*, 2 December. Online. Available: http://english.peopledaily.com.cn/200212/02/eng20021202_107752.shtml (accessed 16 December 2016).

Wong, A. (2005) 'The reappropriation of *tongzhi*', *Language in Society*, 34: 763–93.

Wong, D.F.K., Li, C.Y., and Song, H.X. (2007) 'Rural migrant workers in urban China: Living a marginalised life', *International Journal of Social Welfare*, 16, 1: 32–40.

Wong, F.Y., Huang, Z.J., He, N., Smith, B.D., Ding, Y., Fu, C., and Young, D. (2008) 'HIV risks among gay- and non-gay-identified migrant money boys in Shanghai, China', *AIDS Care*, 20, 2: 170–80.

Wong, L. (2011) 'Chinese migrant workers: Rights attainment deficits, rights consciousness and personal strategies', *China Quarterly*, 208: 870–92.

World Health Organization (1992) *The ICD-10 classification of mental and behavioural disorders – Clinical descriptions and diagnostic guidelines*, Geneva: World Health Organization.

World Health Organization Regional Office for the Western Pacific (WHO/WPR) (2006) Joint UNFPA/WHO Meeting on 100% Condom Use Programme, Manila, 3–5 October.

World Health Organization (2014) Consolidated Guidelines on HIV Prevention, Diagnosis, Treatment and Care for Key Populations, July.

World Health Organization (2015) Tool to Set and Monitor Targets for HIV Prevention, Diagnosis, Treatment and Care for Key Populations, July.

World Health Organization Regional Office for the Western Pacific (WHO/WPR) (2004) *Experiences of 100% condom use programme in selected countries of Asia*, Geneva: World Health Organization.

World Health Organization Regional Office for the Western Pacific (WHO/WPR) (2004) *Experience of 100% condom use programme in selected countries of Asia*, Geneva: World Health Organization.

World Health Organization Regional Office for the Western Pacific (WHO/WPR) (2006) Joint UNFPA/WHO Meeting on 100% Condom Use Programme, Manila, 3–5 October.

World Health Organization Regional Office for the Western Pacific (WHO/WPR) and the Chinese Center for Disease Control and Prevention (CDC) (2004) *100% condom use programme: Experience from China (2001–2004)*, Manila, Philippines: WHO/WPR.

Wu, D. (2011a) 'Zhu Dake: zhechang taolun youzhuyu gaishan tongxinglian shou qishi de diwei' [Zhu Dake: This debate will improve the status of homosexuals, a group that faces discrimination], *Ifeng.com*, 7 July. Online. Available: http://ent.ifeng.com/idol-news/special/lvlipingantihomo/zuixin/detail_2011_07/07/7495019_0.shtml (accessed 16 December 2016).

Wu, D. (2011b) 'Chen Danqing: mei Lü Liping zheyinong wei tongxinglian shuohua de shengyin chubulai' [Chen Danqing: Homosexuality is out in the open because of the Lü Liping case], *Ifeng.com*, 13 July. Online. Available: www.china.com.cn/info/2011-07/08/content_22948585.htm (accessed 29 March 2016).

Wu, F. (2008) 'Xuanshi yongtao: falü zai ganga de shanxiao' [Condom pledge: A legal mockery], *Dahe Bao*, 2 December, p. A04.

Wu, J. (1987) 'Kaizhan qingchunqi xingzhishi he xingdaode jiaoyu keburonghuan' [There is a pressing need for sex education and moral guidance for adolescent youth], *Zhongguo Xinli Weisheng Zazhi*, 3: 97–101.

Wu, J. (2010) 'Zhongguo liudongrenkou de xing yu shengzhijiankang' [Current status of sexual and reproductive health among internal migrants in China], *Guoji Shengzhi Jiankang/Jihuashengyu Zazhi*, 29, 6: 414–21.

Wu, J., and Lijun, J. (2008) 'Anquantao shipin guanggao zaici liujin ditie [Condom video advertisements appear on subway trains again], *Dongfang Zaobao*, 25 March, p. A09.

Wu, J., Zongmin, J., Dongbao, Y., Kai, S., and Pengfei, Z. (2006) 'Liudongrenkou zhong nongmingong de aizibing fangzhi zhengce yu jianyi' [AIDS policies and proposals for rural-to-urban migrant workers], *Zhongguo Aizibing Xingbing*, 12, 6: 575–6.

Wu, R., Guochang, C., and Dingdu, Y. (2010) 'Zhongguo guan'ai tongxinglian jiankang zazhi 'Pengyou' yin jingfei wenti tingkan' [China's homosexual health magazine 'Friend

Exchange' stops publishing for financial reasons], *Xinhuanet*, 22 July. Online. Available: http://news.xinhuanet.com/2010-07/22/c_12363387.htm (accessed 16 December 2016).

Wu, W., and Fuliang, S. (2012) 'Yixingshi tuijin yaoju 'ling juli' fuwu' [Yixing City promotes 'zero distance' contraceptive services], *Zhongguo Renkoubao*, 13 March, p. 2.

Wu, Y. (2004) 'Zhuazhu shiji jiji tansuo, quanmian tuijin aizibing fangzhi gongzuo' [Seize the opportunity to actively explore and promote AIDS prevention work], National AIDS Prevention Conference, Beijing.

Wu, Z., Rou, K., and Cui, H. (2004) 'The HIV/AIDS epidemic in China: history, current strategies and future challenges', *AIDS Education and Prevention*, 16(3 Suppl A): 7–17.

Wu, Z.Y., Rou, K.M., Jia, M.H., Duan, S., and Sullivan, S.G. (2007) 'The first community-based sexually transmitted disease/HIV intervention trial for female sex workers in China', *AIDS*, 21: S89–94.

Xia, G., and Yang, X. (2005) 'Risky sexual behavior among female entertainment workers in China: Implications for HIV/STD prevention intervention', *AIDS Education and Prevention*, 17, 2: 143–56.

Xia, Guomei (2009) 'Shangyexing xingjiaoyi: lifa de liangnan yu chulu' [The commercial sex trade: Legislative dilemma and solution], *Tansuo yu Zhengming*, 12: 37–41.

Xiao, J. (2008) '<Aizibing Fangzhi Tiaoli> de shizheng yanjiu [An Empirical Study of the Regulations on AIDS Prevention and Treatment], Master thesis, China University of Political Science and Law, Beijing.

Xie, H., and Xing, W. (2010) 'Maiyinnü zhiren xianchang shijian xiangguan zerenren bei zhuize' [The person in charge of 'prostitution at the scene of the incident' will be held responsible], *Guangzhou Ribao*, 27 July, p. A14.

Xie, Q. (2008) 'Fang'airenyuan ling xiaojie xuanshi jinri kaishi yiding yong anquantao' [Female sex workers pledge to HIV prevention officers that they will use condoms from this day forth], *Guangzhou Ribao*, p. A4.

Xin, M. (2012) 'Rural-urban migration in China', First draft prepared for Oxford Companion to the Economics of China, 14 March. Online. Available: http://people.anu.edu.au/xin.meng/companion_migration.pdf (accessed 16 December 2016).

Xiong, R., Xiaodong, W., Fei, Y., Yuan, C., and Zhijun, L. (2010) 'MSM aizibing ziyuan zixun jiance fuwu moshi tansuo' [Exploring the service model of HIV voluntary counseling and testing among men who have sex with men], *Zhongguo Gonggong Weisheng Guanli*, 26, 251–3.

Xu, F. (2009) 'Governing China's peasant migrants: Building *xiaokang* socialism and harmonious society', in E. Jeffreys (ed.) *China's Governmentalities: Governing Change, Changing Government*, Abingdon: Routledge, pp. 38–62.

Xu, L. (2011) 'Poster boys of safe sex', *China Daily*, 19 December, p. 20.

Xu, Y. (2005) 'Hunansheng fushengzhang Xu Yunzhao zai dianshidianhua huiyi shang fayan' [Vice-governor of Hunan Province Xun Yunzhao's speech at a national TV/telephone conference on AIDS prevention], Gov.cn, 28 November, Online. Available: www.gov.cn/zhibo/2005-11/28/content_111205.htm (accessed 16 December 2016).

Yan, H., Ming, Z., Jianjun, L., Wenhui, G., Haiyang, H., Xiaoyan, L., Xiping, H., and Jinkou, Z. (2010) 'Nannan xingjiechuzhe aizibing xingbing ganran zhuangkuang ji xingwei tezheng he ganyu celüe' [Prevalence of sexually transmissible infections and the behavioural characteristics of men who have sex with men in Jiangsu province], *Zhongguo Yufang Yixue Zazhi*, 11, 12: 1249–52.

Yan, Y. (2005) 'Shui geng xuyao mianfei anquantao' [Who needs free condoms the most], *Guangming Ribao*, 27 January. Online. Available: http://news.sina.com.cn/o/2005-01-27/08524962111s.shtml (accessed 16 December 2016).

Yang, D. (1989) 'Zhongguo jingshen jibing fenlei yu zhenduan biaozhun zhiding gongzuo de lishi yu xiangzhuang' [History and current state of the compilation of Chinese psychiatric classification and diagnostic criteria], *Shanghai Jingshen Yixue*, 1: 10–2.

Yang, R. (dir.) and Lennon, T. (prod.) (2006) *The Blood of Yingzhou District*, documentary film 40 minutes, Thomas Lennon Films. Online. Available: www.bloodofyingzhou.com/ (accessed 20 December 2017).

Yang, S., Weiwei, W., and Huan, C. (2002) 'Nide xingxingwei anquan ma?' [Is your sexual behaviour safe?], *Xiandai Xiaofei Daobao*, 8 August, p. 1.

Yang, T.Z., Wang, W., Abdullah, A.S., Beard, J., Cao, C.J., and Shen, M.W. (2009) 'HIV/AIDS-related sexual risk behaviors in male rural-to-urban migrants in China', *Social Behavior and Personality*, 37, 3: 419–32.

Yang, X., Derlega, V.J., and Luo, H. (2007) 'Migration, behaviour change and HIV/STD risks in China', *AIDS Care*, 19, 2: 282–8.

Yang, X.S., and Xia, G.M. (2008) 'Temporary migration and STD/HIV risky sexual behavior: A population-based analysis of gender differences in China', *Social Problems*, 55, 3: 322–46.

Yang, Z. (2008) 'Chi Susheng: "butinghua" de renda daibiao' [Chi Susheng: A "disobedient" People's Congress delegate], *Zhongguo Xinwen Zhoukan*, 9: 27–9.

Ye, G. (2001) 'Yiwangshi – ji Beijing fengbi jiyuan, wei jinü zhenzhi xingbing' [Recalling the past: The closure of brothels in Beijing, and providing STI treatment to prostitutes], *Zhonghua Mafeng Pifubing Zazhi*, 17, 3: 229.

Ye, H. (2010) 'Zhongguo dalu xinggongzuozhe jigou Wuhan jietou changyi hefahua [Chinese sex workers' organization calls for legalization on Wuhan street], Liumangyan de BLOG, weblog, 2 August. Online. Available: http://blog.sina.com.cn/s/blog_4681c8dc0100kzuo.html (accessed 29 March 2016).

Yin, Q., Yong, W., Zuxin, G., Jingmu, M., and Zhanhong, Z. (2009) 'Yihun liudongfunü biyun fangfa xuanze ji yingxiang yinsu fenxi' [Analysis of the factors affecting the choice of contraceptive methods adopted by married female migrants], *Zhongguo Gonggong Weisheng*, 25, 2: 148–9.

'Yiqing baogao' [Epidemic Report] (2009) *Xingbing Qingkuang Jianbao*, 1: 2–29.

'Yi shengming de mingyi' [In the Name of Life] (2005) *China Central Television*, 9 August. Online. Available: www.cctv.com/news/netnews/20050809/100222.shtml (accessed 16 December 2016).

Yi xin de linian kandai aizibing fangzhi gongzuo' [New thinking on the work of AIDS prevention] (2006) *Nanfang Ribao*, 1 December, p. A02.

Youku (2008) 'Laoxiang bang laoxiang' [A fellow villager helping another], *Youku*. Online. Available: http://v.youku.com/v_show/id_XMTMzOTAzNjA4.html (accessed 16 December 2016).

Yu, Fenggao (1996) 'Aizibing: tongxinglianzhe de kuguo – renlei jibing de beijing wenhua zhiyi' [AIDS: The bitter fruit of homosexuality – the background culture of human disease], *Shuwu*, 2: 20–4.

Yu, H.-Q. (2016) 'The biopolitics of China's HIV governance', in D. Bray and E. Jeffreys (eds) *New Mentalities of Government in China*, Abingdon: Routledge, pp. 182–204.

Yu, J. (2009) 'Zhichi yu shufu: chuantong shehui wangluo yu dixia xingchanye zhong de nüxing' [Support and restraint: Women in traditional social networks and the underground sex industry], *Shehui Kexue Luntan*, 7: 35–9.

Yu, X. (2004) 'Anquantao shengchan qiye buru gongyi xuanchuan' [Condom companies involved in public service advertisements], *Keji Ribao*, 15 October, p. 3.

Yu, Y. (2006) Tongxinglianrenqun de shengcun zhuangkuang yanjiu-yi Changsha nantongxinglianrenqun weili [Research into the living conditions of homosexuals using the example of a male homosexual community in Changsha], M.A. thesis, Central South University, Changsha.

Yu, Y.J. (2013) 'Subjectivity, hygiene, and STI prevention: A normalization paradox in the cleanliness practices of female sex workers in post-socialist China', *Medical Anthropology Quarterly*, 27, 3: 348–67.

Zhai, S. (2008) 'You nongmingong shang chunwan xiangdaode' [Some thoughts on seeing migrants workers on the Spring Festival Gala], *Xinhua Ribao*, 9 February.

Zhang, B. (1994) *Tongxing'ai* [Same-sex Love], Ji'nan: Shandong Kexue Jishu Chubanshe.

Zhang, B., Xiufang, L., Tiezhong, H., Dianchang, L., and Ningxiao, C. (2001) '"*Pengyou tongxin*" – dui nannan xingjiechuzhe de aizibing ganyu xiangmu ['Friends Exchange' – an effective HIV/AIDS intervention program for men who have sex with men], *Zhongguo Jiankang Jiaoyu*, 17, 4: 206–10.

Zhang, B.C., and Chu, Q.S. (2005) 'MSM and HIV/AIDS in China', *Cell Research*, 15, 11–12: 858–64.

Zhang, C., Hong, Y., Li, X., Qiao, S., Zhou, Y., and Su, S. (2013) 'Psychological stressors in the context of commercial sex among female sex workers in China', *Health Care for Women International*, 36, 7: 1–15.

Zhang, G. (2006) 'Cong gonggonglixing kandai fang'ai yu saohuang' [A rational look at AIDS prevention and anti-vice campaigns], *Fazhi Ribao*, 17 October. Online. Available: http://news.sina.com.cn/o/2006-10-17/081210252860s.shtml (accessed 16 December 2016).

Zhang, H. (2006) 'Female sex sellers and public policy in the People's Republic of China', in E. Jeffreys (ed.) *Sex and Sexuality in China*, Abingdon: Routledge, pp. 139–58.

Zhang, J. (1991) 'Aizibing zai Zhongguo: xianzhuang wenti yu weilai' [AIDS in China: Current situation and future issues], *Weilai yu Fazhan*, 3: 43–7.

Zhang, J. (1998) 'Woguo xingbing yiqing de xianzai, guoqu yu jianglai [The history and current situation of sexually transmitted infection in China], *Zhonghua Liuxingbingxue Zazhi*, 19, 2: 118–21.

Zhang, J. (1999) 'Zhongguo jinchang' [Prohibiting prostitution in China], *Renmin Gongan*, 18: 54–5.

Zhang, K-L., Mao, S-J., and Xia, D-Y. (2004) 'Epidemiology of HIV and sexually transmitted infections in China', *Sexual Health*, 16: 39–46.

Zhang, L. (1997) 'Xin xingfa weishenme yao quxiao liumangzui [Why hooliganism will be deleted from the new Criminal Law], *Fazhi yu Jingji*, 5: 40.

Zhang, L. (2001) 'Migration and privatization of space and power in late socialist China', *American Ethnologist*, 28, 1: 179–205.

Zhang, L. (2002) 'Yulechangsuo de anquantao xingdong' [Condom action in entertainment and leisure venues], *Nanfang Zhoumo*, 28 November. Online. Available: http://culture.163.com/editor/021128/021128_68011.html (accessed 16 December 2016).

Zhang, Y. (2006) 'Haerbin ban xinggongzuozhe peixunban yinfa anchang hefahua zhizheng' [Harbin sex worker training class triggers debate about legalizing prostitution], *Nanfang Zhoumo*, 16 October. Online. Available: http://news.qq.com/a/20061019/001508.htm (accessed 16 December 2016).

Zhang, Y. (2015) 'Fewer crimes to be subject to death penalty', *China Daily*, 31 August. Online. Available: www.chinadaily.com.cn/china/2015-08/31/content_21742870.htm (accessed 16 December 2016).

Zhang, Y., Kang, G., Yucui, M., Yinzhu, Z., Liyan, H., and Yimin, C. (2010) 'Weihun liudong funü xingjiankang xingwei xianzhuang diaocha' [Investigation of sexual health behaviours among unmarried female migrants], *Zhongguo Gonggong Weisheng*, 26, 8: 963–4.

Zhao, J. (2007) *Chengfa de bianjie-maiyin xingshi zhengce shizheng yanjiu* [The Boundaries of Punishment – Empirical Research on Criminal Policy on Prostitution], Beijing: Zhongguo Fazhi Chubanshe.

Zhao, X., Guangju, M., and Chunlin, Z., (2004) 'Beida Qinghua jujue gongkai fafang anquantao' [Beijing University and Tsinghua University refuse to distribute condoms openly on campus], *Beijing Qingnianbao*, 24 November 2004, p. A4.

Zhao, Y. (2000) 'Watchdogs on party leashes? Contexts and implications of investigative journalism in post-Deng China', *Journalism Studies*, 1, 4: 577–97.

Zheng, L. (2000a) 'Tongxinglianrenqun aizibing sinüe de jiaoluo' [Homosexual community ravaged by AIDS], *Jiankangbao*, 28 August, p. 1.

Zheng, L. (2000b) 'Tongxinglian aizibing wenti zhide guanzhu' [The issue of homosexuality and AIDS deserves attention], *Jiankangbao*, 22 November, p. 1.

Zheng, T. (2006) 'Cool masculinity: Male clients' sex consumption and business alliance in urban China's sex industry', *Journal of Contemporary China*, 15, 46: 161–82.

Zheng, T. (2009a) *Ethnographies of Prostitution in Contemporary China: Gender Relations, HIV/AIDS, and Nationalism*, New York: Palgrave Macmillan.

Zheng, T. (2009b) 'The culture politics of condoms in the time of AIDS in China', *China Perspectives*, 1: 55–66.

Zheng, T. (2009c) *Red Lights: The Lives of Sex Workers in Postsocialist Chin*a, Minneapolis: The University of Minnesota Press.

Zheng, T. (2010) 'Vilifying and promoting condoms: Condom debate during the time of AIDS in China', *The New York Sociologist*, 4: 50–74.

Zheng, Y. (2007) 'Zhongguo aizibing gongzuochangsuo jiaoyu xiangmu' qidong' [China launches 'AIDS education in workplaces project'], *Gongren Ribao*, 30 January, p. 7.

'Zhengxie weiyuan jianyi: xingjiaoyi zhong shiyong anquantao ying jianqing chufa' [Suggestion from members of the Chinese People's Political Consultative Conference: punishment should be lenient when condoms are used in the sex trade] (2003) *Nanfang Dushibao*, 9 March. Online. Available: http://news.sina.com.cn/c/2003-03-09/122567767s.shtml (accessed 16 December 2016).

Zhong, X. (2014) 'Wenming dixian burong xiedu' [The bottom line of civilization should not be breached], *Renmin Ribao*, 14 February, p. 4.

'Zhonggong fabu zui yan dangji lie chu 6 lei fumian qingdan (quanwen)' [Chinese Communist Party issues the most stringent list of disciplinary regulation, listing 6 categories of violations (full text)] (2015) *Xinhua*, 21 October. Online. Available: http://news.sina.com.cn/c/nd/2015-10-21/doc-ifxizwti6817718.shtml (accessed 16 December 2016)

Zhonggong zhongyang bangongting, guowuyuan bangongting, zhongyang junwei bangongting [Central Committee of the Communist Party of China, the State Council and the Central Military Commission (1992) 'Zhonggong zhongyang bangongting, guowuyuan bangongting, zhongyang junwei bangongting guanyu jiaqiang dangzhengjun jiguan suoshu lüguan guanli yanjin maiyinpiaochang huodong de tongzhi' [Notice of the Central Committee of the Communist Party of China, the State Council and the Central Military Commission, on strengthening management of political authority-owned hotels and prohibiting prostitution]. Online. Available: www.pkulaw.cn/fulltext_form.aspx?db=chl&gid=10169 (accessed 16 December 2016).

Zhonggong zhongyang guanyu shehuizhuyi jingshen wenming jianshe zhidao fangzhen de jueyi [Resolution of the Central Committee of the Communist Party of China on guidelines for strengthening the construction of socialist spiritual civilization] (1986) Twelfth Plenary Meeting of the Sixth Central Committee of the Communist Party of China, 18

February. Online. Available: http://cpc.people.com.cn/GB/64162/64168/64565/65381/4429515.html (accessed 16 December 2016).

Zhonggong zhongyang bangongting, guowuyuan bangongting yinfa 'dang zheng jiguan guonei gongwu jiedai guanli guiding' [The Central Committee of the Communist Party of China and the State Council issue 'Regulations on Domestic Official Hospitality for Party and Government Organs'] (2013) *Xinhua*, 8 December. Online. Available: http://news.xinhuanet.com/politics/2013-12/08/c_118467426.htm (accessed 16 December 2016).

Zhonggong zhongyang xuanchuanbu, weishengbu [Publicity Department of the Central Committee of the Chinese Communist Party and Ministry of Health] (2004) 'Aizibing fanzhi gongzuo xuanchuan tigang de tongzhi' [Notice on the Guidelines on AIDS Prevention Publicity Work], 26 July. Online. Available: www.healthpolicy.cn/news/zfxx/201112/t20111231_1389634.shtml (accessed 16 December 2016).

Zhongguo jibing yufang kongzhi zhongxin [Chinese Center for Disease Control and Prevention] (2004) *Yulechangsuo fuwu xiaojie yufang aizibing xingbing ganyu gongzuo zhinan* [Guidelines for AIDS and STI Prevention Work for Female Service Providers (*fuwu xiaojie*) in Entertainment and Leisure Venues], June, Beijing. Online. Available: www.chinacdc.cn/jkzt/crb/azb/jszl_2219/201103/U020110414480075964141.pdf (accessed 1 February 2017).

Zhongguo jibing yufang kongzhi zhongxin [Chinese Center for Disease Control and Prevention] (n.d.) 'Yufang aizi: wo you yi "tao"' Preventing AIDS: I have a 'method/condom'], Chinese Center for Disease Control and Prevention and Qingdao-London Durex Company Ltd.

Zhongguo jibing yufang kongzhi zhongxin, xingbing aizibing yufang kongzhi zhongxin [Chinese Center for Disease Control and Prevention, National Center for AIDS/STD Control and Prevention] (2007) *Nannanxingxingweirenqun aizibing gaoweixingwei ganyu gongzuo zhinan* [Guidelines for interventions into AIDS-related high-risk behaviours among men who have sex with men], September.

Zhongguo jibing yufang kongzhi zhongxin, xingbing aizibing yufang kongzhi zhongxin [Chinese Center for Disease Control and Prevention, National Center for AIDS/STD Control and Prevention] (2016a) *Nannanxingxingweirenqun yufang aizibing ganyu gongzuo zhinan* [Guidelines for interventions to prevent AIDS among men who have sex with men], May. Online. Available: www.chinaaids.cn/jszn/201609/W020160913346815395954.pdf (accessed 30 January 2017).

Zhongguo jibing yufang kongzhi zhongxin, xingbing aizibing yufang kongzhi zhongxin [Chinese Center for Disease Control and Prevention, National Center for AIDS/STD Control and Prevention] (2016b) *Yixing xingchuanbo gaoweirenqun yufang aizibing ganyu gongzuo zhinan* [Guidelines for interventions to prevent AIDS among groups at high-risk through heterosexual sexual transmission], May. Online. Available: www.chinacdc.cn/jkzt/crb/zl/azb/jszl_2219/201609/W020160922471323174286.pdf (accessed 30 January 2017).

Zhongguo nongxuehui [China Association of Agricultural Science Societies] (2009) *Hua' shuo fang'ai* [Picturing AIDS Prevention], Beijing: Zhongguo Nongye Kexue Jishu Chubanshe.

Zhongguo renkou yu jihua shengyu [China Population and Family Planning Commission of China] (n.d.) Aizibing yufang xiangmu [AIDS Prevention Programs]. Online. Available: http://shehui.haitegaoxin.net/pdfbook/XRQFQFBABAAFFM.pdf (accessed 16 December 2016).

Zhongguo xingbing aizibing fangzhi xiehui [Chinese Association of STD/AIDS Prevention and Control] and UNAIDS (n.d.) *Hua shuo 'aizi'* [Picturing AIDS], Beijing: 27 Nanwei Rd, Xuanwu District.

Zhonghua renmin gongheguo gonganbu ling: di 88 hao [Order No. 88 of the Ministry of Public Security] (2006) 'Gongan jiguan banli xingzheng anjian chengxu guiding' [Regulations on the Procedures for Handling Administrative Cases by Public Security Organs], passed on 29 March 2006 effective 24 August 2006. Online. Available: www.gov.cn/flfg/2006-09/07/content_380611.htm (accessed 12 December 2016).

Zhonghua renmin gongheguo gonganbu ling: di 125 hao [Order No.125 of the Ministry of Public Security] (2012) 'Gongan jiguan banli xingzheng anjian chengxu guiding' [Regulations on the Procedures for Handling Administrative Cases by Public Security Organs], passed on 19 December 2012 effective 1 January 2013. Online. Available: www.mps.gov.cn/n2254314/n2254409/n2254443/n2254452/c3708279/content.html (accessed 12 December 2016).

Zhonghua renmin gongheguo guojia weisheng he jihua shengyu weiyuanhui [Ministry of Health and National Population and Family Planning Commission of the People's Republic of China] (2004) Guanyu yufang aizibing tuiguang shiyong anquantao (biyuntao) de shishi yijian [Guidelines on preventing AIDS and promoting condom use], 7 July. Online. Available: www.moh.gov.cn/mohyzs/pzcxx/200804/32049.shtml (accessed 25 January 2017).

Zhonghua renmin gongheguo xingfa [Criminal Law of the People's Republic of China] (1979) Adopted by the Second Session of the Fifth National People's Congress on 1 July 1979, promulgated by Order No. 5 of the Chairman of the Standing Committee of the National People's Congress on 6 July 1979, effective 1 January 1980. Online. Available: www.npc.gov.cn/wxzl/wxzl/2000-12/06/content_4379.htm (accessed 12 December 2016).

Zhongyangdianshitai dajia lanmu [China Central Television Station Master Program] (2005) *Dayi jingcheng-book one* [Doctors with High Skill and Morality], Beijing: Shangwu Yinshuguan.

Zhou, B. (2010) 'Si bumen fawen yaoqiu jiaoyu wanjiu maiyinnü jinzhi youjie shizhong gongkai baoguang' [Four departments dispatch a notice on educating and rescuing female sex sellers and prohibiting the public parading of apprehended suspects], *Fazhi Ribao*, 12 December, p. 1.

Zhou, B. (2011) 'Cong tongxinglian fenzheng kan wenhua kuanrong' [Dispute over homosexuality highlights a culture of tolerance], *21Shiji Jingji Baodao*, 5 July, p. 2.

Zhou, J. (2006) 'Dalu dixia xingchanye 'hefahua' fengbo' [Controversy over legalizing the underground sex industry in mainland China], *Fenghuang Zhoukan*. Online. Available: www.sachina.edu.cn/Htmldata/news/2006/04/1220.html (accessed 12 December 2016).

Zhou, L. (1993) 'Zhongguo jianjue daji maiyinpiaochang huodong' [China resolves to strike hard against prostitution], *Liaowang*, 21: 18–9.

Zhou, L., and Zhengyan, X. (2006) 'Maiyin hefahua' zai Zhongguo de 'maodun' yujing' [The 'contradiction' of talking about the 'legalization of prostitution' in the Chinese context], *Xinhuawang Yunnan Pindao*. Online. Available: http://tieba.baidu.com/p/1442760425 (accessed 12 December 2016).

Zhou, R. (2006a) 'Dixia xingchanye xuyao yangguang guanli' [The underground sex industry should be brought into the open], *Jiancha Fengyun*, 4: 60–1.

Zhou, R. (2006b) 'Lianghui daibiao bufang yiyi dixia xingchanye' [Delegates at the National People's Congress and the Chinese People's Political Consultative Conference might as well discuss the underground sex industry], *People's Daily*, 19 January.

Online. Available: http://opinion.people.com.cn/GB/35560/4042747.html (accessed 12 December 2015).

Zhou, X. (2006) 'Fang'ai yu saohuang de ganga: wei fang xingbing aizibing hashi wei "xiaojie" peixun' [Preventing AIDS and anti-vice campaign embarrassment: Harbin runs 'working girl training classes' to combat STI and AIDS], *Dongfang Jinbao*, 11 October. Online. Available: http://news.sina.com.cn/c/2006-10-16/011710242626s.shtml (accessed 23 February 2017).

Zhu, A. (2006) '"100% anquantao" – shijieweishengzuzhi gonggongchangsuo fafang anquantao Jingjiang shidian xiangmu huigu ['100 Per Cent Condom Use' – a review of the Jingjiang pilot project of the World Health Organization's condom distribution in public venues program], *Lanling*, 5: 13–5.

Zhu, Q., Jianming, L., Chuang, Y., Fan, L., and Jing, X. (1994) 'Tichang zunshou xingdaode haishi shiyong biyuntao yufang aizibing' [Preventing AIDS: [Should we be] promoting condoms or sexual morality?], *Zhongguo Jiankang Jiaoyu*, 11, 10: 25–31.

Zhu, W. (2002) 'Yingxiang gonggong zhengce de anquantao xingdong' [The condom action that affected public policy], *Sanlian Shenghuo Zhoukan*, 16 October.

Zhu, Y. (2001) 'Tongxinglian bu zai shu xingbiantai' [Homosexuality is no longer treated as sexual perversion], *Xinhua Meiri Dianxun*, 16 April, p. 5.

Zhuang, X., Wu, Z.Y., Poundstone, K., Yang, C.Q., Zhong, Y.Q., and Jiang, S.Y. (2012) 'HIV-related high-risk behaviors among Chinese migrant construction laborers in Nantong, Jiangsu', *Plos One*, 7, 3: 1–6.

Zou, H., Xue, H., Wang, X., and Lu, D. (2012) 'Condom use in China: Prevalence, policies, issues and barriers', *Sexual Health*, 9, 1: 27–33.

Zuigao renmin fayuan, zuigao renmin jianchayuan [Supreme People's Court and Supreme People's Procuratorate] (1984) 'Zuigao renmin fayuan, zuigao renmin jianchayuan guanyu dangqian banli liumanganjian zhong juti yingyong falü de ruogan wenti de jieda' [Supreme People's Court and Supreme People's Procuratorate: answers on questions about the current handling of cases of hooliganism according to law], 2 November. Online. Available: www.chinalawedu.com/news/1200/21994/22009/2006/3/li79920231013600214-0.htm (accessed 12 December 2016).

Index

Page numbers in italic indicate a figure on the corresponding page.

100% CUP *see* 100 Per Cent Condom Use Program
100 Per Cent Condom Use Program (China): Centers for Disease Control and Prevention (China), 32–3, 34; implementation 14–15, 18, 19–20, 25–46; media coverage 36–53; National Population and Family Planning Commission 20, 26, 32, 33
100 Per Cent Condom Use Program (Thailand), 14–15, 19, 21–5

Acquired Immunodeficiency Syndrome *see* HIV/AIDS
AIDS *see* HIV/AIDS

CCP *see* Chinese Communist Party
CDC *see* country-specific Centers for Disease Control and Prevention
Centers for Disease Control and Prevention (American), 2–3
Centers for Disease Control and Prevention (Chinese): 100 Per Cent Condom Use Program 32–3, 34; disease response coordination 11, 13, 16; health intervention in prostitution 63, 71, 74–85, 92; homosexual AIDS prevention 95, 96–7, 105–11, 108; migrant labourer AIDS education 124; transgender AIDS prevention 144–5
China's Action Plan for the Containment and Prevention of HIV/AIDS (2001–2005), 11, 28, 37, 47, 127
China's Action Plan for the Containment and Prevention of HIV/AIDS (2006–2010), 33, 73, 83, 90, 124, 127
China's Action Plan for the Containment and Prevention of HIV/AIDS (2011–2015), 73, 90, 127–8, 138
China's Action Plan for the Containment and Prevention of HIV/AIDS (2016–2020), 73, 96, 126, 128, 138, 142, 150
Chinese Communist Party: censorship of prostitution in society 63–5; Medium- and Long-Term Strategic Plan for HIV/AIDS Prevention and Control 11, 44, 62–3, 65–6, 127; response to prostitution 5–8, 55–60, 64, 73n1; venereal disease 5, 7, 19–20, 58, 68; *see also* China's Action Plan for the Containment and Prevention of HIV/AIDS
Chi Susheng 87–8, 89
condom: media coverage 12, 13, 36–53; promoting disease control 62, 65–8, 67, 72; usage in homosexual population 94–5, 95, 104, 106–7, 110–11; usage in migrant labourer population 119, 124–6, 129, 132, 138–9; usage in prostitute population 55–6, 62–3, 65–72, 75–92; *see also* 100 Per Cent Condom Use Program
Consolidated Guidelines on HIV Prevention, Diagnosis, Treatment and Care for Key Populations 142–9

focal population groups 117
Foucault, Michel 2, 112, 140–1

governmentality 2, 4, 75, 140–1

Hacking, Ian 4, 141
HIV *see* HIV/AIDS

HIV/AIDS: 100 Per Cent Condom Use Program 18–53; 100 Per Cent Condom Use Program infection statistics 19, 20, 21, 26, 34; baseline infection statistics 3, 9, 10, 16, 62, 144; celebrity outreach 134–8; condom usage in homosexual population 94–5, 95, 104, 106–7, 110–11; condom usage in migrant labourer population 119, 124–6, 129, 132, 138–9; condom usage in prostitute population 55–6, 62–3, 65–72, 75–92; disease identification 2–5; education resources for homosexuals 106–10; education resources for migrant labourers 129–34, 133; education resources for prostitutes 57, 75–6, 79–84, 92; future trend of infection statistics 142, 144, 150; homosexual AIDS prevention 94–115, 95, 108; homosexual infection statistics 94, 96, 103–5, 107; initial spread through China 8–11; intervention strategies for homosexuals 105–11, 108; intervention strategies for migrant labourers 127–9; intervention strategies for prostitutes 18–53, 74–93; Joint United Nations Programme on HIV/AIDS, 3–5, 10–11, 25, 36, 79–82, 109–10, 117–18, 135, 140–50; media coverage 11–14, 15, 36–53, 63–4, 83–7, 111–15; Medium- and Long-Term Strategic Plan for HIV/AIDS Prevention and Control 11, 44, 62–3, 65–6, 127; migrant labourer infection statistics 117, 118, 120; migrant labourers 117–39, 133; promoting condom as disease control 62, 65–68, 72; prostitution AIDS prevention 5–8, 15–17, 18–53, 74–93; prostitution infection statistics 72, 90, 92; Thailand 14–15, 19, 21–5; transgender population 144–5, 147–9; venereal disease 5, 7, 20, 58; *see also* Joint United Nations Programme on HIV/AIDS; World Health Organization
homosexual AIDS prevention 94–115, 95, 108; Centers for Disease Control and Prevention (Chinese), 95, 96–7, 105–11, 108; emergence of homosexuality 97 100; HIV/AIDS education resources 106–10; HIV/AIDS intervention strategies 105–11, 108; homosexual infection statistics 94, 96, 103–5, 107; homosexuality as public health issue 100–15, 108; Li Yinhe 99, 111, 113; media coverage 111–15; Men's World 101–2; money boy 105, 107; non-governmental organizations 102–4, 107, 110, 114, 116n1; prostitution 104–5, 107–9; serosorting 95–6; strategic positioning 95–6; surveys and interviews 110–11; Wan Yanhai 101–2
Human Immunodeficiency Virus *see* HIV/AIDS

intervention strategies: for homosexuals 105–11, 108; for migrant labourers 127–9; for prostitutes 18–53, 74–93; public health monitor role 76–9, 83–6, 90–3

jinü 68, 70, 80, 104
Joint United Nations Programme on HIV/AIDS, 3–5, 10–11, 25, 36, 79–82, 109–10, 117–18, 135, 140–50; Consolidated Guidelines on HIV Prevention, Diagnosis, Treatment and Care for Key Populations 142–9; global blueprint for ending AIDS, 142–3; transgender population 147–9

Li Yinhe 99, 111, 113

maiyinnü 69–70, 85, 89
media coverage of HIV/AIDS 11–14, 15, 36–53, 63–4, 83–7, 111–15
Medium- and Long-Term Strategic Plan for HIV/AIDS Prevention and Control 11, 44, 62–3, 65–6, 127
Men's World 101–2
migrant labourers 117–39, 133; China's Action Plan for the Containment and Prevention of HIV/AIDS, 124, 127–8, 138; condom usage 119, 124–6, 129, 132, 138–9; factors in HIV/AIDS vulnerability 117–19, 123–7; HIV/AIDS celebrity outreach 134–8; HIV/AIDS education resources 129–34, 133; HIV/AIDS intervention strategies 127–9; infection statistics 117, 118, 120; population characteristics 122–3; population mobility 117–18, 119–22, 122; Wang Baoqiang 135–7; Xiao Zhang 132, 133
Ministry of Health: AIDS education 130, 134, 135; homosexual sexual activity 96, 100, 101–2, 104, 112; initial spread of HIV, 9, 13; prostitution 74,

93; sexually transmissible infection surveillance 61, 63
Ministry of Public Security: homosexual sexual activity 102; prostitution 7, 8, 49, 55, 60, 63, 89
money boy 105, 107

National Center for AIDS/STD Control and Prevention: focal population groups 117; HIV/AIDS surveillance 11; homosexual sexual activity 13, 95, 96, 97, 103, 108, 110
National Population and Family Planning Commission: 100 Per Cent Condom Use Program 20, 26, 32, 33; migrant labourer AIDS education 128, 130
NCAIDS *see* National Center for AIDS/STD Control and Prevention
NGO *see* non-governmental organizations
non-governmental organizations: AIDS prevention resources 3, 12; homosexual AIDS prevention 102–4, 107, 110, 114, 116n1; prostitute AIDS prevention 23, 28, 50, 77–8, 88, 92, 145
NPFPC *see* National Population and Family Planning Commission

population mobility 117–18, 119–22, 122
prostitution: 100 Per Cent Condom Use Program 18–53; advocacy for legalization 86–9; censorship of in society 63–5; Chi Susheng 87–8, 89; HIV/AIDS education resources 57, 75–6, 79–84, 92; HIV/AIDS intervention strategies 18–53, 74–93; homosexual AIDS prevention 104–5, 107–9; infection statistics 72, 90, 92; jinü 68, 70, 80, 104; maiyinnü 69–70, 85, 89; media coverage 36–53, 63–4, 83–7; Medium- and Long-Term Strategic Plan for HIV/AIDS Prevention and Control 11, 44, 62–3, 65–6, 127; Ministry of Health 74, 93; Ministry of Public Security 7, 8, 49, 55, 60, 63, 89; money boy 105, 107; non-governmental organizations 23, 28, 50, 77–8, 88, 92, 145; public health monitors 76–9, 83–6, 90–3; renaming profession 68–72; response to 5–8, 15–16, 55–60, 64, 73n1; Thailand 14–15, 19, 21–5; xiaojie 68–70, 71, 74, 80; xinggongzuozhe 69–70, 71, 88; Ye Haiyan 88–9; Zhou Ruijin 86–7, 89
public health monitors: intervention strategies 76–9, 83–6, 90–3; prostitute HIV/AIDS intervention strategies 76–9, 83–6, 90–3

sexually transmissible infection: 100 Per Cent Condom Use Program 18–53; 100 Per Cent Condom Use Program infection statistics 19, 20, 21, 26, 34; baseline infection statistics 3, 9, 10, 16, 62; celebrity outreach 134–8; condom usage in homosexual population 94–5, 95, 104, 106–7, 110–11; condom usage in migrant labourer population 119, 124–6, 129, 132, 138–9; disease identification 2–5; education resources for homosexuals 106–10; education resources for migrant labourers 129–34, 133; education resources for prostitutes 57, 75–6, 79–84, 92; future trend of infection statistics 142, 144, 150; homosexual AIDS prevention 94–115, 95, 108; homosexual infection statistics 94, 96, 103–5, 107; initial spread through China 8–11; intervention strategies for homosexuals 105–11, 108; intervention strategies for migrant labourers 127–9; intervention strategies for prostitutes 18–53, 74–93; Joint United Nations Programme on HIV/AIDS, 3–5, 10–11, 25, 36, 79–82, 109–10, 117–18, 135, 140–50; media coverage 11–14, 15, 36–53, 63–4, 83–7, 111–15; Medium- and Long-Term Strategic Plan for HIV/AIDS Prevention and Control 11, 44, 62–3, 65–6, 127; migrant labourer infection statistics 117, 118, 120; migrant labourers 117–39, 133; prostitution AIDS prevention 5–8, 15–17, 18–53, 74–93; prostitution infection statistics 72, 90, 92; Thailand 14–15, 19, 21–5; transgender population 144–5, 147–9; *see also* Joint United Nations Programme on HIV/AIDS; World Health Organization
sexually transmitted disease *see* sexually transmissible infection
sex worker *see* prostitution
STD *see* sexually transmissible infection
STI *see* sexually transmissible infection
syphilis 5, 58, 111

Tool to Set and Monitor Targets for HIV Prevention, Diagnosis, Treatment and Care for Key Populations 142–9

UNAIDS *see* Joint United Nations Programme on HIV/AIDS

venereal disease 5, 7, 20, 58, 68

Wang Baoqiang 135–7
Wan Yanhai 101–2
WHO *see* World Health Organization
World Health Organization: 100 Per Cent Condom Use Program (China), 14, 18, 19–20, 25–46; 100 Per Cent Condom Use Program (Thailand), 19, 21–5; AIDS surveillance 3–5, 9, 13, 17, 141–9; China–WHO Country Cooperation Strategy 2016–2020, 142; Consolidated Guidelines on HIV Prevention, Diagnosis, Treatment and Care for Key Populations 142–9; global blueprint for ending AIDS, 142–3; Tool to Set and Monitor Targets for HIV Prevention, Diagnosis, Treatment and Care for Key Populations 142–9; transgender population 147–9

xiaojie 68–70, 71, 74, 80
Xiao Zhang 132, 133
xinggongzuozhe 69–70, 71, 88

Ye Haiyan 88–9

Zhou Ruijin 86–7, 89

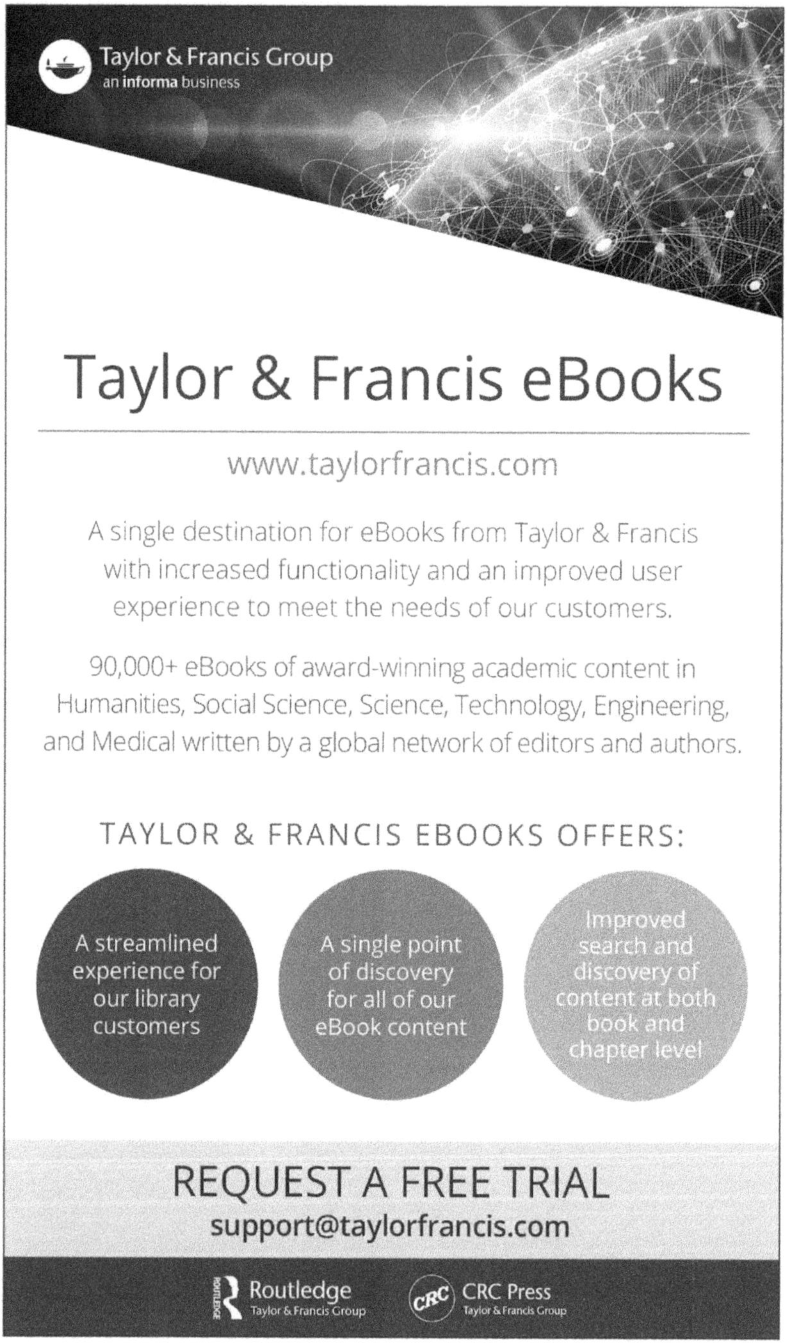